ESOPHAGEAL CANCER – CELL AND MOLECULAR BIOLOGY, BIOMARKERS, NUTRITION AND TREATMENT

Edited by **Ferdous Rastgar Jazii**

Esophageal Cancer - Cell and Molecular Biology, Biomarkers, Nutrition and Treatment
http://dx.doi.org/10.5772/1196
Edited by Ferdous Rastgar Jazii

Contributors

Shinichi Miyamoto, Shuko Morita, Manabu Muto, Yusuke Sato, Satoru Motoyama, Junichi Ogawa, Irene Vegh, Ana Isabel Flores, Michael Gibson, Yoshihiro Komatsu, Mingzhou Guo, Yan Jia, Wenji Yan, Malek Safa, Hassan Reda, Guiju Sun, Tingting Wang, Guiling Huang, Shaokang Wang, Fukang Liu, Jiasheng Wang, Ming Su, Ferdous Rastgar Jazii, Maryam Zare, Mehdi Moghanibashi, Hajime Orita, Malcolm Brock, Koichi Sato, Hirokazu Yokoyama, Toshifumi Hlbi, Haruko Yokoyama

Notice

First published in Croatia, 2012 by INTECH d.o.o.
eBook (PDF) Published by IN TECH d.o.o.
Place and year of publication of eBook (PDF): Rijeka, 2019.
IntechOpen is the global imprint of IN TECH d.o.o.
Printed in Croatia

Legal deposit, Croatia: National and University Library in Zagreb

Additional hard and PDF copies can be obtained from orders@intechopen.com

Esophageal Cancer - Cell and Molecular Biology, Biomarkers, Nutrition and Treatment
Edited by Ferdous Rastgar Jazii

p. cm.

ISBN 978-953-51-0223-6

eBook (PDF) ISBN 978-953-51-6999-4

Meet the editor

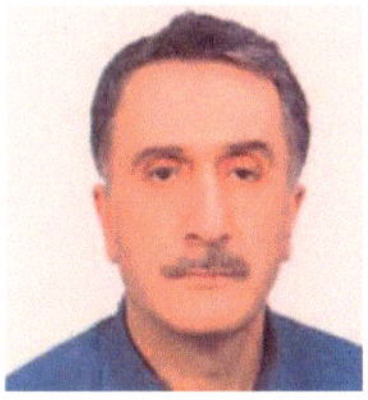

Dr Ferdous Rastgar Jazii is associate professor in the National Institute of Genetic Engineering and Biotechnology (NIGEB) of Iran. He did both his PhD and master's programs in biochemistry and bachelor's in biology. His postdoctoral studies in the Hospital for Sick Children (Sickkids) in Toronto were done on the role of mRNA binding proteins in translational control of protein synthesis in metabolic diseases. His research activities are focused on the cancer, and primarily molecular etiology of esophageal cancer. Proteomics combined with cell and molecular biology is applied in his studies in the etiology and identification of cancer specific tumor markers. Investigations on the role and contribution of structural proteins e.g. beta-tropomyosin, their significance, and regulation by signal transduction pathways are among major research interests of his group in cancer biology and molecular etiology.

Contents

Preface IX

Chapter 1 **Molecular Biology Character of Esophageal Cancer 1**
Mingzhou Guo, Yan Jia and Wenji Yan

Chapter 2 **Growth Factors, Signal Transduction Pathways, and Tumor Suppressor Genes in Esophageal Cancer 21**
Maryam Zare, Mehdi Moghanibashi and Ferdous Rastgar Jazii

Chapter 3 **Biomarkers, Stem Cells and Esophageal Cancer 49**
Irene Vegh and Ana I. Flores

Chapter 4 **Proteomics and Esophageal Cancer 79**
Mehdi Moghanibashi, Maryam Zare and Ferdous Rastgar Jazii

Chapter 5 **The Interaction Between the Metabolism of Retinol and Ethanol in Esophageal Mucosa – A Possible Mechanism of Esophageal Cancer in Alcoholics 101**
Hirokazu Yokoyama, Haruko-Shiraishi Yokoyama and Toshifumi Hibi

Chapter 6 **Study on the Dietary Factors of Esophageal Cancer 127**
Guiju Sun, Tingting Wang, Guiling Huang, Ming Su, Jiasheng Wang, Shaokang Wang and Fukang Liu

Chapter 7 **Current Therapy for Esophageal Adenocarcinoma 153**
Yoshihiro Komatsu and Michael K. Gibson

Chapter 8 **Nonsurgical Management of Esophageal Cancer 171**
Malek M. Safa and Hassan K. Reda

Chapter 9 **Emerging Therapies for Esophageal Cancer 207**
Hajime Orita, Malcolm Brock and Koichi Sato

Chapter 10 **Multiple Early-Stage Malignant Melanoma of the Esophagus with a Long Follow-Up Period After Endoscopic Treatment: Report of a Case and a Literature Review 227**
Shin'ichi Miyamoto, Shuko Morita and Manabu Muto

Chapter 11 **Pulmonary Edema Induced by Esophagectomy 239**
Yusuke Sato, Satoru Motoyama and Junichi Ogawa

Preface

With particular distribution in the world and hundreds fold variation in the incidence rate between the high and low risk regions it is well established that both environmental factors as well as genetic predisposition are involved in tumorigenesis of esophageal cancer. As a result environmental, nutritional, habitual, and socio-economic factors, as well as cell and molecular alterations have to be subject of investigations in the etiology of this type of cancer. At molecular level, while a large number of alterations have so far been proposed for esophageal carcinogenesis, however several specific events were attributed to be more significant and key players of the role in the process of esophageal carcinogenesis. These events are specific molecular mechanisms and pathways involved in the regulation of the both oncogenes and tumor suppressor genes.

The present book covers recent achievements in the cell and molecular, nutritional, in addition to clinical features of esophageal cancer. The first two chapters of the book describe fundamental features including genetic, cellular and molecular aspects of esophageal cancer. Chapter three and four have aimed candidate molecular markers of esophageal cancer. Chapter three describes the present molecular marker in addition to the role of stem cell biology in the identification of biomarkers. Chapter four has focused on the application of proteomic in the etiology and identification of tumor markers regarding esophageal cancer; the present identified marker and future prospects.

Chapter five and six have oriented toward dietary and metabolic pathways. In chapter five our present knowledge of structural and functional features of retinoic acid and effect of ethanol metabolic pathway on retinoic acid supply in pathogenesis of esophageal cancer is discussed. Chapter six has focused on a long term case-control cohort study on the role of different nutritional factors, minerals, vitamins in esophageal cancer.

The last five chapters are dedicated to the clinical features of esophageal cancer. Chapter seven and eight have focused on the histo-pathological features, diagnosis as well as current therapies of esophageal cancer and chapter nine on the application of recent achievements in the cell and molecular biology based targeted cancer therapy. Chapter ten and eleven have briefly focused on the two especial features of esophageal cancer which have received less attention in the literatures. In chapter ten a case report of primary malignant melanoma of the esophagus (PMME), a rare disease diagnosed in the advanced stage years after the first diagnosis is discussed and finally the last chapter has focused on the importance of recognition and monitoring Extravascular Lung Water using PiCCO system during preoperative managements of esophagectomy with extensive lymph node dissection for thoracic esophageal cancer.

Dr Ferdous Rastgar Jazii
Associate Professor, Faculty at the National Institute
of Genetic Engineering and Biotechnology of Iran (NIGEB),
Iran
Research Fellow, Department of Molecular Structure and Function,
Hospital for Sick Children Research Institute, Toronto,
Canada

1

Molecular Biology Character of Esophageal Cancer

Mingzhou Guo, Yan Jia and Wenji Yan
Department of Gastroenterology & Hepatology,
Chinese PLA General Hospital
China

1. Introduction

Esophageal cancer (EC) is the eighth most common cancer and the sixth most common cause of cancer death worldwide. Esophageal squamous cell carcinoma (ESCC) and adenocarcinoma (EAC) are two major histopathological type of esophageal cancer. The incidence of EC was increased in the past 3 decades. Five-year survival of advanced cancer is still very poor, even though improved surgical techniques and adjuvant chemoradiation therapy. It is very important to understand esophageal cancer biology.

2. Genetic changes in esophageal cancer

Genetic change is one of the major events in transforming normal esophageal epithelia to malignant cells. Mutations and genetic polymorphisms in coding gene sequences may cause functional alteration of genes. Functional mutation and single nucleotide polymorphism (SNP) (eg.p53, SULT1A1, CYP3A5, ALDH2, ADH1B1 and ECRG1) is related to susceptibility of esophageal cancer.

2.1 Effects of mutations and SNPs in esophageal cancer

P53 is involved in multiple cellular pathways including apoptosis, transcriptional regulation, and cell cycle control. Alterations in p53 have been reported to occur at an early stage of EC. P53 mutation was observed in exon 5 and accounted for about 77% of ESCC patients (Hu, Huang et al., 2001). Fanconi gene family is another interesting example. The risk of ESCC is associated with both heterozygous and homozygous mutations in several Fanconi anemia-predisposing genes, such as heterozygous insertion/deletion mutations in FANCD2 (p.Val1233-del), FANCE (p.Val311SerfsX2) and FANCL (p.Thr367AsnfsX13) (Akbari et al., 2011).

SNPs in p53 pathway also play important roles in EC tumorigenesis. SNP in p53 gene (Arg72Pro) decreased apoptosis and was associated with increased risk, earlier age of onset, reduced response to chemotherapy and early recurrence in esophageal cancers (Pietsch et al., 2006). T309G is located in the promoter region of MDM2, which is the regulator of p53 pathway. Transcription factor may easily bind to the G variant of MDM2, increase MDM2 expression and reduce apoptosis in response to DNA damage (Bond et al., 2004). MDM2 T309G G/G was associated with an increased risk of death in ESCC (Cescon et al., 2009).

SNPs in key genes are associated with EC, such as genes involved in nucleotide excision repair (NER) and base excision repair (BER) pathways. The increasing number of variant alleles in SNPs of NER showed a significant trend to EAC, including XPD Lys751Gln, ERCC1 8092 C/A and ERCC1 118C/T (Tse et al., 2008). Esophageal cancer related gene 1 (ECRG1) is reported as a novel tumor suppressor. ECRG1 is normally expressed in esophagus, but reduced in ESCC. ECRG1 (Arg290Gln) was identified as the susceptible SNP of ESCC (Li et al., 2006). It has been found that the increased risk of ESCC relates to combined SULT1A12*2 genotype and CYP3A5 heterozygous genotypes, especially in tobacco smokers (Dandara et al., 2006). SNP of ATP-binding cassette sub-family B (MDR/TAP) member 1 gene (ABCB1) was reported to be associated with lymph node and distant metastases in EC (Narumiya et al., 2011). SNP also impacted disease-free survival (DFS) of ECs. The MDM2 T/G and CDH1 GA/GA genotype confer risk of death in EAC patients (Boonstra et al., 2011). Vascular endothelial growth factor (VEGF) 936C/T is associated with an improved overall survival compared with wild type genotype in EC (Bradbury et al., 2009).

2.2 Effects of chromosomal abnormalities in esophageal cancer

Genomic alterations, such as amplification, deletion, translocation and loss of heterozygosity (LOH) play an important role in initiation and progression of cancer. Recently a panel of chromosome instability biomarkers, including LOH and DNA content, has been reported to identify patients at high and low risk of progression from Barrett's esophagus (BE) to EAC (Paulson et al., 2009).

Chromosomal aberrations have been discovered in BE and EAC, including frequent gain of chromosomes 6p (10-37%), 7q (17-37%), 7p (30-60%), 8q (50-80%), 10q (20-50%), 15q (10-40%), 17q (30-50%), and 20q (50-80%); and frequent loss of chromosomes 4q (20-50%), 5q (20-50%), 9p (20-50%), 14q (30-40%), 16q (36-40%), 17p (30%), 18q (20-60%) and Y (60-76%). The proto-oncogenes are often duplicated, such as MYC (8q), EGFR (7p) and ERBB2 (17q). But tumor suppressor genes are usually deleted in BE and EAC, including APC, CDKN2A, p53, and SMAD4 (Akagi et al., 2009). Genomic instability varied widely across chromosomal arms, with the highest frequency of LOH on 9p, CN (copy numbers) loss on 3p, and CN gain on 3q in ESCC (Hu et al., 2009).

ERBB2 and Topoisomerase (DNA) II alpha (TOP2A) genes are located in 17q12-q21.2 region which was reported to be amplified in EACs. Amplification of ERBB2 was found in 10% to 70% of EAC samples. Antagonist of ERBB2, Trastuzumab/Herceptin, inhibits growth of OE19 EAC cell line, which exhibits high expression of ERBB2. TOP2A gene is associated with cell proliferation, and amplified TOP2A has been reported in ESCC (Akagi et al., 2009). The epidermal growth factor receptor (EGFR) I, a tyrosine kinase (TK) involved in several tumor progression and may serve as an important therapeutic target (Erlotinib, Cetuximab). Homogeneous EGFR amplification defines a subset of aggressive Barrett's adenocarcinoma with poor prognosis (Marx et al., 2010). Numerous studies have been reported that chromosomal abnormalities (aneuploidy and tetraploidy) and loss of heterozygosity (LOH) may be used as biomarkers to predict progression of Barrett's esophagus to EAC (Reid et al., 2000). It was demonstrated that a number of SNPs was highly correlated with chromosomal abnormalities in Barrett's esophagus and EAC (Li et al., 2008).

3. Epigenetic changes in esophageal cancer

The term epigenetics refers to the study of heritable changes in gene expression without changes in gene sequence. In addition to genetic alteration, epigenetic modifications are recognized as a common molecular alteration in human cancers. DNA methylation and histone modifications are important epigenetic changes during tumor initiation and progression (Sadikovic et al., 2008). Non-coding RNA (ncRNA) is another kind of epigenetic regulation factor, especially microRNA (miRNA) was recently regarded as the important gene expression regulator. Epigenetic regulation was involved in different pathways including cell cycle, apoptosis, DNA repair et al (W. Zhang et al., 2008; X. Zhang et al., 2010).

3.1 DNA methylation

DNA methylation leads to gene silencing either by directly block the transcriptional factors binding to DNA, or by MBP which recruits chromatin remodeling co-repressor complexes (Klose & Bird, 2006). Promoter region methylation was reported frequently in human esophageal cancer. DNMT1, DNMT3A and DNMT3B have been identified as DNA methytransferases in eukaryotic cells. DNMT1 is involved in maintaining DNA methylation, DNMT3A and DNMT3B are responsible for *de novo* methylation. Overexpression of these DNMTs were reported to be involved in a variety of cancers including EC (Kassis et al., 2006). DNMT3L and DNMT2 were reported recently related to DNA methylation. DNMT3L is required for the methylation of imprinted genes in germ cells, and interacts with DNMT3a and 3b in *de novo* methyltransferase activity (Chen et al., 2005). And the function of DNMT2 remains unclear, its strong binding to DNA suggests that it may mark specific sequences in the genome.

Methylation profile is different in ESCC and EAC. Adenomatous polyposis coli (APC) is frequently methylated in EAC, but infrequently in ESCC (Zhang & Guo, 2010). CDKN2A/p16^{INK4a} methylation is a frequent and early event both in ESCC and EAC (Wang et al., 2009). Caudal type homeobox 2 (CDX2) is expressed in gut epithelia and plays an important role in establishing intestinal phenotype during development. CDX2 is frequently methylated in ESCC (49%), but rarely in EAC (5%) (Guo et al., 2007). Inactivation of CDX2 in EC associated with DNA methylation may be an important determinant of squamous or non-adenomatous phenotype. Multiple genes methylation increases during progression from esophageal mucosa to EC [Figure1] (Fang et al., 2007; Guo et al., 2006). No RARβ2 methylation was observed in normal esophagus but increased methylation was found with the progression of esophageal carcinogenesis. Hypermethylation of p16 and APC is related to high-grade dysplasia or cancer in BE patients.

There is considerable epidemiological evidence suggesting that alcohol, tobacco, diets deficient in vitamins/protective antioxidants, carcinogens and thermal injuries are important in the pathogenesis of EC. Cigarette smoke is a key factor in esophageal carcinogenesis. It was reported that cigarette smoking is a cause of SSBP2 promoter methylation and that SSBP2 harbors a tumor suppressive role in ESCC through inhibition of Wnt signaling pathway (Huang et al., 2011). A previous study demonstrated that duration of tobacco smoking is correlated significantly with DNA methylation of HOXA9, MT1M, NEFH, RSPO4, and UCHL1 in the background esophageal mucosa of EC patients (Oka et al., 2009).

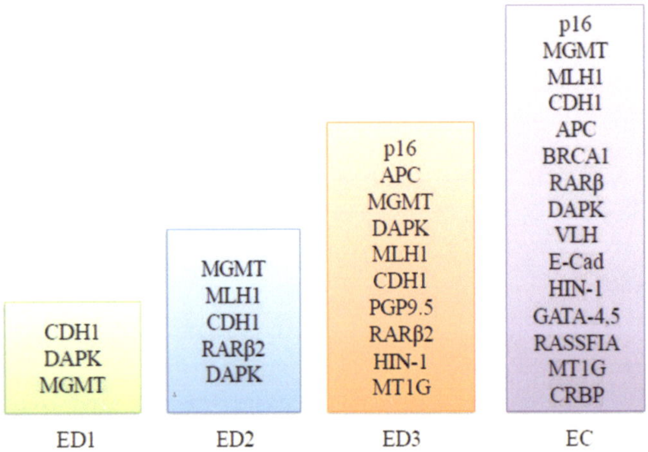

ED: esophageal dysplasia; EC: esophageal cancer

Fig. 1. Accumulated methylation of genes in the progression of esophageal cancer.

3.2 Histone modification

Histone modification (acetylation, methylation, phosphorylation, ubiquitylation, et al.) has important functions in many biological processes including heterochromatin formation, X-chromosome inactivation and transcriptional regulation. In mammals histone arginine methylation is found on residues 2, 8, 17 and 26 of histone H3 and residue 3 of histone H4. Histone lysine methylation occurs on histones H3 and H4 and can be mono-, di- or trimethylated. Similar to histone lysine methylation, arginine methylation occurs in mono-methyl, symmetrical di-methyl or asymmetrical di-methyl state, and contributes to both active and repressive effects on chromatin function (Martin & Zhang, 2005). Methylation on the same site can lead to different outcomes depending on the number of methyl groups added. However the functional relevance of these modification states remains poorly understood. Although there is no evidence that lysine methylation directly affects chromatin dynamics, acetylation of lysine residues in histones is reported to antagonize folding of chromatin in vitro (Hansen, 2002). In mice, for example, it has been shown that pericentric heterochromatin is specifically enriched in trimethyl-H3-K9 and H4-K20, and the effect is silencing of transcription; while mono- and dimethyl-H3-K9 and H4-K20 are found in euchromatin, and play activating transcriptional function, even though there some argues (Peters et al., 2003; Schotta et al., 2004). The main sites of lysine methylation that have been associated with gene activity include K4, K36 and K79 of histone H3. Trimethylation of lysine 27 on histone H3 (H3K27me3) is an silencing epigenetic marker.

Acetylation neutralizes the positive charge of lysine, it has been suggested that this modification might operate through an electrostatic mechanism and histone acetylation is associated with active gene transcription. DNA methylation and histone modifications have recently been reported to cooperate in controlling gene expression (Johnson et al., 2002). Methylation of histone H3 lysine 9 was triggered by DNA methylation. DNA methyltransferases have been shown to interact with histone deacetylases (HDAC), histone methyltransferases, and methyl-cytosine-binding proteins in complex network (Fuks et al., 2000). Histone modifications and DNA methylation are epigenetic phenomena that play a critical role in neoplastic processes.

H3K18Ac and H3K27triMe was correlated with worse survival of ESCC, especially in early stages patients (Langer et al., 2009). Zester homolog 2 (EZH2) is reported to be overexpressed and correlates with poor prognosis in human cancers. The expression frequency and expression levels of H3K27me3 were significantly higher in ESCCs than in normal tissues by immunohistochemistry. Expression of H3K27me3 was significantly correlated with WHO grade, tumor size, T status, locoregional progression and EZH2 expression. High expression level of H3K27me3 was significantly associated with poor locoregional progression-free survival (LPFS) in ESCC (He et al., 2009). A study of 237 ESCC patients showed that histone modifications have significant effects on recurrence-free survival (RFS) after esophagectomy in ESCC, such as acetylation of histone H3 lysine9 (H3K9Ac), histone H3 lysine 18 (H3K18Ac), and histone H4 lysine 12 (H4K12Ac), and the dimethylation of histone H3 lysine 9 (H3K9diMe) and histone H4 arginine 3 (H4R3diMe). 1% increased global level of H3K18Ac in pathologic stage III worsened RFS at 1.009 times, after adjusting for age, sex, and operative method (I et al., 2010). Global levels of histone modifications in ESCC may be an independent prognostic factor of RFS.

3.3 Non-coding RNA

Non-coding RNAs (ncRNAs) are functional RNA molecules that do not code for proteins. Based on size, they are divided into different classes: long ncRNAs (lncRNAs), Piwi-interacting RNAs (piRNAs), small interfering RNAs (siRNAs), microRNAs (miRNAs), etc (Brosnan & Voinnet, 2009). NcRNAs were regarded as important factors of cancer. MiRNA is only well-studied ncRNAs in different disease, including esophageal cancer. MiRNAs are a class of single stranded, evolutionarily conserved non-coding RNAs, only 17-25 ribonucleotides long, involved in a wide spectrum of basic cellular activities through their negative regulation of gene expression.

MiRNAs play important roles in cellular activities such as proliferation, apoptosis and differentiation (Bartel, 2004). MiRNAs are involved in the development, progression and prognosis of esophageal cancers (Feber et al., 2011). As shown in Table 1, expression of miRNAs is different in EAC and ESCC. It was reported that miR-25, miR-151 and miR-424 were up-regulated, whereas miR-29c, miR-99a and miR-100 were reduced in EC. The pattern of these miRNAs may be used to distinguish malignant from normal esophagus. Low level of miR-103/107 expression showed a strong correlation with high overall and disease-free survival periods for EC patients, which may be used for the diagnosis of esophageal cancer. Higher level of miR-196a was observed in EAC, BE and dysplastic lesions compared with normal mucosa. MiR-145, miR-133a and miR-133b inhibited cell proliferation and invasion in ESCC. MiR-200a has been linked to the etiology and prognosis of ESCC. Expression levels of mature miR-21 and mature miR-145 were significantly higher in ESCC than those in normal epithelium, and were significantly associated with lymph node positive, recurrence and metastasis in ESCC (Akagi et al., 2011; Guo et al., 2008; Kano et al., 2010; Maru et al., 2009).

Patho-logical type	Overexpression	Downregulation	Predicted targets of miRNAs	Reference
EAC	miR-215, miR-560, miR-615-3p, miR-192, miR-326, miR-147	miR-100, miR-23a, miR-605, miR-99a, miR-205, let-7c,miR-203	HMGA2 (let-7c), ZEB1 and ZEB2 (miR-205)	(Fassan et al., 2010)
ESCC	miR-145, miR-133a, miR-133b	Let-7	FSCN1(miR-145,miR-133a, miR-133b) HMGA2 (Let-7)	(Kano et al., 2010; Liu et al., 2011)
ESCC, EAC	miR-21	miR-375	PDCD4, NFIB, PTEN, TPM1 (miR-21); PDK1 (miR-375)	(Mathe et al., 2009; Matsushima et al., 2010)
ESCC	miR-93	miR203,miR205	FUS1, E2F1, TP53INP1 (miR-93); ΔNp63 (miR-203)	(Feber et al., 2008; Yuan et al., 2011)
ESCC	miR-373, miR-129	miR-10a	Rab11, APC, LATS2 (miR-373); LATS2 (miR-129) HOX family (miR-10a)	(Matsushima et al., 2010)

EAC: esophageal adenocarcinoma; ESCC: esophageal squamous cell carcinoma

Table 1. MiRNAs expression profile in EAC and ESCC.

In the progression from low-grade dysplasia (LGD) to high-grade dysplasia (HGD) of esophagus, miR-513, miR-125b, miR-101 and miR-197 were up-regulated; miR-23b, miR-20b, miR-181b, miR-203, miR-193b, and miR-636 were down-regulated. MiR-345, miR-494, miR-193a, let-7a, let-7b were down-regulated in progression from HGD to EAC (Yang et al., 2009). MiR-196a level is increased with the progression from normal mucosa to EAC (Maru et al., 2009).

In the past few years, increasing evidence has indicated that a substantial number of miRNAs were regulated by DNA methylation in cancers. Like protein-coding genes, hypermethylation in promoter region of miRNAs was recognized as the mechanism of miRNA regulation in cancers. For example, miR-375, miR-34a, miR-34b/c and miR-129-2 were down-regulated by hypermethylation in EC, and frequent methylation of miR-129-2 was regarded as early detection biomarker of ESCC (Chen et al., 2011; Li et al., 2011).

4. Biology of esophageal precancerous lesion

Most tumors are adenocarcinomas in western societies, squamous cell cancers constitute over 80% of EC in the world. The development of human esophageal cancer is a multistep, progressive process. An early indicator of this process is an increased proliferation of esophageal epithelial cells morphologically including basal cell hyperplasia, different grades of dysplasia, carcinoma in situ (CIS) and advanced esophageal squamous cell carcinoma (ESCC) (Guo et al., 2008). The widely studied precancerous lesion is Barrett's esophagus.

Barrett's esophagus (BE) is an acquired condition in response to chronic gastro-esophageal reflux. EAC was developed through progression from normal epithelium to metaplasia, and different grade of dysplasia (Flejou, 2005). Barrett's esophagus is defined as replacement of normal squamous epithelium with intestinal column epithelium in distal portion of esophagus. The incidence rate of HGD or cancer per patient-year for non-dysplastic Barrett's esophagus was 0.49%. 13.4% of LGD will become HGD or cancer in one year. 10% or greater of high-grade dysplasia may develop to invasive cancer per patient-year (Curvers et al., 2010; Shaheen & Richter, 2009). Barrett's esophagus is thought to be a precancerous lesion with the following changes: augmentation of cell cycle and proliferation, increased angiogenesis and aneuploidy, decreased antiproliferative signaling and apoptosis. The molecular basis of the development of EAC, although extensively studied (Brabender et al., 2004; McManus et al., 2004), is still remains unclear. Better understanding of the molecular alterations during its development might improve prevention and treatment.

In the last three decades, the incidence of Barrett's esophagus-associated esophageal adenocarcinoma (BEAC) is increasing very fast in western world (Blot & McLaughlin, 1999). Despite improvements in treatments of EAC, the prognosis is still poor (Falk, 2002). Therapeutic advances in BEAC have lagged behind other cancers due to its paucity of reliable models in vitro and in vivo. Although Bic-1 and OE33 cells have been established as BEAC-derived cell lines, molecular character remains unclear. BEACs have been shown to undergo loss of heterozygosity at chromosome 18q, the location of smad2 and smad4, in up to 69% of patients, and in as many as 46% of patients with non-dysplastic BE (Barrett et al., 1996; Wu et al., 1998). For the treatment, 2-methoxyestradiol (2-ME(2)) is increasingly recognized as a novel chemotherapy drug to activate a wide array of anti-cancer targets with a relative sparing of normal tissues (Dahut et al., 2006; Sweeney et al., 2005). 2-ME(2) was reported to play an important role in chemoprevention and therapy of BEAC (Kambhampati et al., 2010).

Bile acids may play an important role in progression from BE to EAC. It is reported that bile acid reflux present in patients with BE may increase cell proliferation via activation of PI-PLCγ2, ERK2 MAP kinase, and NADPH oxidase NOX5-S, thereby causing DNA damage and gene mutation, which contribute to the development of EAC (Hong et al., 2010). Trefoil factor 3 (TFF3) was identified as a promising biomarker to screen asymptomatic patients for Barrett's esophagus (Lao-Sirieix et al., 2009). Increased expression of cyclinD has been implicated in predisposition to transform from metaplastic epithelium to cancer (Trudgill et al., 2003).

5. Key protein and pathway involved in esophageal cancer

More than 500,000 patients are diagnosed as esophageal cancer annually. Molecular factors are including aberrant regulation of cyclooxygenase-2 (COX-2), TNF-α and several pathways such as Wnt signaling pathway, TGF-β signaling pathway, NF-κB signaling pathway and so on.

5.1 Wnt signaling pathway

Wnt/β-catenin signaling pathway plays crucial roles in regulation of cellular activity during embryonic development and human diseases including cancers (Logan & Nusse, 2004). Numerous Wnt signaling components, including WNT, secreted frizzled-related proteins (SFRPs), β-catenin, are also of pivotal importance in carcinogenesis of esophageal cancers (Clement et al., 2006).

Epigenetic regulation of key genes in Wnt signaling pathway was described above. Aberrant activation of Wnt signaling pathway has significant effect on the development of esophageal cancer from Barrett's esophagus. WNT2 is upregulated along the progression from LGD to EAC, its expression was higher in dysplasia and EAC than in BE, with 77% of EAC showing high expression of WNT2 (Clement et al., 2006). β–catenin has emerged as a key regulator of Wnt signaling pathway, which plays an important role in development and progression to cancers. Accumulation of nuclear β–catenin in esophagus squamous epithelium might be the crucial step for the carcinogenesis of ESCC (Veeramachaneni et al., 2004). Reduced membranous β-catenin expression has been associated with progression, invasion and poor prognosis in EC (Krishnadath et al., 1997). SRY-box containing gene 17 (SOX17) is reported to play critical roles in regulation of development and stem/precursor cell function through repression of Wnt pathway activity (Gubbay et al., 1990). Hypermethylation of SOX17 was found frequently in ESCC (Zhang et al., 2008). Several studies have reported nuclear accumulation of β-catenin is an indicator of activation of Wnt/β-catenin signaling, and nuclear translocation of β-catenin was observed during progression of BE towards EAC (Osterheld et al., 2002).

5.2 TGF-β pathway

Transforming growth factor-β (TGF-β) was initially identified and named on the basis of its ability to stimulate fibroblast growth in soft agar, but it is now the best-studied growth inhibitory protein. TGF-β family has emerged as a major source of signals that control cell growth and differentiation (Massague, 2000). TGF-β signaling pathway is reported to be frequently involved in gastrointestinal carcinogenesis (Blaker et al., 2002).

TGF-β is regarded as both tumor suppressor and oncogene (Pardali & Moustakas, 2007). In human prostate cancer, overexpression of TGF-β1 enhanced angiogenesis around the tumor, which increased metastasis of prostate cancer. On the other hand, gallbladder tumors secrete TGF-β, which inhibits angiogenesis and results in reduced tumor growth. Thrombospondin1 (THBS1), cystene-rich protein 61 (Cyr61) and connective tissue growth factor (CTGF) are all involved in TGF-β signaling pathway, which plays an important role in tumorigenesis. In human breast cancer THBS1 reduces tumor growth, metastasis and angiogenesis (Sheibani & Frazier, 1995). TGF-β signaling pathway can be activated by THBS1 through its interaction with latent TGF-β binding proteins (LTBP), so that TGF-β is capable of binding to its receptors and stimulating Smad pathway (Crawford et al., 1998). Smad proteins bind to Cyr61 and CTGF promoters, which leads to transcription of Cyr61 and CTGF and activation of angiogenesis and tumor growth (Bartholin et al., 2007; Holmes et al., 2001). It has been reported that THBS1 expression in stroma of ESCC was correlated with lymph node metastasis and Cyr61 expression in Barrett's tissue of EAC was significantly higher than that in Barrett's esophagus with no cancer (Di Martino et al., 2006; Oshiba et al., 1999). Recently, CTGF expression was found to be upregulated in ESCC and significantly related to survival of ESCC patients (Koliopanos et al., 2002). Moreover, CTGF, CYR61 and THBS1 were overexpressed in ESCC, and Cyr61 and CTGF could serve as independent prognostic markers for ESCC (Zhou et al., 2009). Expression level of Smad4 was profoundly reduced at all stages of progression from Barrett's dysplasia to esophageal carcinoma. And 70% of EACs had hypermethylation of Smad4 gene. In Barrett's metaplasia-dysplasia-adenocarcinoma sequence, downregulation of Smad4 occurs due to several mechanisms, including methylation, deletion, and protein modification. And the resulting functional effects of impaired TGF-β signaling are profound throughout this carcinogenesis (Onwuegbusi et al., 2006).

TGF-β signaling has been shown to be paradoxical in tumorigenesis. In addition to inhibitors of TGF-β signaling, as tumor suppressor, many factors may activate TGF-β signaling, such as HDAC inhibitor, SAHA and synthetic terpenoid. It is a good strategy to block the initiation of tumorigenesis through the development of TGF-β mimics in order to achieve chemoprevention.

5.3 NF-κB signaling pathway

NF-κB signaling pathway plays important roles in regulation of cell growth and motility. The NF-κB family is composed of p50, p52, RelA/p65, c-rel, and Rel B. The homodimers and heterodimers are sequestered in cytoplasm as an inactive form by the inhibitor of kappa B (IκB). Upon stimulation, the IκB kinase complex (IKK) phosphorylates κB inhibitor, which releases NF-κB and allows its phosphorylation, nuclear translocation, and subsequent activation of target genes involved in the regulation of cell proliferation, survival, angiogenesis and metastasis (Brown et al., 1995). Constitutively active NF-κB is commonly detected in human cancer cell lines and tumor tissues including ESCC, but is rare in normal cells (Sethi et al., 2008). There is strong evidence of NF-κB being involved in cancer progression, thus NF-κB and its downstream signaling may serve as therapeutic targets (Basseres & Baldwin, 2006). However, the role of NF-κB signaling pathway is not quite understood during esophageal carcinogenesis. It is reported that inhibition of NF-κB can increase the chemosensitivity of EC cells in vitro (Li et al., 2006).

NF-κB inhibitors (Bay11-7082 and sulfasalazine) were found to reduce proliferation, induce apoptosis, increase chemosensitivity (5-fluorouracil, and cisplatin), inhibit migration and invasion of ESCC cell lines. More importantly, Bay11-7082 had significant antitumor effects on ESCC xenografts in nude mice by promoting apoptosis, and inhibiting proliferation and angiogenesis, as well as reduced the metastasis of ESCC cells to lungs without significant toxic effects. NF-κB inhibitors may be potential therapeutic agents for patients with esophageal cancer (Li et al., 2009).

5.4 Proteins involves in the other pathways

Except to signaling pathways mentioned above, there are other key proteins were also involved in esophageal carcinogenesis. Short survival and disappointing prognosis of EC is due to its resistance to many clinical therapies such as chemotherapy and radiotherapy

(Toshimitsu et al., 2004). Aurora-A kinase, a serine/threonine protein kinase, is a potential oncogene. Amplification and overexpression of Aurora-A have been found in ESCC. Overexpression of Aurora-A lead to resistance to cisplatin-induced apoptosis and promoted proliferation in esophageal cancer cell lines (Tanaka et al., 2005).

RARβ2 is reported to be a putative tumor suppressor and is necessary for growth inhibiton of retinoic acid (RA) (Chambon, 1996). Loss of RARβ expression was an early event associated with esophageal carcinogenesis and the status of squamous differentiation (Qiu et al., 1999). Frequent methylation and loss of RARβ2 expression was found in ESCC. DNA methylation of RARβ2 and tumor grade were correlated significantly in EC. And the correlation of methylation and loss of RARβ2 expression was only found in G2 stage. RARβ2 expression was restored and cell growth was inhibited by 5-aza-dc treatment (Liu et al., 2005).

Extensively study of key proteins and signaling pathways will help further understanding the mechanisms of esophageal carcinogenesis, and may improve traditional therapy.

6. Biomarker for esophageal cancer diagnosis and prognosis

Esophageal cancer is one of the most common malignancy worldwide. The overall 5-year survival rates are 10% to 15% due to late diagnosis, metastasis, and resistance to radiotherapy and chemotherapy. Novel early detection marker is urgently needed.

6.1 Potential markers for clinical application in esophageal cancer

Increasing number of studies are focused on EC early detection and promising results were obtained. CDC25B-Abs were reported to be a possible prognostic serological marker for poor survival in advanced ESCC. Expression of HIWI in ESCC is significantly associated with poorer prognosis. WDHD1 is a potential therapeutic target and a candidate biomarker for patients with EC. IGF2 LOI may be a clinically relevant molecular marker of risk for EAC and imprinting status is associated with post-operative outcome following esophageal resection. As shown in Table 2, methylation of HLA-I, CDH1, Integrin α4, RUNX3 and Claudin-4 is associated with poor prognosis, whereas methylation of APC and FHIT is related to better prognosis in ESCC.

Frequent methylation of CDKN2A/p16^{INK4a}, O^{6}-methylguanine-DNA methyltransferase (MGMT), E-cadherin (CDH1) and RARβ2 was found in esophageal cancer. Accumulation of gene methylation was detected in the progression of esophageal cancer (Guo et al., 2006). HIN-1 (High in normal-1) is a tumor suppressor gene that is highly expressed in many normal tissues. Loss of HIN-1 expression and promoter region methylation was found in 13 (72%) of esophageal cancer cell lines. And methylation of HIN-1 was present in 0% of normal mucosa, 31% of grade I dysplasia, 33% of grade II dysplasia, 44% of grade III dysplasia, and 50% of esophageal cancer specimens (Guo et al., 2008). Methylation of HIN-1 is an early event in dysplastic transformation to esophageal cancer.

Cytokeratin (CK) is an essential cytoskeletal component involved in fixation of nucleus and maintenance of cell morphology. No expression of CK18 or CK8 was found in non-cancerous squamous epithelium. CK18 and CK8 were found of 42.9% and 40.5% positive respectively in esophageal carcinoma. Prognosis is poorer in patients with CK18-positive than in negative ESCC. CK18 expression was reported to be an independent prognostic factors in ESCC. And CK18/CK8 correlated with progression of ESCC (Makino et al., 2009).

Gene	Histological type	Prognostic value	Follow-up period	Reference
HLA-I	ESCC	poor prognosis, lymph node metastasis	Shorter in 3 years	(Qifeng et al., 2011)
APC	ESCC	superior prognosis, decreased metastatic lymph nodes	35 months	(Kim et al., 2009)
FHIT	ESCC	superior prognosis	35 months	(Kim et al., 2009)
CDH1	ESCC	increased recurrence and poor RFS after surgery in stage I cancer	3.3 years	(Lee et al., 2008)
Integrin α4	ESCC	increased recurrence and poor RFS in stage II cancer	3.3 years	(Lee et al., 2008)
RUNX3	ESCC	poor prognosis	Shorter in 4 years	(Tonomoto et al., 2007)
Claudin-4	ESCC	poor prognosis	31.5 months (median)	(Sung et al., 2011)

EAC: esophageal adenocarcinoma; ESCC: esophageal squamous cell carcinoma;
BE: Barrett's esophageal; ED: esophageal dysplasia; RFS: recurrence-free survival

Table 2. Prognostic value of gene methylation in esophageal cancer.

Increased β-catenin expression was noted in 18.2% ESCC samples. Reduced expression of Axin, β-TrCP and APC was observed in 46.0%, 24.4%, and 48.2% specimens, respectively. Axin is a negative regulator of Wnt signalling pathway, and genetic alterations of AXIN1 have been suggested to be an important factor in carcinogenesis. Reduced Axin expression was observed in 46% of ESCC. Expression of Axin was found to be correlated inversely with depth of invasion, lymph node metastasis, and lymphatic invasion in ESCC. Reduced Axin protein expression, lymph node involvement, and distant metastasis were significant negative predictors for overall survival and disease-free survival (Li et al., 2009; Nakajima et al., 2003).

MiRNA expression profiling could provide prognostic utility in staging esophageal cancer and treatment plan by endoscopic and neoadjuvant therapies. The alterations of specific miRNAs may further elucidate the metastatic mechanism and allow development of targeting therapy (Feber et al., 2011). Elevated levels of miR-21, miR-155, miR-146b, and miR-181b and reduced expression level of miR-223 were significantly associated with poor prognosis (Mathe et al., 2009).

7. Conclusion

The major goal of molecular biology study is curing of esophageal cancer. Although the molecular biological character was described above, the mechanism of esophageal carcinogenesis remains unclear. Esophageal cancer is still one of the most lethal diseases even though the improved approaches of diagnosis, prevention and treatment. Therefore, greater effort is desired to comprehensively understand the molecular biology of esophageal carcinogenesis. The insight into cancer biology could be translated into practical approaches for the prevention, diagnosis and treatment of esophageal cancer. Due to the complexity of cancers, the early detection of esophageal cancer is more important at present time.

8. References

Akagi, I., Miyashita, M., Ishibashi, O., Mishima, T., Kikuchi, K., Makino, H., Nomura, T., Hagiwara, N., Uchida, E., & Takizawa, T. (2011). Relationship between altered expression levels of MIR21, MIR143, MIR145, and MIR205 and clinicopathologic features of esophageal squamous cell carcinoma. *Dis Esophagus*. Mar 31.

Akagi, T., Ito, T., Kato, M., Jin, Z., Cheng, Y., Kan, T., Yamamoto, G., Olaru, A., Kawamata, N., Boult, J., Soukiasian, H., Miller, C., Ogawa, S., Meltzer, S., & Koeffler, H. (2009). Chromosomal abnormalities and novel disease-related regions in progression from Barrett's esophagus to esophageal adenocarcinoma. *Int J Cancer* 125(10): 2349-2359.

Akbari, M., Malekzadeh, R., Lepage, P., Roquis, D., Sadjadi, A., Aghcheli, K., Yazdanbod, A., Shakeri, R., Bashiri, J., Sotoudeh, M., Pourshams, A., Ghadirian, P., & Narod, S. (2011). Mutations in Fanconi anemia genes and the risk of esophageal cancer. *Human genetics* 129(5): 573-582.

Barrett, M., Schutte, M., Kern, S., & Reid, B. (1996). Allelic loss and mutational analysis of the DPC4 gene in esophageal adenocarcinoma. *Cancer Res* 56(19): 4351-4353.

Bartel, D. (2004). MicroRNAs: genomics, biogenesis, mechanism, and function. *Cell* 116(2): 281-297.

Bartholin, L., Wessner, L., Chirgwin, J., & Guise, T. (2007). The human Cyr61 gene is a transcriptional target of transforming growth factor beta in cancer cells. *Cancer Lett* 246(1-2): 230-236.

Basseres, D. & Baldwin, A. (2006). Nuclear factor-kappaB and inhibitor of kappaB kinase pathways in oncogenic initiation and progression. *Oncogene* 25(51): 6817-6830.

Blaker, H., von Herbay, A., Penzel, R., Gross, S., & Otto, H. (2002). Genetics of adenocarcinomas of the small intestine: frequent deletions at chromosome 18q and mutations of the SMAD4 gene. *Oncogene* 21(1): 158-164.

Blot, W. & McLaughlin, J. (1999). The changing epidemiology of esophageal cancer. *Semin Oncol* 26(5 Suppl 15): 2-8.

Bond, G., Hu, W., Bond, E., Robins, H., Lutzker, S., Arva, N., Bargonetti, J., Bartel, F., Taubert, H., Wuerl, P., Onel, K., Yip, L., Hwang, S., Strong, L., Lozano, G., & Levine, A. (2004). A single nucleotide polymorphism in the MDM2 promoter attenuates the p53 tumor suppressor pathway and accelerates tumor formation in humans. *Cell* 119(5): 591-602.

Boonstra, J., van Marion, R., Tilanus, H., & Dinjens, W. (2011). Functional polymorphisms associated with disease-free survival in resected carcinoma of the esophagus. *J Gastrointest Surg* 15(1): 48-56.

Brabender, J., Marjoram, P., Salonga, D., Metzger, R., Schneider, P., Park, J., Schneider, S., Holscher, A., Yin, J., Meltzer, S., Danenberg, K., Danenberg, P., & Lord, R. (2004). A multigene expression panel for the molecular diagnosis of Barrett's esophagus and Barrett's adenocarcinoma of the esophagus. *Oncogene* 23(27): 4780-4788.

Bradbury, P., Zhai, R., Ma, C., Xu, W., Hopkins, J., Kulke, M., Asomaning, K., Wang, Z., Su, L., Heist, R., Lynch, T., Wain, J., Christiani, D., & Liu, G. (2009). Vascular endothelial growth factor polymorphisms and esophageal cancer prognosis. *Clin Cancer Res* 15(14): 4680-4685.

Brosnan, C. & Voinnet, O. (2009). The long and the short of noncoding RNAs. *Curr Opin Cell Biol* 21(3): 416-425.

Brown, K., Gerstberger, S., Carlson, L., Franzoso, G., & Siebenlist, U. (1995). Control of I kappa B-alpha proteolysis by site-specific, signal-induced phosphorylation. *Science* 267(5203): 1485-1488.

Cescon, D., Bradbury, P., Asomaning, K., Hopkins, J., Zhai, R., Zhou, W., Wang, Z., Kulke, M., Su, L., Ma, C., Xu, W., Marshall, A., Heist, R., Wain, J., Lynch, T., Christiani, D., & Liu, G. (2009). p53 Arg72Pro and MDM2 T309G polymorphisms, histology, and esophageal cancer prognosis. *Clin Cancer Res* 15(9): 3103-3109.

Chambon, P. (1996). A decade of molecular biology of retinoic acid receptors. *FASEB J* 10(9): 940-954.

Chen, X., Hu, H., Guan, X., Xiong, G., Wang, Y., Wang, K., Li, J., Xu, X., Yang, K., & Bai, Y. (2011). CpG island methylation status of miRNAs in esophageal squamous cell carcinoma. *Int J Cancer*. May 5.

Chen, Z., Mann, J., Hsieh, C., Riggs, A., & Chedin, F. (2005). Physical and functional interactions between the human DNMT3L protein and members of the de novo methyltransferase family. *J Cell Biochem* 95(5): 902-917.

Clement, G., Braunschweig, R., Pasquier, N., Bosman, F., & Benhattar, J. (2006). Alterations of the Wnt signaling pathway during the neoplastic progression of Barrett's esophagus. *Oncogene* 25(21): 3084-3092.

Crawford, S., Stellmach, V., Murphy-Ullrich, J., Ribeiro, S., Lawler, J., Hynes, R., Boivin, G., Bouck, N. (1998). Thrombospondin-1 is a major activator of TGF-beta1 in vivo. *Cell* 93(7): 1159-1170.

Curvers, W., ten Kate, F., Krishnadath, K., Visser, M., Elzer, B., Baak, L., Bohmer, C., Mallant-Hent, R., van Oijen, A., Naber, A., Scholten, P., Busch, O., Blaauwgeers, H., Meijer, G., & Bergman, J. (2010). Low-grade dysplasia in Barrett's esophagus: overdiagnosed and underestimated. *Am J Gastroenterol* 105(7): 1523-1530.

Dahut, W., Lakhani, N., Gulley, J., Arlen, P., Kohn, E., Kotz, H., McNally, D., Parr, A., Nguyen, D., Yang, S., Steinberg, S., Venitz, J., Sparreboom, A., & Figg, W. (2006). Phase I clinical trial of oral 2-methoxyestradiol, an antiangiogenic and apoptotic agent, in patients with solid tumors. *Cancer Biol Ther* 5(1): 22-27.

Dandara, C., Li, D., Walther, G., Parker, M. (2006). Gene-environment interaction: the role of SULT1A1 and CYP3A5 polymorphisms as risk modifiers for squamous cell carcinoma of the oesophagus. *Carcinogenesis* 27(4): 791-797.

Di Martino, E., Wild, C., Rotimi, O., Darnton, J., Olliver, R., & Hardie, L. (2006). IGFBP-3 and IGFBP-10 (CYR61) up-regulation during the development of Barrett's oesophagus

and associated oesophageal adenocarcinoma: potential biomarkers of disease risk. *Biomarkers* 11(6): 547-561.
Falk, G. (2002). Barrett's esophagus. *Gastroenterology* 122(6): 1569-1591.
Fang, M., Chen, D., & Yang, C. (2007). Dietary polyphenols may affect DNA methylation. *J Nutr* 137 (1 Suppl): 223S-228S.
Fassan, M., Volinia, S., Palatini, J., Pizzi, M., Baffa, R., De Bernard, M., Battaglia, G., Parente, P., Croce, C., Zaninotto, G., Ancona, E., & Rugge, M. (2010). MicroRNA expression profiling in human Barrett's carcinogenesis. *Int J Cancer*. Dec 2.
Feber, A., Xi, L., Luketich, J., Pennathur, A., Landreneau, R., Wu, M., Swanson, S., Godfrey, T., & Litle, V. (2008). MicroRNA expression profiles of esophageal cancer. *J Thorac Cardiovasc Surg* 135(2): 255-260; discussion 260.
Feber, A., Xi, L., Pennathur, A., Gooding, W., Bandla, S., Wu, M., Luketich, J., Godfrey, T., & Litle, V. (2011). MicroRNA prognostic signature for nodal metastases and survival in esophageal adenocarcinoma. *Ann Thorac Surg* 91(5): 1523-1530.
Flejou, J. (2005). Barrett's oesophagus: from metaplasia to dysplasia and cancer. *Gut* 54 Suppl 1: i6-12.
Fuks, F., Burgers, W., Brehm, A., Hughes-Davies, L., & Kouzarides, T. (2000). DNA methyltransferase Dnmt1 associates with histone deacetylase activity. *Nat Genet* 24(1): 88-91.
Gubbay, J., Collignon, J., Koopman, P., Capel, B., Economou, A., Munsterberg, A., Vivian, N., Goodfellow, P., Lovell-Badge, R. (1990). A gene mapping to the sex-determining region of the mouse Y chromosome is a member of a novel family of embryonically expressed genes. *Nature* 346(6281): 245-250.
Guo, M., House, M., Suzuki, H., Ye, Y., Brock, M., Lu, F., Liu, Z., Rustgi, A., & Herman, J. (2007). Epigenetic silencing of CDX2 is a feature of squamous esophageal cancer. *Int J Cancer* 121(6): 1219-1226.
Guo, M., Ren, J., Brock, M., Herman, J., & Carraway, H. (2008). Promoter methylation of HIN-1 in the progression to esophageal squamous cancer. *Epigenetics* 3(6): 336-341.
Guo, M., Ren, J., House, M., Qi, Y., Brock, M., & Herman, J. (2006). Accumulation of promoter methylation suggests epigenetic progression in squamous cell carcinoma of the esophagus. *Clin Cancer Res* 12(15): 4515-4522.
Guo, Y., Chen, Z., Zhang, L., Zhou, F., Shi, S., Feng, X., Li, B., Meng, X., Ma, X., Luo, M., Shao, K., Li, N., Qiu, B., Mitchelson, K., Cheng, J., & He, J. (2008). Distinctive microRNA profiles relating to patient survival in esophageal squamous cell carcinoma. *Cancer Research* 68(1): 26-33.
Hansen, J. (2002). Conformational dynamics of the chromatin fiber in solution: determinants, mechanisms, and functions. *Annu Rev Biophys Biomol Struct* 31: 361-392.
He, L., Liu, M., Li, B., Rao, H., Liao, Y., Guan, X., Zeng, Y., & Xie, D. (2009). Prognostic impact of H3K27me3 expression on locoregional progression after chemoradiotherapy in esophageal squamous cell carcinoma. *BMC cancer* 9: 461.
Holmes, A., Abraham, D., Sa, S., Shiwen, X., Black, C., & Leask, A. (2001). CTGF and SMADs, maintenance of scleroderma phenotype is independent of SMAD signaling. *J Biol Chem* 276(14): 10594-10601.

Hong, J., Behar, J., Wands, J., Resnick, M., Wang, L., Delellis, R., Lambeth, D., & Cao, W. (2010). Bile acid reflux contributes to development of esophageal adenocarcinoma via activation of phosphatidylinositol-specific phospholipase Cgamma2 and NADPH oxidase NOX5-S. *Cancer Res* 70(3): 1247-1255.

Hu, N., Huang, J., Emmert-Buck, M., Tang, Z., Roth, M., Wang, C., Dawsey, S., Li, G., Li, W., Wang, Q., Han, X., Ding, T., Giffen, C., Goldstein, A., & Taylor, P. (2001). Frequent inactivation of the TP53 gene in esophageal squamous cell carcinoma from a high-risk population in China. *Clin Cancer Res* 7(4): 883-891.

Hu, N., Wang, C., Ng, D., Clifford, R., Yang, H., Tang, Z., Wang, Q., Han, X., Giffen, C., Goldstein, A., Taylor, P., & Lee, M. (2009). Genomic characterization of esophageal squamous cell carcinoma from a high-risk population in China. *Cancer research* 69(14): 5908-5917.

Huang, Y., Chang, X., Lee, J., Cho, Y., Zhong, X., Park, I., Liu, J., Califano, J., Ratovitski, E., Sidransky, D., & Kim, M. (2011). Cigarette smoke induces promoter methylation of single-stranded DNA-binding protein 2 in human esophageal squamous cell carcinoma. *Int J Cancer* 128(10): 2261-2273.

I, H., Ko, E., Kim, Y., Cho, E., Han, J., Park, J., Kim, K., Kim, D., & Shim, Y. (2010). Association of global levels of histone modifications with recurrence-free survival in stage IIB and III esophageal squamous cell carcinomas. *Cancer Epidemiol Biomarkers Prev* 19(2): 566-573.

Johnson, L., Cao, X., & Jacobsen, S. (2002). Interplay between two epigenetic marks. DNA methylation and histone H3 lysine 9 methylation. *Curr Biol* 12(16): 1360-1367.

Kambhampati, S., Banerjee, S., Dhar, K., Mehta, S., Haque, I., Dhar, G., Majumder, M., Ray, G., Vanveldhuizen, P., & Banerjee, S. K. (2010). 2-methoxyestradiol inhibits Barrett's esophageal adenocarcinoma growth and differentiation through differential regulation of the beta-catenin-E-cadherin axis. *Mol Cancer Ther* 9(3): 523-534.

Kano, M., Seki, N., Kikkawa, N., Fujimura, L., Hoshino, I., Akutsu, Y., Chiyomaru, T., Enokida, H., Nakagawa, M., & Matsubara, H. (2010). miR-145, miR-133a and miR-133b: Tumor suppressive miRNAs target FSCN1 in esophageal squamous cell carcinoma. *Int J Cancer* 127(12): 2804-2814.

Kassis, E., Zhao, M., Hong, J., Chen, G., Nguyen, D., & Schrump, D. S. (2006). Depletion of DNA methyltransferase 1 and/or DNA methyltransferase 3b mediates growth arrest and apoptosis in lung and esophageal cancer and malignant pleural mesothelioma cells. *J Thorac Cardiovasc Surg* 131(2): 298-306.

Kim, Y., Park, J. , Jeon, Y., Park, S. , Song, J., Kang, C. , Sung, S., & Kim, J. (2009). Aberrant promoter CpG island hypermethylation of the adenomatosis polyposis coli gene can serve as a good prognostic factor by affecting lymph node metastasis in squamous cell carcinoma of the esophagus. *Dis Esophagus* 22(2): 143-150.

Klose, R. & Bird, A. (2006). Genomic DNA methylation: the mark and its mediators. *Trends Biochem Sci* 31(2): 89-97.

Koliopanos, A., Friess, H., di Mola, F., Tang, W., Kubulus, D., Brigstock, D., Zimmermann, A., Buchler, M. (2002). Connective tissue growth factor gene expression alters tumor progression in esophageal cancer. *World J Surg* 26(4): 420-427.

Krishnadath, K., Tilanus, H., van Blankenstein, M., Hop, W., Kremers, E., Dinjens, W., Bosman, F. (1997). Reduced expression of the cadherin-catenin complex in oesophageal adenocarcinoma correlates with poor prognosis. *J Pathol* 182(3): 331-338.

Langer, R., Ott, K., Feith, M., Lordick, F., Siewert, J. R., & Becker, K. (2009). Prognostic significance of histopathological tumor regression after neoadjuvant chemotherapy in esophageal adenocarcinomas. *Mod Pathol* 22(12): 1555-1563.

Lao-Sirieix, P., Boussioutas, A., Kadri, S., O'Donovan, M., Debiram, I., Das, M., Harihar, L., & Fitzgerald, R. (2009). Non-endoscopic screening biomarkers for Barrett's oesophagus: from microarray analysis to the clinic. *Gut* 58(11): 1451-1459.

Lee, E., Lee, B., Han, J., Cho, E., Shim, Y., Park, J., & Kim, D. H. (2008). CpG island hypermethylation of E-cadherin (CDH1) and integrin alpha4 is associated with recurrence of early stage esophageal squamous cell carcinoma. *Int J Cancer* 123(9): 2073-2079.

Li, A., Hsu, P., Tzao, C., Wang, Y., Hung, I., Huang, M., & Hsu, H. (2009). Reduced axin protein expression is associated with a poor prognosis in patients with squamous cell carcinoma of esophagus. *Ann Surg Oncol* 16(9): 2486-2493.

Li, B., Li, Y., Tsao, S., & Cheung, A. (2009). Targeting NF-kappaB signaling pathway suppresses tumor growth, angiogenesis, and metastasis of human esophageal cancer. *Mol Cancer Ther* 8(9): 2635-2644.

Li, J., Minnich, D., Camp, E., Brank, A., Mackay, S., & Hochwald, S. (2006). Enhanced sensitivity to chemotherapy in esophageal cancer through inhibition of NF-kappaB. *J Surg Res* 132(1): 112-120.

Li, X., Galipeau, P., Sanchez, C., Blount, P., Maley, C., Arnaudo, J., Peiffer, D., Pokholok, D., Gunderson, K., & Reid, B. J. (2008). Single nucleotide polymorphism-based genome-wide chromosome copy change, loss of heterozygosity, and aneuploidy in Barrett's esophagus neoplastic progression. *Cancer prevention research* 1(6): 413-423.

Li, X., Lin, R., & Li, J. (2011). Epigenetic Silencing of MicroRNA-375 Regulates PDK1 Expression in Esophageal Cancer. *Digestive diseases and sciences.* Apr 30

Li, Y., Zhang, X., Huang, G., Miao, X., Guo, L., Lin, D., Lu, S. (2006). Identification of a novel polymorphism Arg290Gln of esophageal cancer related gene 1 (ECRG1) and its related risk to esophageal squamous cell carcinoma. *Carcinogenesis* 27(4): 798-802.

Liu, Q., Lv, G., Qin, X., Gen, Y., Zheng, S., Liu, T., & Lu, X. (2011). Role of microRNA let-7 and effect to HMGA2 in esophageal squamous cell carcinoma. *Mol Biol Rep.* May 20

Liu, Z., Zhang, L., Ding, F., Li, J., Guo, M., Li, W., Wang, Y., Yu, Z., Zhan, Q., & Wu, M. (2005). 5-Aza-2'-deoxycytidine induces retinoic acid receptor-beta(2) demethylation and growth inhibition in esophageal squamous carcinoma cells. *Cancer Lett* 230(2): 271-283.

Logan, C. & Nusse, R. (2004). The Wnt signaling pathway in development and disease. *Annu Rev Cell Dev Biol* 20: 781-810.

Makino, T., Yamasaki, M., Takeno, A., Shirakawa, M., Miyata, H., Takiguchi, S., Nakajima, K., Fujiwara, Y., Nishida, T., Matsuura, N., Mori, M., & Doki, Y. (2009).

Cytokeratins 18 and 8 are poor prognostic markers in patients with squamous cell carcinoma of the oesophagus. *Br J Cancer* 101(8): 1298-1306.

Martin, C. & Zhang, Y. (2005). The diverse functions of histone lysine methylation. *Nat Rev Mol Cell Biol* 6(11): 838-849.

Maru, D., Singh, R., Hannah, C., Albarracin, C., Li, Y., Abraham, R., Romans, A., Yao, H., Luthra, M., Anandasabapathy, S., Swisher, S., Hofstetter, W., Rashid, A., & Luthra, R. (2009). MicroRNA-196a is a potential marker of progression during Barrett's metaplasia-dysplasia-invasive adenocarcinoma sequence in esophagus. *The American journal of pathology* 174(5): 1940-1948.

Marx, A., Zielinski, M., Kowitz, C., Dancau, A., Thieltges, S., Simon, R., Choschzick, M., Yekebas, E., Kaifi, J., Mirlacher, M., Atanackovic, D., Brummendorf, T., Fiedler, W., Bokemeyer, C., Izbicki, J., & Sauter, G. (2010). Homogeneous EGFR amplification defines a subset of aggressive Barrett's adenocarcinomas with poor prognosis. *Histopathology* 57(3): 418-426.

Massague, J. (2000). How cells read TGF-beta signals. *Nat Rev Mol Cell Biol* 1(3): 169-178.

Mathe, E., Nguyen, G., Bowman, E., Zhao, Y., Budhu, A., Schetter, A., Braun, R., Reimers, M., Kumamoto, K., Hughes, D., Altorki, N., Casson, A., Liu, C., Wang, X., Yanaihara, N., Hagiwara, N., Dannenberg, A., Miyashita, M., Croce, C., & Harris, C. (2009). MicroRNA expression in squamous cell carcinoma and adenocarcinoma of the esophagus: associations with survival. *Clin Cancer Res* 15(19): 6192-6200.

Matsushima, K., Isomoto, H., Kohno, S., & Nakao, K. (2010). MicroRNAs and esophageal squamous cell carcinoma. *Digestion* 82(3): 138-144.

McManus, D., Olaru, A., & Meltzer, S. (2004). Biomarkers of esophageal adenocarcinoma and Barrett's esophagus. *Cancer Res* 64(5): 1561-1569.

Nakajima, M., Fukuchi, M., Miyazaki, T., Masuda, N., Kato, H., & Kuwano, H. (2003). Reduced expression of Axin correlates with tumour progression of oesophageal squamous cell carcinoma. *Br J Cancer* 88(11): 1734-1739.

Narumiya, K., Metzger, R., Bollschweiler, E., Alakus, H., Brabender, J., Drebber, U., Holscher, A., & Warnecke-Eberz, U. (2011). Impact of ABCB1 C3435T polymorphism on lymph node regression in multimodality treatment of locally advanced esophageal cancer. *Pharmacogenomics* 12(2): 205-214.

Oka, D., Yamashita, S., Tomioka, T., Nakanishi, Y., Kato, H., Kaminishi, M., & Ushijima, T. (2009). The presence of aberrant DNA methylation in noncancerous esophageal mucosae in association with smoking history: a target for risk diagnosis and prevention of esophageal cancers. *Cancer* 115(15): 3412-3426.

Onwuegbusi, B., Aitchison, A., Chin, S., Kranjac, T., Mills, I., Huang, Y., Lao-Sirieix, P., Caldas, C., & Fitzgerald, R. (2006). Impaired transforming growth factor beta signalling in Barrett's carcinogenesis due to frequent SMAD4 inactivation. *Gut* 55(6): 764-774.

Oshiba, G., Kijima, H., Himeno, S., Kenmochi, T., Kise, Y., Tanaka, H., Nishi, T., Chino, O., Shimada, H., Machimura, T., Tsuchida, T., Nakamura, M., Ueyama, Y., Tanaka, M., Tajima, T., & Makuuchi, H. (1999). Stromal thrombospondin-1 expression is correlated with progression of esophageal squamous cell carcinomas. *Anticancer Res* 19(5C): 4375-4378.

Osterheld, M., Bian, Y., Bosman, F., Benhattar, J., & Fontolliet, C. (2002). Beta-catenin expression and its association with prognostic factors in adenocarcinoma developed in Barrett esophagus. *Am J Clin Pathol* 117(3): 451-456.

Pardali, K., & Moustakas, A. (2007). Actions of TGF-beta as tumor suppressor and pro-metastatic factor in human cancer. *Biochim Biophys Acta* 1775(1): 21-62.

Paulson, T., Maley, C., Li, X., Li, H., Sanchez, C., Chao, D., Odze, R., Vaughan, T., Blount, P., & Reid, B. (2009). Chromosomal instability and copy number alterations in Barrett's esophagus and esophageal adenocarcinoma. *Clin Cancer Res* 15(10): 3305-3314.

Peters, A., Kubicek, S., Mechtler, K., O'Sullivan, R., Derijck, A., Perez-Burgos, L., Kohlmaier, A., Opravil, S., Tachibana, M., Shinkai, Y., Martens, J., & Jenuwein, T. (2003). Partitioning and plasticity of repressive histone methylation states in mammalian chromatin. *Mol Cell* 12(6): 1577-1589.

Pietsch, E., Humbey, O., & Murphy, M. (2006). Polymorphisms in the p53 pathway. *Oncogene* 25(11): 1602-1611.

Qifeng, S., Bo, C., Xingtao, J., Chuanliang, P., & Xiaogang, Z. (2011). Methylation of the promoter of human leukocyte antigen class I in human esophageal squamous cell carcinoma and its histopathological characteristics. *J Thorac Cardiovasc Surg* 141(3): 808-814.

Qiu, H., Zhang, W., El-Naggar, A., Lippman, S., Lin, P., Lotan, R., & Xu, X. (1999). Loss of retinoic acid receptor-beta expression is an early event during esophageal carcinogenesis. *Am J Pathol* 155(5): 1519-1523.

Reid, B., Levine, D., Longton, G., Blount, P., & Rabinovitch, P. (2000). Predictors of progression to cancer in Barrett's esophagus: baseline histology and flow cytometry identify low- and high-risk patient subsets. *Am J Gastroenterol* 95(7): 1669-1676.

Sadikovic, B., Al-Romaih, K., Squire, J., & Zielenska, M. (2008). Cause and consequences of genetic and epigenetic alterations in human cancer. *Curr Genomics* 9(6): 394-408.

Schotta, G., Lachner, M., Sarma, K., Ebert, A., Sengupta, R., Reuter, G., Reinberg, D., & Jenuwein, T. (2004). A silencing pathway to induce H3-K9 and H4-K20 trimethylation at constitutive heterochromatin. *Genes Dev* 18(11): 1251-1262.

Sethi, G., Sung, B., & Aggarwal, B. (2008). Nuclear factor-kappaB activation: from bench to bedside. *Exp Biol Med (Maywood)* 233(1): 21-31.

Shaheen, N. & Richter, J. (2009). Barrett's oesophagus. *Lancet* 373(9666): 850-861.

Sheibani, N., & Frazier, W. (1995). Thrombospondin 1 expression in transformed endothelial cells restores a normal phenotype and suppresses their tumorigenesis. *Proc Natl Acad Sci U S A* 92(15): 6788-6792.

Sung, C., Han, S., & Kim, S. (2011). Low expression of claudin-4 is associated with poor prognosis in esophageal squamous cell carcinoma. *Ann Surg Oncol* 18(1): 273-281.

Sweeney, C., Liu, G., Yiannoutsos, C., Kolesar, J., Horvath, D., Staab, M., Fife, K., Armstrong, V., Treston, A., Sidor, C., & Wilding, G. (2005). A phase II multicenter, randomized, double-blind, safety trial assessing the pharmacokinetics, pharmacodynamics, and efficacy of oral 2-methoxyestradiol capsules in hormone-refractory prostate cancer. *Clin Cancer Res* 11(18): 6625-6633.

Tanaka, E., Hashimoto, Y., Ito, T., Okumura, T., Kan, T., Watanabe, G., Imamura, M., Inazawa, J., & Shimada, Y. (2005). The clinical significance of Aurora-A/STK15/BTAK expression in human esophageal squamous cell carcinoma. *Clin Cancer Res* 11(5): 1827-1834.

Tonomoto, Y., Tachibana, M., Dhar, D., Onoda, T., Hata, K., Ohnuma, H., Tanaka, T., & Nagasue, N. (2007). Differential expression of RUNX genes in human esophageal squamous cell carcinoma: downregulation of RUNX3 worsens patient prognosis. *Oncology* 73(5-6): 346-356.

Toshimitsu, H., Hashimoto, K., Tangoku, A., Iizuka, N., Yamamoto, K., Kawauchi, S., Oga, A., Furuya, T., Oka, M., & Sasaki, K. (2004). Molecular signature linked to acquired resistance to cisplatin in esophageal cancer cells. *Cancer Lett* 211(1): 69-78.

Trudgill, N., Suvarna, S., Royds, J., & Riley, S. (2003). Cell cycle regulation in patients with intestinal metaplasia at the gastro-oesophageal junction. *Mol Pathol* 56(6): 313-317.

Tse, D., Zhai, R., Zhou, W., Heist, R., Asomaning, K., Su, L., Lynch, T., Wain, J., Christiani, D., Liu, G. (2008). Polymorphisms of the NER pathway genes, ERCC1 and XPD are associated with esophageal adenocarcinoma risk. *Cancer causes & control* : CCC 19(10): 1077-1083.

Veeramachaneni, N., Kubokura, H., Lin, L., Pippin, J., Patterson, G., Drebin, J., & Battafarano, R. (2004). Down-regulation of beta catenin inhibits the growth of esophageal carcinoma cells. *J Thorac Cardiovasc Surg* 127(1): 92-98.

Wang, J., Guo, M., Montgomery, E., Thompson, R., Cosby, H., Hicks, L., Wang, S., Herman, J., & Canto, M. (2009). DNA promoter hypermethylation of p16 and APC predicts neoplastic progression in Barrett's esophagus. *Am J Gastroenterol* 104(9): 2153-2160.

Wu, T., Watanabe, T., Heitmiller, R., Zahurak, M., Forastiere, A. & Hamilton, S. (1998). Genetic alterations in Barrett esophagus and adenocarcinomas of the esophagus and esophagogastric junction region. *Am J Pathol* 153(1): 287-294.

Yang, H., Gu, J., Wang, K., Zhang, W., Xing, J., Chen, Z., Ajani, J., & Wu, X. (2009). MicroRNA expression signatures in Barrett's esophagus and esophageal adenocarcinoma. *Clin Cancer Res* 15(18): 5744-5752.

Yuan, Y., Zeng, Z., Liu, X., Gong, D., Tao, J., Cheng, H., & Huang, S. (2011). MicroRNA-203 inhibits cell proliferation by repressing DeltaNp63 expression in human esophageal squamous cell carcinoma. *BMC Cancer* 11: 57.

Zhang, W., Glockner, S., Guo, M., Machida, E., Wang, D., Easwaran, H., Van Neste, L., Herman, J., Schuebel, K., Watkins, D., Ahuja, N., & Baylin, S. B. (2008). Epigenetic inactivation of the canonical Wnt antagonist SRY-box containing gene 17 in colorectal cancer. *Cancer Res* 68(8): 2764-2772.

Zhang, X. & Guo, M. (2010). The value of epigenetic markers in esophageal cancer. *Frontiers of medicine in China* 4(4): 378-384.

Zhou, Z., Cao, W., Xie, J., Lin, J., Shen, Z., Zhang, Q., Shen, J., Xu, L., & Li, E. (2009). Expression and prognostic significance of THBS1, Cyr61 and CTGF in esophageal squamous cell carcinoma. *BMC Cancer* 9: 291.

2

Growth Factors, Signal Transduction Pathways, and Tumor Suppressor Genes in Esophageal Cancer

Maryam Zare[1,2], Mehdi Moghanibashi[1,3] and Ferdous Rastgar Jazii[1,4]
[1]*Department of Biochemistry, National Institute of Genetic Engineering & Biotechnology (NIGEB), Tehran,*
[2]*Department of Biology, Payam-Noor University, Tehran,*
[3]*Islamic Azad University, Kazerun Branch, School of Medicine, Kazerun, Shiraz,*
[4]*Department of Molecular Structure and Function, Research Institute, Hospital for Sick Children (Sickkids), Toronto, ON,*
[1,2,3]*Iran*
[4]*Canada*

1. Introduction

Esophageal cancer is the eighth common cancers in the world and the sixth most common cause of cancer-related death throughout the world [1, 2]. Histologically, esophageal cancer can be divided into adenocarcinoma and squamous cell carcinoma (SCCE). Esophageal cancer is among the most malignant type of cancers which rapidly invade into the surrounding tissues, metastases to the surrounding lymph nodes, and distant organs. Since clinical symptoms of esophagus cancer appear in the advanced stages of carcinogenesis, the majority of patients are diagnosed and receive medical attention only when the tumor has already gained substantial volume, spread into surrounding tissues, and cause obstruction when food is swallowed. Despite large improvements in the detection of cancers, surgical procedures and treatments, the prognosis of esophageal cancer remains poor and the 5-year survival rate is still low [3]. Therefore, early detection, seeking new strategies for treatment, comprehensive understanding of the molecular and genetic alterations of esophageal carcinogenesis are essential.

In addition to molecular alterations environmental and nutritional factors, as well as cultural habits are thought to be contributing factors in the development of esophageal cancer. The two major habitual risk factors are tobacco smoking and alcohol consumption. Chronic irritation and inflammation of the esophageal mucosa, which might be caused by substantial alcohol intake, achalasia, and frequent consumption of extremely hot beverages, increases the incidence rate of squamous cell carcinoma of the esophagus. In addition, a clear link between squamous cell carcinoma of esophagus and low socioeconomic status has also been established.

While the major risk factors for esophageal adenocarcinoma are the two altered physiological conditions: gastroesophageal reflux disease (GERD) and Barrett's esophagus [3], such association have not been proposed for squamous cell carcinoma of esophagus. In turn, a large number of molecular events were found to be involved in the development and progression of squamous cell carcinoma of esophagus. These events include genetic and epigenetic alterations in oncogenes, tumor suppressor genes, cell adhesion molecules, DNA repair genes, cell cycle regulatory genes, genetic instability as well as telomerase activation, and aberrant regulation of growth factors and their receptors. Recent studies have indicated that activation of cyclin D1, *erbB-2*, and *c-myc* oncogenes and inactivation of *p53*, *Rb*, *APC*, and *p16* tumor suppressor genes are frequently involved in esophageal cancers [3-6].

2. Growth factors

The significant role of growth factors and growth factor-mediated signaling pathways in the tumorigenesis of esophagus has been well established and similar to many other types of cancers as a preferred target for esophageal cancer therapy [4].

Growth factors regulate growth and development of cells. They might be supplied by distant glands and tissues, neighboring cells, or *in situ* by tumor cells themselves. Thus growth factors might be provided by endocrine, paracrine or autocrine mechanisms among which autocrine mechanism is thought to play a significant role in the growth of cancer cells [7, 8]. Most growth factors are polypeptides that regulate numerous cellular responses, notably cell proliferation. They exert their effects by binding to specific receptor on the cell surface; which most often is associated with an intrinsic tyrosine kinase activity, or by forming a complex with an intracellular tyrosine kinase [9]. Following to binding of growth factors to their corresponding receptors the tyrosine kinase activity is induced and phosphorylation of specific residue(s) in the intracellular domain of receptors occurs. Such phosphorylated cytoplasmic domains serve as docking sites for downstream signal transduction molecules and trigger signaling pathways that induce expression of cyclin D1, promoting cellular proliferation and survival (Fig 1, Fig 2) [10]. Aberrant regulation of growth factors and their corresponding receptors in addition to structural alterations in receptors play important role in tumorigenesis of esophageal cancer [4].

2.1 Epidermal Growth Factor Receptor (EGFR)

The epidermal growth factor receptor (EGFR) family and their ligands including epidermal growth factor (EGF) and transforming growth factor-α (TGF-α) are implicated in the development of esophageal cancer [7, 11-17]. The EGFR family composes of four members: EGFR (HER-1, erbB-1), HER2 (erbB-2, Neu), HER3 (erbB-3) and HER4 (erbB-4) [4, 18], all of which are tyrosine kinase receptors that are activated by ligand-induced homo or hetero dimerization. Overexpression of EGFRs is common in esophageal cancer and has been reported in several cell lines of SCCE, 29-92% of tumor samples of SCCE [19, 20] and 80% of patients with adeno and squamous cell carcinoma [21, 22]. EGFR upregulation correlates with poor prognosis, low survival rate and minimal response to chemotherapy [20, 23-25]. Amplification of EGFR gene has been found approximately in 8-30% of esophageal adenocarcinomas [21, 26]. Additionally, expression of EGF or TGF-α ligands along with overexpression of EGFR is correlated with esophageal cancer [7, 11, 12, 14-17]. EGF overexpression has also been detected in Barrett's-associated adenocarcinomas [13, 27, 28].

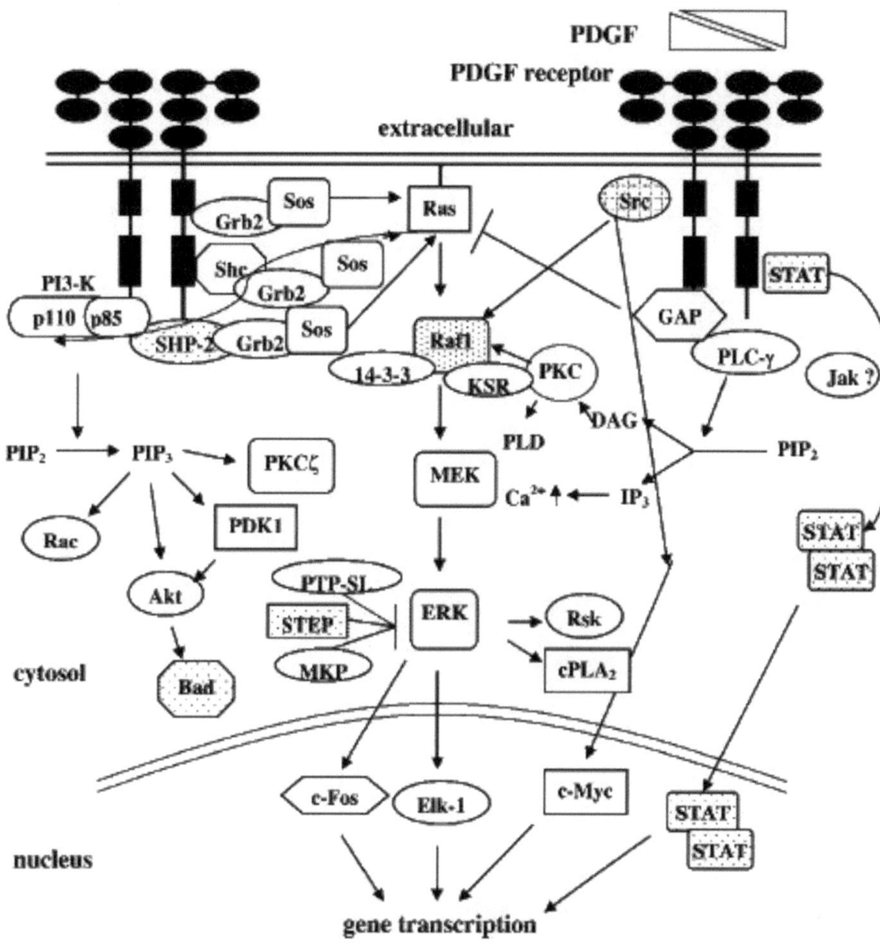

Fig. 1. Schematic presentation of growth factor-mediated signaling pathways. The picture illustrates signaling pathways downstream of PDGF receptors, activated by ligand-induced dimerization. Other tyrosine kinase receptors induce similar pathways. Arrows indicate activation; inhibitory interactions are indicated by blunted lines [4].

EGF may also serve growth inhibitory effect that shown to be mediated by STAT-1 (signal transducer and activator of transcription1) pathway and its mediation in the upregulation of p21 cyclin dependent kinase inhibitor [4, 29, 30].

EGFR activation is associated with metastasis as it modulates cell adhesion, angiogenesis, invasion and migration. Since EGFR activation increases expression of matrix metaloproteases (MMPs) it causes degradation of extracellular matrix and promotes invasion and metastasis in esophageal cancer [31, 32]. In addition, it has also been shown that EGF is implicated in relocalization of E-cadherin from the lateral adherent sides to cell surface, resulting in cell morphology change and increased invasiveness [33].

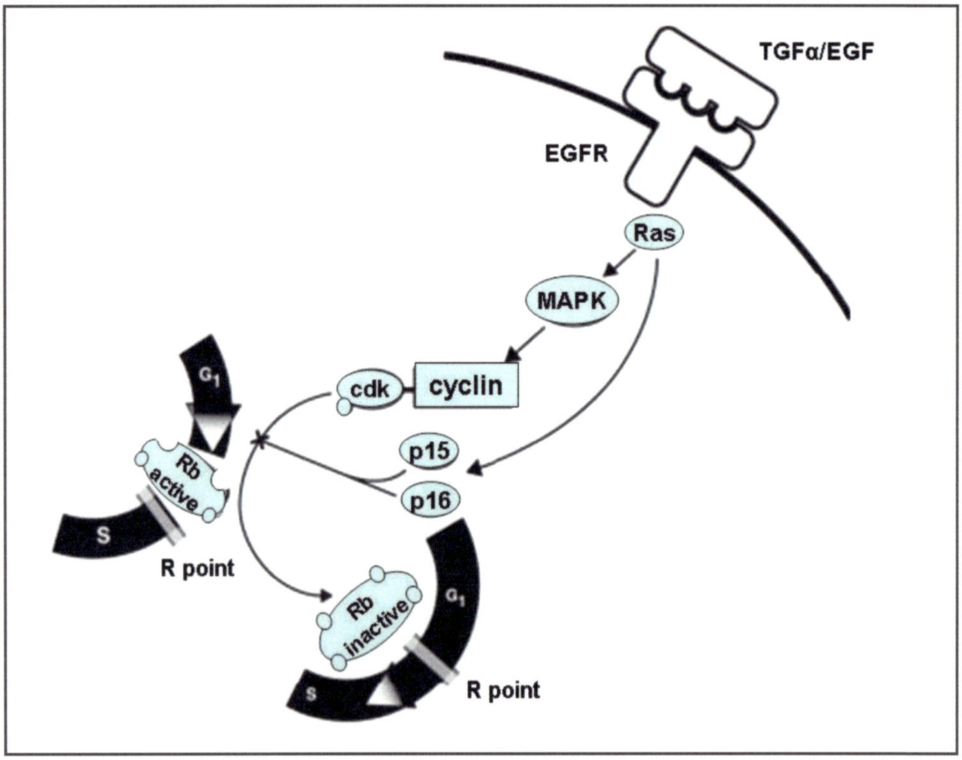

Fig. 2. Growth factors, Ras signaling and cell cycle regulation. Binding of growth factors TGF-α and EGF with EGFR (a tyrosine kinase receptor) promotes cell cycle progression by activating Ras and MAPK. MAPK signaling induces the expression of cyclins which bind CDKs and inactivate Rb. Activation of Ras also induces growth inhibitory effectors including p16 and p15. Similar to p53, p16 and p15 induce G1 arrest by inhibiting the function of cyclins and CDKs, thereby preventing cell cycle progression through the R-point [27]. By definition restriction point (R-point) is a point or event in G1 of a cell cycle at which cell becomes committed to progress cell cycle without requirement to extracellular proliferation stimulant.

2.2 Human Epidermal Growth Factor Receptor 2 (HER2)

Activation of certain tyrosine kinase receptors, such as EGF receptors and HER2 (erbB-2) results in phosphorylation of catenins and prevention of their binding to cadherins [34-36]. Regarding to this notion, overexpression of EGFR and HER2 (erbB-2) in esophageal cancer could possibly lead to sequestration of β-catenin, which result in the altered cell adhesion and increased tumor aggressiveness [27].

The role of HER-2 overexpression in esophageal cancer has been reported in 9%-60% of cases; depending on the stage of disease, tumor histology, or the applied methodology [4, 8, 11, 37-41]. There is no known ligand for HER-2, as it does its function by forming heterodimer with other tyrosine kinase receptors. In fact, *HER-2* (*erbB-2*) is an oncogenic form of the normal receptor tyrosine kinase and overexpression of erbB-2 by tumor cells is associated with hyperproliferation [4, 42]. Moreover, HER-2 expression may change during tumor progression [4, 43-45]. Although some studies demonstrate that HER-2 overexpression correlates with invasion, lymph node metastasis, and chemoresistance in esophageal cancer [46-48], others have shown that its expression is associated with favorable response to chemo or radiotherapy in esophagus cancer [49].

2.3 Insulin-like Growth Factor-1 (IGF-1) and IGF-1 receptor (IGF-1R)

Insulin-like growth factor-1 (IGF-1) and its tyrosine kinase receptor: IGF-1R, contribute to esophageal cancer. Tumor growth upon overexpression of IGF-1R, prevention of apoptosis via IGF-1 autocrine loop, and mitogenic effects of IGF-1 and IGF-2 has been reported in esophageal cancer as well as Barrett's-associated neoplasia [7, 50-52]. In addition, IGF binding protein-3 (IGFBP3); the major regulator of IGF-1 or IGF-2, is frequently overexpressed in SCCE in parallel with EGFR overexpression [53]. IGFBP3 has been shown to promote transforming growth factor β1-mediated epithelial to mesenchymal transition and motility in esophageal cancer [54]. Furthermore, the level of serum IGF-1 and IGFBP3 significantly increases in esophageal cancer patients, which correlates with tumor invasion, poor prognosis, and low survival rate of patients [55] .

Platelet-derived growth factor (PDGF) comprise a family of dimeric isoforms including the related A, B, C, and D polypeptides chains which bind to α- and β-tyrosine kinase receptors [56]. The significance of PDGF and its receptors in esophageal cancer is unclear. In physiological condition, normally, there is no expression of PDGF receptors in epithelial cells, while a number of studies have indicated the expression of different PDGF isoforms in esophageal cancer. It was found that PDGF-BB isoform promotes the growth of human esophageal carcinoma cell line and prevents apoptosis of cancer cells [57]. Additionally, overexpression of PDGFR-β receptor has been shown in tumor tissues of esophageal cancer [23, 58].

2.4 Vascular Endothelial Growth Factor (VEGF) and other angiogenesis factors

Vascular endothelial growth factor (VEGF) is composed of a family of closely related members, including VEGF-A, VEGF-B, VEGF-C, and VEGF-D as well as placental growth factor, among which VEGF-A is usually known as VEGF which is the main growth factor of endothelial cells. VEGF contributes to the vascular permeability, proliferation, as well as prevention of endothelial cell apoptosis. VEGFs utilize tyrosine kinase receptors of VEGFR family, including VEGFR-1 and VEGFR-2, and VEGFR-3, in which VEGFR-1 and VEGFR-2 transmit growth signals for blood vascular endothelial cells while, VEGFR-3 is involved in the regulation of lymphatic endothelial cells [59-61].

Overexpression of VEGF has been found in 30-60% of esophagus cancer cases. It is significantly correlated with advanced stage of disease, extent of microvessel density, distant metastasis, and poor survival rate in patients [62-64]. Upregulation of VEGF along with fibroblast growth factor has been shown in Barrett's esophagus and adenocarcinomas of esophagus as well as gastroesophageal junction tumor [65]. Since VEGF overexpression is associated with malignant potential of esophageal carcinoma and a higher level of which could be observed in serum (S-VEGF) of esophageal cancer patients; it could be considered as a significant and independent prognostic factor and a useful clinical biomarker for evaluation of patient's prognosis [66].

The major role of VEGF is in the process of angiogenesis where it plays an essential role in growth and metastasis of esophageal carcinoma. Among VEGF family, VEGF-C has shown to be correlated with the process of lymphangiogenesis leading to lymph node micrometastasis (LMN). It is considered as one of the most important prognostic factors of esophagus squamous cell carcinoma [67-69]. The association between VEGF-C expression with angiolymphatic invasion, lymph node metastasis and lower survival rate has been shown in esophageal adenocarcinoma as well [70]. Moreover, bone marrow micrometastases in esophageal cancer correlates with an increased level of plasma VEGF [71]. It has been shown that VEGF-C, and VEGF-D are involved in the early stages of esophageal carcinogenesis since they are also expressed in dysplastic lesions of both types of esophageal carcinomas [72, 73].

In addition to VEGF, other factors such as heparin-binding growth factor (midkine), fibroblast growth factor, thymidine phosphorylase, and hepatocyte growth factor contribute to tumor angiogenesis as well [66].

Overexpression and release of fibroblast growth factor (FGF-2) by stromal fibroblasts correlates with tumor recurrence and short survival in esophageal cancer patients [66, 74]. Stromal fibroblasts are also involved in tumor progression through degradation of extracellular matrix, secretion of growth factors, and regulation of epithelial cell behavior. It has also been shown that FGF receptor 2-positive fibroblasts provide a suitable microenvironment for tumor development and progression through stimulation of cancer cell proliferation, induction of angiogenesis, cell mobility, inhibition of cell adhesion, and promotion of epithelial-mesenchymal transition [75].

While many studies indicate an anti angiogenesis role for TGF-β, one study by using 3D in vitro model, has shown the role of fibroblasts and TGF-β in VEGF-induced angiogenesis in esophageal cancer, in which the paracrine TGF-β secretion by SCCE cells leads to the activation of stromal fibroblasts, which undergo a myofibroblastic transdifferentiation and expression of VEGF. Secretion of VEGF from activated fibroblasts, known as carcinoma-associated fibroblasts (CAFs), subsequently stimulate endothelial cells migration and vascular network formation (Fig 3) [76].

Midkine (MK) is a heparin-binding growth factor which overexpresses in esophageal carcinoma and plays a role in tumor angiogenesis and invasion [77]. Serum MK (S-MK) is an independent prognostic factor and may be a useful tumor marker for esophageal carcinoma, since the level of S-MK is increased in patients with esophageal carcinoma. It is also associated with tumor size, immunoreactivity, and poor survival of patients [66, 78, 79].

Hepatocyte growth factor (HGF), also known as scatter factor, is another factor that derives from specialized cancer-associated fibroblasts (CAFs) in the extracellular matrix that acts in a paracrine way to promote SCCE invasion via activation of VEGF and IL8 expression [80, 81]. It has been found that HGF and its tyrosine kinase receptor, c-Met, play significant role in esophageal carcinogenesis. Increased levels of HGF in serum, correlates positively with VEGF of serum, and significantly associates with the advanced stage of metastasis and low survival; provide an independent prognostic factor as well [66, 80]. Moreover, increased expression of c-Met tyrosine kinase receptor is significantly correlated with the reduced survival rate, distant metastasis, and local recurrence of cancer in esophageal cancer patients [80, 82, 83]. Grugan *et al.* have shown activation of HGF/Met signaling in human SCCE

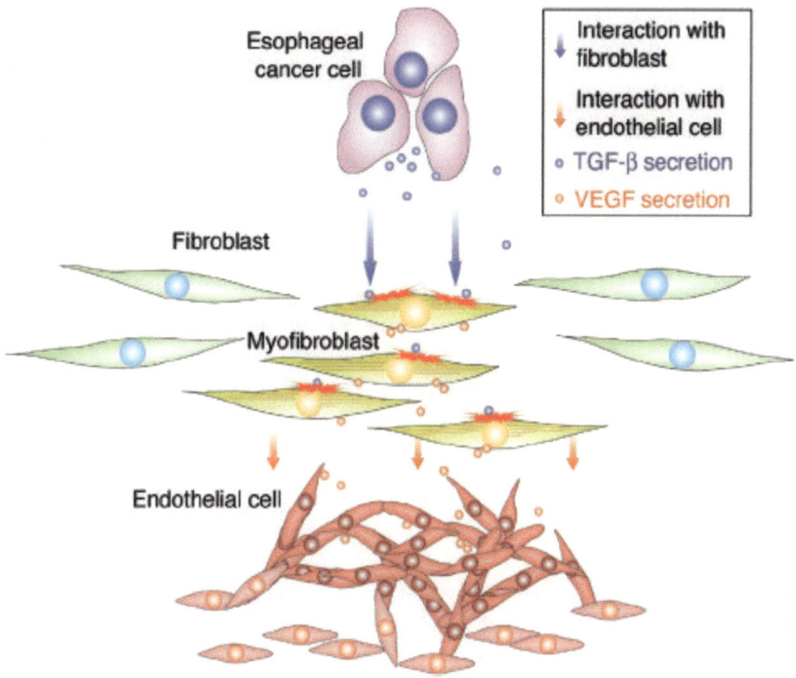

Fig. 3. Schematic illustration of SCCE cells and fibroblasts involvement in the vascular network formation. Esophageal cancer cells produce TGF-β to activate stromal normal fibroblasts. Tumor stromal fibroblasts become transdifferentiated into myofibroblasts that secrete VEGF, which in turn induce endothelial cell migration and the formation of a microcapillary network [76].

tissues and SCCE cell lines upon EGFR and p53 overexpression. Secretion of HGF by stromal fibroblasts induces the transformed esophageal epithelial cells to invade extracellular matrix; however, other unidentified factors may also cooperate with HGF in this process, which further highlight the significance of this pathway in esophageal carcinoma invasion and progression [84].

Recently another growth factor: connective tissue growth factor (CTGF, CCN2), has been introduced by Li and colleagues to be involved in the development and progression of SCCE in addition to poor survival of SCCE patients. It is suggested to be an independent factor for SCCE patients' prognosis as well as diagnosis of the precancerous lesions; as a result early detection of SCCE [85].

3. Signal transduction pathways

3.1 Ras signaling

Activation of the Ras pathway takes place upon a wide range of stimuli that could initiate its signaling. Ras activation begins with a vast array of upstream activated receptors including receptor tyrosine kinases, serpentine receptors, heterotrimeric G-proteins, integrins and cytokine receptors [86]. Among these activators, the best described mean of Ras stimulation is via receptor tyrosine kinases such as EGF receptor (Fig 4). Binding of growth factors to their cognate receptors promote cellular proliferation through signal transduction cascades, initiated by the activation of membrane associated Ras proteins. Ras/Raf/mitogen activated protein kinase (MAPK) is one of the key Ras dependent growth-stimulating signaling cascade activated when growth factors bind their tyrosine kinase receptors, which ultimately leads to the induction of cyclin D1 [87, 88].

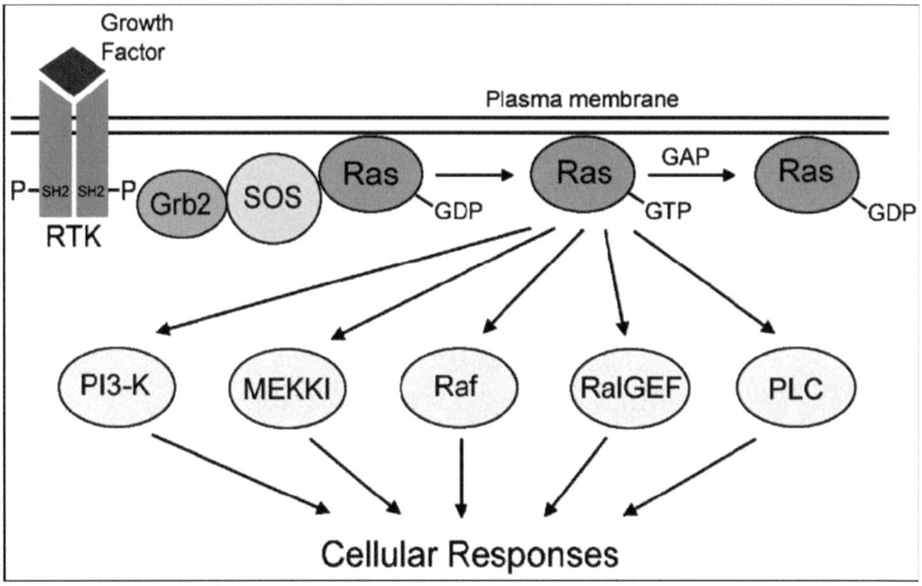

Fig. 4. A simplified overview of Ras activation and signaling cascade. Activation of a receptor tyrosine kinase (RTK) by an appropriate growth factor stimulates autophosphorylation of SH2 domains that recruit Grb2. Guanine nucleotide exchange factors (GEF) such as SOS are localized to the membrane by Grb2, which then stimulate Ras to exchange GDP for GTP. The activated Ras interacts with multiple signaling pathways, including phosphoinositide 3Vkinase (PI3-K), MEKKI, Raf kinase, RalGEFs and phospholipase C (PLC) to induce cellular responses. Ras signaling is terminated when GTPase activating proteins such as p120 and NF-1 stimulate Ras to hydrolyze GTP to GDP [86].

Ras pathway can also inhibit proliferation by inducing expression of p16 and p15 that are members of the INK4 family (Fig 2). These proteins block the Rb phosphorylation induced by cyclin D1/CDK complex, which results in cell cycle arrest in G1 [88]. Several lines of evidence have addressed the importance of Ras effectory pathways in the carcinogenesis of esophagus cancer; most notably through contribution of growth factors and their tyrosine kinase receptors, and in particular EGF and EGFR which are commonly deregulated and/or found at high level of expression in esophageal cancer [4, 5, 21, and 89].

In addition, mitogen activated protein kinase (MAPK) signal transduction pathway including Ras-Raf-MEK-ERK, PI3K/Akt, and JNK were found to be hyperactivated in esophageal cancer. This pathway modulates cell proliferation, invasion and metastasis, and resistance to chemotherapeutic agents, and ionizing radiation in esophageal cancer cells [24,

91-93]; in which, inhibition of MAPK signaling could enhance sensitivity of esophageal cancer cells to chemotherapeutic agents [94-96].

Lawler *et al.* [97] have also shown that mobility and invasiveness of metastatic esophageal cancer cells are potentiated by shear stress through the Rho kinase (ROCK) and Ras-signaling pathways, suggesting a novel physiological role for Rock and Ras in metastatic behavior of cancer cells [97].

The contribution of Ras/ERK signaling has been demonstrated by Senmaru *et al.* They have shown a dominant negative H-*ras* mutant (N116Y) inhibits EGF-stimulated activation of Erk2 in esophageal cancer cells. Furthermore, using adenoviral vectors and increased expression of this mutant significantly reduces the growth of human squamous cell carcinoma of esophagus cells *in vitro* and *in vivo* [98].

Furthermore, the significance of Ras signaling and its downstream pathways has also been recently indicated in tumorigenesis of esophageal cancer. Since, it was found that activation of MEK/ERK and PI3K/Akt effectory pathways play important role in downregulation of tropomyosin-1, which is a member of tropomyosin family and actin cytoskeleton-related proteins, in squamous cell carcinoma of esophagus [99].

Due to the importance of Ras dependent signaling drugs blocking these pathways were used in chemotherapy. Among such drugs are statins; a type of popular cholesterol-lowering agents including drugs such as Lipitor, were shown to inhibit tumor growth and proliferation of cancer cells as well as stimulation of apoptosis in esophageal cancer cell lines. These effects are achieved by inhibiting the Ras, ERK and protein kinase B (Akt) signaling pathways [90].

3.2 Wnt signaling

Wnt/β-catenin pathway initiates a signaling cascade critical for the normal development. The aberrant activity of this signaling pathway is associated with several forms of human carcinomas [100, 101]. Wnt ligands begin intracellular signaling pathways by binding to the G-protein -coupled receptors frizzleds (Fzs) [102]. In the absence of Wnt signals, GSK-3 phosphorylates cytosolic β-catenin within a destruction complex comprised of adenomatous polyposis coli (APC), Axin-1, casein kinase-1 (CK-1), and other proteins, the end result of which is targeting β-catenin for ubiquitin-mediated degradation (Fig 5a).

Upon Wnt binding to the Frizzled receptor and low-density lipoprotein receptor-related protein (LRP) co-receptors, the cytoplasmic Dishevelled (Dsh) protein becomes activated which in turn antagonizes the effects of GSK-3 through prevention of destruction complex formation and thus β-catenin phosphorylation. This in turn leads to the stabilization and accumulation of cytoplasmic β-catenin. GSK-3 could also be inactivated through phosphorylation by PI3-K (Fig 5c). As a result, accumulated cytoplasmic β-catenin enters into the nucleus where it binds to the T cell factor/TCF/LEF (T-cell factor/lymphoid enhancer-binding factor 1) transcription factor family and stimulates transcription of target genes including *c-myc, cyclin D1, c-jun,* and *fra-1* (Fig 5b), which plays critical roles in cell growth, proliferation, and differentiation [101-104]. Aberrant expression and function of Wnt signaling components result in aberrant nuclear accumulation of β-catenin which in turn contributes to the tumorigenesis of esophageal cancer through increased expression of cyclin D1 [105].

In addition to its role in Wnt signaling, β-catenin is also involved in cell adhesion, providing a link between actin cytoskeleton and cadherin(s) cell adhesion molecules [106, 107]. E-cadherin and β-catenin are primarily found in the cell membrane of the normal squamous mucosa of esophagus and the nondysplastic, specialized intestinal metaplasia of Barrett's esophagus [108, 109]. Immunohistochemical studies of dysplastic Barrett's esophagus has shown that membrane E-cadherin and β-catenin are decreased, while their level is increased in cytoplasm and nucleus [110].

Loss of APC tumor suppressor gene plays important role in the development of esophageal cancer, since loss of heterozygosity (LOH) of 5q21, the APC locus, occurs commonly in adenocarcinomas of esophagus [111-113]. Mutations in β-catenin and/or APC gene also alter degradation of β-catenin, as a result, its aberrant accumulation leads to the increased transcription of target genes. However, it has been shown that mutations of APC and β-catenin genes, unlike in colorectal carcinoma, involve in only a small subset of esophageal and esophagogastric junction carcinomas [114], or somehow are rare in esophageal cancer [115]. However some studies have confirmed that mutations of APC gene occur in human esophageal cancer [116, 117].

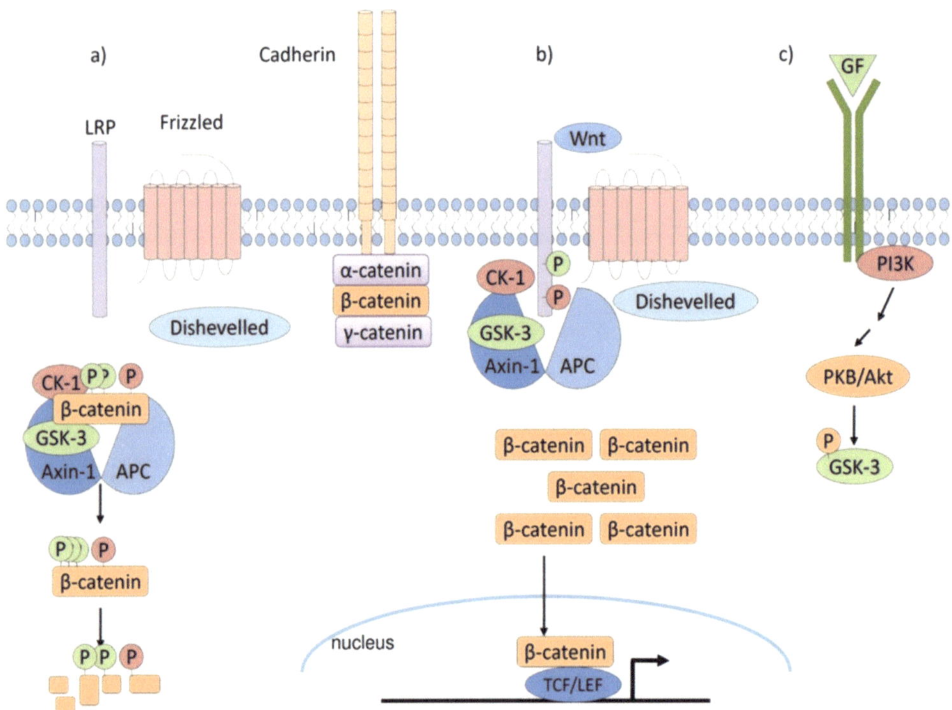

Fig. 5. The role of Wnt signaling in the activation of gene expression through mediation of β-catenin induced transcription. The non-phosphorylated form of β-catenin is active while the phosphorylated form of which is doomed to the inactivation and proteasomal degradation (a). Dishevelled antigonises β-catenin phosphorylation by GSK-3 (b) and PI3K does the same function by phosphorylating GSK-3 and thus inhibition GSK-3 mediated phosphorylation of β-catenin (c) [118].

Although mutations in *APC* or *β-catenin* are rare in esophageal cancer, alterations of upstream components, such as overexpression of Wnt2 ligand and Frizzled receptors or downregulation of Wnt antagonists and inactivation of secreted frizzeled-related protein (SFRP) genes by promoter methylation have been reported to play a dominant role in the activation of the Wnt pathway during esophageal carcinogenesis [119, 120].

Nonetheless, inactivation of APC by promoter methylation is involved in esophageal cancer, where it occurs in 83-92% of Barrett's high grade dysplasia and esophageal adenocarcinoma as well as 40-50% of Barrett's metaplasia without dysplasia [121, 122]. Higher level of promoter methylation of *APC* was also found by Clement, *et al.* in 100% of barrett's esophagus samples and in 95% of esophageal adenocarcinomas as well [119]. Several lines of evidence have also shown the role of *APC* promoter hypermethylation in squamous cell carcinoma of esophagus, as it was observed in about 50% of cases, to contribute in the progression of dysplasia to carcinoma in SCCE carcinogenesis along with low survival rate of patients [122-124]. Moreover, methylated *APC* DNA has been detected in the plasma of patients with esophageal adenocarcinoma and squamous cell carcinoma. Methylated APC promoter has shown to be associated with a significantly low patient survival [122], suggesting the capability of hypermethylated *APC* tumor suppressor gene to be a potential biomarker in esophageal cancer.

Wang *et al.* have recently shown a prominent role of Wnt signaling in SCCE carcinogenesis. They identified that Wnt2/β-catenin signaling pathway is activated in SCCE cells, as sodium nitroprusside (SNP) and siRNA against β-catenin not only inhibit expression of β-catenin and its major downstream effectors including c-myc and cyclin D1, but also induce cell cycle arrest and apoptosis, suggesting that Wnt2/β-catenin pathway may be a potential molecular target for SCCE therapy [125]. Inactivation of GSK3β, observed by higher phosphorylation of Ser9 GSK3β, has been found in most cancers with epithelial origin, including esophagus cancer [126, 127].

3.3 Dopamine and cyclic-AMP-regulated phosphoprotein

Recently, the role of t-DARPP (Dopamine and cyclic-AMP-regulated phosphoprotein) in the regulation of β-catenin has been investigated in esophageal cancer. DARPP-32 is a major regulator of dopaminergic neurotransmission in brain. It is the key factor for the functioning of the dopaminoceptive neurons [128]. DARPP-32 and t-DARPP, a truncated isoform of DARPP-32, are suggested as novel cancer-related genes [129].

Overexpression of t-DARPP has been reported in gastrointestinal malignancies as well as esophageal adenocarcinomas [130, 131], which leads to activation of Wnt signaling and increased cell proliferation through phosphorylation of GSK-3β, nuclear accumulation of β-catenin, and upregulation of *cyclin D1* and *c-myc* target genes. It has also been shown that t-DARPP mediated GSK-3β phosphorylation is AKT-dependent [132].

3.4 PI3K signaling

The involvement of phosphatidylinositol 3-kinase (PI3K)/AKT pathway in esophageal tumorigenesis was also subject of investigations. Phosphatidylinositol 3-kinases (PI3Ks) are a ubiquitous family of lipid kinases that catalyse the phosphorylation of phosphatidylinositol

(PI), PI(4)P and PI(4,5)P2 that leads to formation of PI(3)P, PI(3,4)P2 and PI(3,4,5)P3, respectively [133]. These phosphorylated lipid products are then able to activate a variety of downstream targets, such as protein kinase B (PKB/AKT), that regulate a wide range of important cellular processes, including cell proliferation, survival, migration, apoptosis, oncogenic transformation and intracellular trafficking of proteins [134].

Constitutive activation of PI3K and AKT is common in cancers including esophageal cancer [135-137]. Amplification of the *PIK3CA*, the gene coding for the $p110_{\alpha}$ catalytic subunit of PI3K, has been reported in SCCE [136] and in a low percentage of adenocarcinoma [138]. In addition, mutation of *PIK3CA* has been found to be an important event in the etiology of esophageal cancer [139].

Recent studies have indicated that inhibition of PI3K reduces proliferation and enhances radiosensitivity of esophageal cancer cells [92, 140]. In addition, the level of p-AKT expression in SCCE increases during chemotherapy, and a high expression of p-AKT correlates with poor prognosis [141].

3.5 Hedgehog signaling

The Hh (Hedgehog) signaling is critical for embryonic development which initiates following to binding of Hh to patched (Ptch) receptor, which releases smoothened (Smo), a potential G protein-coupled receptor (GPCR), from Ptch mediated repression. Smo signal transduction eventually leads to increased expression and activation of Gli, a transcription factor that regulates corresponding target genes [142-144]. Deregulation of this pathway leads to abnormal proliferation and transformation of cells in different tumors, such as small cell lung cancer, pancreatic cancer, prostate cancer and digestive tract cancer, including esophageal cancer [145-149] Hyperactive Hh signaling has been reported to be implicated in esophageal cancer [146, 147]. It has also been shown that PI3K/AKT pathway plays a critical role in epidermal growth factor (EGF), Gβγ and Shh-induced Hh signaling. Conversely, PI3K/AKT and MAPK signaling cooperate with the Shh pathway to promote esophageal cancer cell survival and proliferation [150].

3.6 Role of Id-1

Overexpression of Id-1, the inhibitor of differentiation or DNA binding, has also been shown in esophageal squamous cell carcinoma. Id-1 promotes proliferation [151], tumorigenicity and metastasis of human esophageal cancer cells through activation of PI3K/AKT signaling pathway [152-154]. Id-1 is a helix-loop-helix protein, which heterodimerizes with the basic helix-loop-helix transcription factors and inhibits them from DNA binding, therefore regulating gene transcription [155].

4. Tumor suppressor genes

4.1 P53

Tumor suppressor genes' inactivation occur by the genetic or epigenetic events such as mutations, allele deletions (LOH), promoter hypermethylation, abnormal splicing, and posttrancriptional silencing by microRNAs [156] in cancers. Alterations in multiple tumor suppressor genes including *Rb*, *p53*, *APC*, *p16*, and *MCC* implicated in carcinogenesis of esophageal cancer. The majority of tumor suppressor genes are involved in the regulation of cell cycle. Cell cycle is controlled precisely through two major regulatory mechanisms, the p53 (p14-MDM2-p53-p21) and pRb (p16-cyclinD1-pRb). Deregulation of both mechanisms play critical role in the development of most human cancers including esophageal cancer.

The *p53* tumor suppressor gene regulates cell cycle progression, apoptosis and DNA repair. It also inhibits vascular endothelial growth factor. *p53* is the most frequent mutated gene in all human malignancies. P53 is normally expressed at low level but accumulates in the nucleus of the damaged cell and transactivates target genes including genes involved in G1 cell-cycle arrest (*p21/WAF1*) and apoptosis (*BAX*) [157-161]. In fact, it plays a role as a genomic policeman to prevent replication of damaged DNA; either by arresting cells in G1 and facilitating DNA repair or by apoptotic elimination of damaged cells [162]. *p53* mutations are common in esophageal cancer which occur in approximately 50-80% of esophageal cancers. More than 92% of these mutations occur in the four conserved domains of the *p53* gene; exon 5 to exon 8, with hot spots at Arg175, Cys176, Arg248, Arg273, and Arg282, 80% of which are point mutations including 46% transition and 36% transversion [5]. Several studies have indicated that alteration of *p53* gene in esophageal cancer occurs in the early stage of carcinogenesis and is associated with tumor progression; suggesting that loss of p53 function is critical for the development of this type of cancer [5, 156].

Although the presence of mutant *p53* have shown to be correlated with the poor prognosis [163, 164], other studies have not found such correlation [165, 166]. It has also been shown that measurement of circulating anti p53 antibody in serum of patients with SCCE is useful for detection of *p53* mutations, and as a tumor marker or prognostic marker [167-169].

4.2 p21/WAF1

The *p21/WAF1* gene is located on chromosome 6p21.2 and encodes a cyclin-dependent kinase inhibitor. Induced by wild-type p53, it mediates G1 arrest following to DNA damage [170]. Mutations and deletions of the *p21/WAF1* gene are less common in human cancers [171]. However, polymorphisms in exon 2 of the *p21/WAF1* gene has been documented to play important role in esophageal tumorigenesis [172]. Moreover, induction of *p21/WAF1* may occur via *p73* [173], a transcription factor that also regulates *p21/WAF1* expression [174] in esophageal cancer. The role of *p21/waf1/CIP1* expression in SCCE prognosis seems to be controversial. Several studies have indicated reduced expression of p21 as an indicator of poor esophageal cancer prognosis [175, 176], while others have found no significant correlation [173, 177]. Conversly others have claimed that p21 overexpression is correlated with a poorer prognosis [165, 178].

4.3 p16/INK4a and p15/INK4b

p16/INK4a, which is located on chromosome 9p21 is another member of cyclin dependent kinase inhibitors and is involved in *p53* independent G1 arrest through inhibition of D type cyclin dependent kinases (CDK4/CDK6) in the Rb phosphorylation [179, 180] and inacivation. Inactivation of *p16/INK4a* is a common event in esophageal cancer and occurs through homozygous deletion, point mutation and/or hypermethylation [181-184]. In

SCCE, homozygous deletion and promoter methylation are the major causes of *p16/INK4a* gene silencing, while somatic mutation is a rare event [185]. *p16/INK4a* methylation or loss of heterozygosity (LOH) occurs in the early stages of SCCE tumor progression [186, 187], while homozygous deletion of its locus is a late event [188]. The two common mechanisms of *p16/INK4a* inactivation in esophageal adenocarcinoma were found to be promoter hypermethylation, which occurs in the early stages of carcinogenesis and loss of heterozygosity [189, 190]; while homozygous deletion have not been documented to play significant role. In addition, loss of *p16/INK4a* expression together with overexpression of cyclin D1 may also be correlated with poor prognosis [191]. Detection of hypermethylated *p16/INK4a* could provide an appropriate biomarker for esophageal cancer screening as it could be observed in the early stages of carcinogenesis [192-194].

p15/INK4b, a homolog of INK4 family whose locus is close to INK4a locus could be subject of stimulation by TGF-β and activate G1 arrest [195]. Changes in *p15/INK4b* has been studied less often in esophageal cancer; however it has been found that inactivation of *p15/INK4b* occurs through homozygous deletion or abnormal methylation at the same time as *p16/INK4a*, which leads to the loss of Rb-regulated restriction point and plays an essential role in esophageal carcinogenesis [188].

4.4 Retinoblastoma (Rb)

The retinoblastoma protein (pRb or commonly known as Rb) is a nuclear phosphoprotein that plays essential role in the regulation of cell cycle. It negatively regulates transcription by forming complex with E2F transcription factor. Phosphorylation of Rb by the cyclin/CDK complex, results in E2Fs release, expression of target genes and cell division [196-198]. While deletions or mutations of *Rb* or inactivation by HPV infection are rare in SCCE, however several studies have indicated that alteration in *p16* and *p53* lead to the blockage of Rb function [199-201]. However, loss of heterozygosity of the retinoblastoma locus plays essential role in the inactivation of *Rb* gene and is associated with p53 alterations in esophageal cancer. It is suggested that association of *Rb* with *p53* inactivation may be the major event in the development and progression of esophageal cancer [199, 202].

5. Other novel tumor suppressor genes

In addition to the well established role of well-known tumor suppressor genes such as *p53*, *Rb*, *APC*, *p21*, and *p16* in the carcinogenesis of esophagus cancer; there are other novel tumor suppressor genes which also play role in the development of esophageal cancer.

ECRG4 (esophageal cancer related gene 4) is a novel candidate tumor suppressor gene for SCCE, which is downregulated through promoter hypermethylation. *ECRG4* is significantly associated with lymph node metastasis, tumor size, and tumor stage in SCCE, providing a candidate prognostic marker for SCCE [203].

ING (Inhibitor of growth gene) family, *ING1* to *ING5*, are new class of candidate tumor suppressor genes that are implicated in the cell cycle control, senescence, apoptosis, DNA repair, and chromatin remodeling. Downregulation of *ING1* was observed to be implicated in esophagus cancer [204].

The tetraspanin cell surface receptor uroplakin 1A (*UPK1A*) has been identified as another candidate tumor suppressor gene, which is downregulated by promoter hypermethylation in SCCE cells. *UPK1A* downregulation correlates with lymph node metastasis, tumor stage, and overall survival of patients, as well [205].

Expression of MAL (T-lymphocyte maturation associated protein), which is a component of protein machinery for apical transport in epithelial polarized cells, remarkably reduces in esophageal cancer. In addition, DNA methylation has shown to be associated with its downregulation [206].

*DLC*1 (deleted in lung cancer 1) is a putative tumor suppressor gene located on chromosome 3 (3p21.3) is supposed to act as a downstream gene in the serine/threonine kinase pathway. Its aberrant splicing was found in one third of esophageal, lung and renal cancers which plays a critical role in the carcinogenesis of these tissues [207].

The *WWOX* (WW domain containing oxireductase) gene located on chromosome 16 (16q23.3-24.1) is a candidate tumor suppressor gene for esophageal carcinoma. Both of *WWOX* alleles were seen to become inactivated in squamous carcinoma of the esophagus through combination of events among which mutations and LOH [208].

Annexin1, a member of annexin family which are calcium and phospholipid-binding proteins have also been shown to be lost or downregulated in esophageal cancer [209]. Additionally, its translocation from plasma membrane in normal cells to the nuclear membrane in malignant cells has proposed to be correlated with the tumorigenesis of esophageal cancer [210].

APC and *MCC* are the two tumor suppressor genes located on chromosome 5 (5q21) which are involved in the development of esophageal cancers through LOH of their corresponding genetic loci [111-113]. It has also been shown that mutations in *APC* and *MCC* genes take place in esophageal cancer as well as promoter hypermethylation [116, 122, and 124].

DCC (deleted in colorectal cancer) is a putative tumor suppressor gene whose loss has been implicated in colorectal tumorigenesis. Decreased or loss of *DCC* expression through promoter hypermethylation [211] as well as point mutations and LOH which are correlated with the degree of lymph node metastasis and differentiation [212], have been shown in esophageal cancer.

The involvement of tropomyosins (TMs) which are a family of cytoskeletal proteins and stabilizers of the actin microfilaments have been indicated in carcinogenesis of esophageal cancer; in which downregulation of β-TM (TM1), was described as a novel tumor suppressor gene [213]. The same role were also observed for TM2 and TM3 in esophageal squamous cell carcinoma [99, 214].

E-cadherin (*CDH1*), one of the most important molecules in cell to cell adhesion in epithelial tissues, localized on the surfaces of epithelial cells was reported to be lost in several cancers including esophageal tumors. Promoter hypermethylation was suggested to be involved in its inactivation as well. Loss of E-cadherin expression correlates with the high grade and advanced stages of disease along with poor prognosis [215, 216].

Downregulation of periplakin (a cell adhesion protein) [217] as well as loss of clusterin (a secreted glycoprotein) both in serum and tissue of esophageal squamous cell carcinoma [218] are among other events that have been correlated to the esophageal tumorigenesis.

6. References

[1] Parkin, D.M., et al., Global cancer statistics, 2002. CA Cancer J Clin 2005; 55(2): 74–108.
[2] Tomizawa, Y. and K.K. Wang, Screening, surveillance, and prevention for esophageal cancer. Gastroenterol Clin North Am 2009; 38(1): 59–73, viii.
[3] Enzinger, P.C. and R.J. Mayer, Esophageal cancer. N Engl J Med 2003; 349(23): 2241–52.
[4] Ekman, S., et al., Activation of growth factor receptors in esophageal cancer-implications for therapy. Oncologist 2007; 12(10): 1165–77.
[5] Kuwano, H., et al., Genetic alterations in esophageal cancer. Surg Today 2005; 35(1): 7–18.
[6] Karpinski, P., M.M. Sasiadek, and N. Blin, Aberrant epigenetic patterns in the etiology of gastrointestinal cancers. J Appl Genet 2008; 49(1): 1–10.
[7] Chen, S.C., et al., Overexpression of epidermal growth factor and insulin-like growth factor-I receptors and autocrine stimulation in human esophageal carcinoma cells. Cancer Res 1991; 51: 1898–1903.
[8] Yoshida, K., et al., EGF- and TGF-alpha, the ligands of hyperproduced EGFR in human esophageal carcinoma cells, act as autocrine growth factors. Int J Cancer 1990; 45: 131–135.
[9] Heldin, C.H., Dimerization of cell surface receptors in signal transduction. Cell 1995; 80: 213–223.
[10] Pawson, T., M. Raina, and P. Nash, Interaction domains: From simple binding events to complex cellular behavior. FEBS Lett 2002; 513: 2–10.
[11] Friess, H., et al., Concomitant analysis of the epidermalgrowth factor receptor family in esophageal cancer: Overexpression of epidermal growth factor receptor mRNA but not of c-erbB-2 and cerbB-3. World J Surg 1999; 23: 1010–1018.
[12] Hunts, J., et al., Hyperproduction and gene amplification of the epidermal growth factor receptor in squamous cell carcinomas. Jpn J Cancer Res 1985; 76: 663– 666.
[13] Jankowski, J., et al., Abnormal expression of growth regulatory factors in Barrett's oesophagus. Clin Sci (Colch) 1991; 81: 663-8.
[14] Jones, G.J., et al., Amplification and expression of the TGF-alpha, EGF receptor and c-myc genes in four human oesophageal squamous cell carcinoma lines. Biosci Rep 1993; 13: 303–312.
[15] Mukaida, H., et al., Expression of human epidermal growth factor and its receptor in esophageal cancer. Jpn J Surg 1990; 20: 275–282.
[16] Ozawa, S., et al., High incidence of EGF receptor hyperproduction in esophageal squamous-cell carcinomas. Int J Cancer 1987; 39: 333–337.
[17] Ozawa, S., et al., Epidermal growth factor receptors in cancer tissues of esophagus, lung, pancreas, colorectum, breast and stomach. Jpn J Cancer Res 1988; 79: 1201–1207.
[18] Bazley, L.A. and W.J. Gullick, The epidermal growth factor receptor family. Endocr Relat Cancer 2005; 12(suppl 1): S17–S27.
[19] Moghal, N. and P.W. Sternberg, Multiple positive and negative regulators of signaling by the EGF-receptor. Curr Opin Cell Biol 1999; 11: 190–6.

[20] Ozawa, S., et al., Prognostic significance of epidermal growth factor receptor in esophageal squamous cell carcinomas. Cancer Epidemiol Biomarkers Prev 1989; 63: 2169–73.

[21] Dragovich, T. and C. Campen, Anti-EGFR-Targeted Therapy for Esophageal and Gastric Cancers: An Evolving Concept. J Oncol 2009; 2009: ID 804108. doi:10.1155/2009/804108.

[22] Takaoka, M., et al., Epidermal growth factor receptor regulates aberrant expression of insulin-like growth factor-binding protein 3. Cancer Research 2004; 64(21): 7711-7723.

[23] Yoshida, K., et al. Expression of growth factors and their receptors in human esophageal carcinomas: Regulation of expression by epidermal growth factor and transforming growth factor alpha. J Cancer Res Clin Oncol 1993; 119: 401- 407.

[24] Gibson, M.K., et al., Epidermal growth factor receptor, p53 mutation, and pathological response predict survival in patients with locally advanced esophageal cancer treated with preoperative chemoradiotherapy. Clin Cancer Res 2003; 9: 6461-6468.

[25] Mukaida, H., et al., Clinical significance of the expression of epidermal growth factor and its receptor in esophageal cancer. Cancer 1991; 68: 142–148.

[26] Rygiel, A.M., et al, Gains and amplifications of c-myc, EGFR, and 20.q13 loci in the no dysplasia-dysplasia-adenocarcinoma sequence of barrett's esophagus. Cancer Epidemiology Biomarkers & Prevention 2008; 17(6): 1380–1385.

[27] Souza, R.F., C.P. Morales, and S.J. Spechler, a conceptual approach to understanding the molecular mechanisms of cancer development in Barrett's oesophagus. Aliment Pharmacol Ther 2001; 15: 1087–1100.

[28] Vissers, K.J., et al., Involvement of cancer-activating genes on chromosomes 7 and 8 in esophageal (Barrett's) and gastric cardia adenocarcinoma. Anticancer Res 2001; 21: 3813–3820.

[29] Watanabe, G., et al., Progression of esophageal carcinoma by loss of EGF-STAT1 pathway. Cancer J 2001; 7: 132–139.

[30] Ichiba, M., et al., Epidermal growth factor inhibits the growth of TE8 esophageal cancer cells through the activation of STAT1. J Gastroenterol 2002; 37: 497–503.

[31] Yoshida, K., et al. Growth factors in progression of human esophageal and gastric carcinomas. Exp Pathol 1990; 40: 291–300.

[32] Xu, H., et al., Difference in responsiveness of human esophageal squamous cell carcinoma lines to epidermal growth factor for MMP-7 expression. Int J Oncol 2003; 23: 469–476.

[33] Shiozaki, H., et al., Effect of epidermal growth factor on cadherin-mediated adhesion in a human oesophageal cancer cell line. Br J Cancer 1995; 71: 250–258.

[34] Behrens. J., et al., Loss of epithelial differentiation and gain of invasiveness correlates with tyrosine phosphorylation of the E-cadherin/beta-catenin complex in cells transformed with a temperature-sensitive v-SRC gene. J Cell Biol 1993; 120:757–66.

[35] Ochiai, A., et al., c-erbB-2 gene product associates with catenins in human cancer cells. Biochem Biophys Res Commun 1994; 205: 73–8.

[36] Shibata. T., et al., Dominant negative inhibition of the association between beta-catenin and c-erbB-2 by N-terminally deleted beta-catenin suppresses the invasion and metastasis of cancer cells. Oncogene 1996; 13: 883–9.

[37] Mimura. K., et al., Frequencies of HER-2/neu expression and gene amplification in patients with oesophageal squamous cell carcinoma. Br J Cancer 2005; 92: 1253-1260.

[38] Dahlberg, P.S., et al., ERBB2 amplifications in esophageal adenocarcinoma. Ann Thorac Surg 2004; 78: 1790 -1800.

[39] Safran, H., et al., Trastuzumab, paclitaxel, cisplatin, and radiation for adenocarcinoma of the esophagus: A phase I study. Cancer Invest 2004; 22: 670–677.

[40] Sunpaweravong, P., et al., Epidermal growth factor receptor and cyclin D1 are independently amplified and overexpressed in esophageal squamous cell carcinoma. J Cancer Res Clin Oncol 2005; 131: 111–119.

[41] Dreilich, M., et al., HER-2 overexpression (3+) in patients with squamous cell esophageal carcinoma correlates with poorer survival. Dis Esophagus 2006; 19: 224 -231.

[42] Alroy, I., Y. Yarden, The ErbB signaling network in embryogenesis and oncogenesis: signal diversication through combinatorial ligand-receptor interactions. FEBS Lett 1997;410: 83–6.

[43] Sauter, E.R., et al., HER-2/neu: A differentiation marker in adenocarcinoma of the esophagus. Cancer Lett 1993; 75: 41- 44.

[44] Hardwick, R.H., et al., c-erbB-2 overexpression in the dysplasia/carcinoma sequence of Barrett's oesophagus. J Clin Pathol 1995; 48: 129 -132.

[45] Walch, A., et al., Coamplification and coexpression of GRB7 and ERBB2 is found in high grade intraepithelial neoplasia and in invasive Barrett's carcinoma. Int J Cancer 2004; 112: 747–753.

[46] Polkowski, W., et al., Prognostic value of Lauren classification and c-erbB-2 oncogene overexpression in adenocarcinoma of the esophagus and gastroesophageal junction. Ann Surg Oncol 1999; 6: 290 -297.

[47] Brien, T.P., et al. HER-2/neu gene amplification by FISH predicts poor survival in Barrett's esophagus-associated adenocarcinoma. Hum Pathol 2000; 31: 35–39.

[48] Akamatsu, M., et al., c-erbB-2 oncoprotein expression related to chemoradioresistance in esophageal squamous cell carcinoma. Int J Radiat Oncol Biol Phys 2003; 57: 1323-1327.

[49] Duhaylongsod, F.G., et al., The significance of c-erb B-2 and p53 immunoreactivity in patients with adenocarcinoma of the esophagus. Ann Surg 1995; 221: 677- 683; discussion 683–684.

[50] Cosaceanu, D., et al., Modulation of response to radiation of human lung cancer cells following insulin-like growth factor 1 receptor inactivation. Cancer Lett 2005; 222: 173–181.

[51] Liu, Y.C., et al., Autocrine stimulation by insulin-like growth factor I is involved in the growth, tumorigenicity and chemoresistance of human esophageal carcinoma cells. J Biomed Sci 2002; 9: 665–674.

[52] Iravani, S., et al., Modification of insulin-like growth factor 1 receptor, c-Src, and Bcl-XL protein expression during the progression of Barrett's neoplasia. Hum Pathol 2003; 34: 975–982.

[53] Takaoka, M., et al., Epidermal growth factor receptor regulates aberrant expression of insulin-like growth factor-binding protein 3. Cancer Res 2004; 64: 7711–23.

[54] Natsuizaka, M., et al., Insulin-like growth factor binding protein-3 promotes transforming growth factor- β1-mediated epithelial-to-mesenchymal transition and motility in transformed human esophageal cells. Carcinogenesis 2010; 31(8): 1344–1353.

[55] Sohda, M., et al., The role of insulin-like growth factor 1 and insulin-like growth factor binding protein 3 in human esophageal cancer. Anticancer Res 2004; 24: 3029 -3034.

[56] Heldin, C.H., A. Ostman, and L. Ronnstrand, Signal transduction via plateletderived growth factor receptors. Biochim Biophys Acta 1998; 1378: F79- F113.

[57] Liu, Y.C., et al., Platelet-derived growth factor is an autocrine stimulator for the growth and survival of human esophageal carcinoma cell lines. Exp Cell Res 1996; 228: 206 -211.

[58] Zhang, X., et al., [Expression and significance of C-kit and platelet-derived growth factor receptor-beta (PDGFRbeta) in esophageal carcinoma.] Ai Zheng 2006; 25(1): 92–95. Chinese.

[59] Ferrara, N. Role of vascular endothelial growth factor in physiologic and pathologic angiogenesis: Therapeutic implications. Semin Oncol 2002; 29(suppl 16): 10 -14.

[60] Ferrara, N., VEGF as a therapeutic target in cancer. Oncology 2005; 69(suppl 3):11–16.

[61] Sato, Y., et al., Properties of two VEGF receptors, Flt-1 and KDR, in signal transduction Ann N Y Acad Sci 2000; 902: 201–205; discussion 205–207.

[62] Shih, C.H., et al. Vascular endothelial growth factor expression predicts outcome and lymph node metastasis in squamous cell carcinoma of the esophagus. Clin Cancer Res 2000; 6: 1161–1168.

[63] Kitadai, Y., et al., Significance of vessel count and vascular endothelial growth factor in human esophageal carcinomas. Clin Cancer Res 1998;4: 2195–2200.

[64] Griffiths L, Stratford I J. Platelet-derived endothelial cell growth factor thymidine phosphorylase in tumor growth and response to therapy. Br J Cancer 1997; 76: 689–93.

[65] Lord, R.V.N., et al., Vascular endothelial growth factor and basic fibroblast growth factor expression in esophageal adenocarcinoma and Barrett esophagus. The Journalof Thoracic and Cardiovascular Surgery 2003; 125: 246–53.

[66] Oshima, Y., et al., Angiogenesis-Related Factors are Molecular Targets for Diagnosis and Treatment of Patients with Esophageal Carcinoma. Ann Thorac Cardiovasc Surg 2010; 16(6): 389–393.

[67] Gu, Y., et al., The number of lymph nodes with metastasis predicts survival in patients with esophageal or esophagogastric junction adenocarcinoma who receive preoperative chemoradiation. Cancer 2006; 106: 1017–1025.

[68] Stacker, S.A., et al., Lymphangiogenesis and cancer metastasis. Nat Rev Cancer 2002; 2: 573–583.

[69] Matsumoto, M., et al., Overexpression of vascular endothelial growth factor-C correlates with lymph node micrometastasis in submucosal esophageal cancer. J Gastrointest Surg 2006; 10: 1016 -1022.

[70] Saad, R.S, Y. El-Gohary, et al., Endoglin (CD105) and vascular endothelial growth factor as prognostic markers in esophageal adenocarcinoma. Hum Pathol 2005; 36: 955–961.

[71] Spence, G.M., A.N. Graham, et al., Bone marrow micrometastases and markers of angiogenesis in esophageal cancer. Ann Thorac Surg 2004; 78: 1944–1949; discussion 1950.

[72] Kitadai, Y., S. Onogawa, et al., Angiogenic switch occurs during the precancerous stage of human esophageal squamous cell carcinoma. Oncol Rep 2004; 11: 315–319.

[73] Auvinen, M.I., et al., Incipient angiogenesis in Barrett's epithelium and lymphangiogenesis in Barrett's adenocarcinoma. J Clin Oncol 2002; 20: 2971-2979.

[74] Barclay, C., A.W. Li, et al., Basic fibroblast growth factor (FGF-2) overexpression is a risk factor for esophageal cancer recurrence and reduced survival, which is ameliorated by co-expression of the FGF-2 antisense gene. Clin Cancer Res 2005; 11: 7683–91.

[75] Zhang, C., L. Fu, et al., Fibroblast growth factor receptor 2-positive fibroblasts provide a suitable microenvironment for tumor development and progression in esophageal carcinoma. Clin Cancer Res 2009; 15: 4017–27.

[76] Noma, K., et al., The essential role of fibroblasts in esophageal squamous cell carcinoma-induced angiogenesis. Gastroenterology 2008; 134(7): 1981–93.

[77] Ren, Y.J. and Q.Y. Zhang., Expression of midkine and its clinical significance in esophageal squamous cell carcinoma. World J Gastroenterol 2006; 12: 2006–10.

[78] Shimada, H., Y. Nabeya, et al., Preoperative serum midkine concentration is a prognostic marker for esophageal squamous cell carcinoma. Cancer Sci 2003; 94: 628–32.

[79] Shimada, H., Y. Nabeya, et al., Increased serum midkine concentration as a possible tumor marker in patients with superficial esophageal cancer. Oncol Rep 2003; 10: 411–4.

[80] Ren, Y., B. Cao, et al., Hepatocyte growth factor promotes cancer cell migration and angiogenic factors expression: a prognostic marker of human esophageal squamous cell carcinomas. Clin Cancer Res 2005; 11: 6190–7.

[81] Iwazawa, T., et al., Primary human fibroblasts induce diverse tumor invasiveness: Involvement of HGF as an important paracrine factor. Jpn J Cancer Res 1996; 87: 1134–1142.

[82] Tuynman, J.B., S.M. Lagarde, et al., Met expression is an independent prognostic risk factor in patients with oesophageal adenocarcinoma. Br J Cancer 2008; 98: 1102–8.

[83] Takada, N., et al., Expression of immunoreactive human hepatocyte growth factor in human esophageal squamous cell carcinomas. Cancer Lett 1995; 97:145–148.

[84] Grugan, K.D., C.G. Miller, et al., Fibroblast-secreted hepatocyte growth factor plays a functional role in esophageal squamous cell carcinoma invasion. Proc Natl Acad Sci USA 2010; 107: 11026–31.

[85] Li, L.Y., et al., Connective tissue growth factor expression in precancerous lesions of human esophageal epithelium and prognostic significance in esophageal squamous cell carcinoma. Dis Esophagus 2010; 24(5): 337–345

[86] Friday, B.B. and A.A. Adjei, K-ras as a target for cancer therapy. Biochim Biophys Acta 2005; 1756(2): 127–44.

[87] Liu, J.J., J.R. Chao, et al., Ras transformation results in an elevated level of cyclin D1 and acceleration of G1 progression in NIH 3T3 cells. Mol Cell Biol 1995; 15: 3654–63.

[88] Malumbres, M., and A. Pellicer, RAS pathways to cell cycle control and cell transformation. Front Biosci 1998; 3: d887–d912.

[89] Meloche, S. and J. Pouyssegur, The ERK1/2 mitogen-activated protein kinase pathway as a master regulator of the G1- to Sphase transition, Oncogene 2007; 26(22): 3227–3239.

[90] Hawk, E.T. and J.L. Viner, Statins in esophageal cancer cell lines: promising lead? Am J Gastroenterol 2008; 103(4): 838–41.

[91] Leu, C.M, C. Chang, and C. Hu, Epidermal growth factor (EGF) suppresses staurosporine-induced apoptosis by inducing mcl-1 via the mitogen-activated protein kinase pathway. Oncogene 2000; 19:1665–1675.

[92] Akimoto, T., T. Nonaka, et al., Selective inhibition of survival signal transduction pathways enhanced radiosensitivity in human esophageal cancer cell lines in vitro. Anticancer Res 2004; 24: 811–819.

[93] Chattopadhyay, I., et al., Gene expression profi le of esophageal cancer in North East India by cDNA microarray analysis. World J Gastroenterol 2007; 13(9): 1438–1444.

[94] Nguyen, D.M, D. Lorang, et al., Enhancement of paclitaxel-mediated cytotoxicity in lung cancer cells by 17- allylamino geldanamycin: In vitro and in vivo analysis. Ann Thorac Surg 2001; 72: 371–378.

[95] Nguyen, D.M., G.A. Chen, et al., Potentiation of paclitaxel cytotoxicity in lung and esophageal cancer cells by pharmacologic inhibition of the phosphoinositide 3-kinase/protein kinase B (Akt)-mediated signaling pathway. J Thorac Cardiovasc Surg 2004; 127: 365–375.

[96] Schrump, D.S. and D.M. Nguyen, Novel molecular targeted therapy for esophageal cancer. J Surg Oncol 2005; 92(3):257–61.

[97] Lawler, K., et al., Mobility and invasiveness of metastatic esophageal cancer are potentiated by shear stress in a ROCK- and Ras-dependent manner. Am J Physiol Cell Physiol 2006; 291(4): C668–77.

[98] Senmaru, N., et al., Suppression of Erk activation and in vivo growth in esophageal cancer cells by the dominant negative Ras mutant, N116Y. Int J Cancer 1998; 78(3): 366–71.

[99] Zare, M., et al., Downregulation of tropomyosin-1 in squamous cell carcinoma of esophagus, the role of Ras signaling and methylation. Molecular Carcinogenesis 2011; DOI: 10.1002/mc.20847,

[100] Logan, C.Y. and R. Nusse., The Wnt signaling pathway in development and disease. Annu. Rev. Cell Dev. Biol 2004; 20: 781–810.

[101] Moon, R.T, A.D. Kohn, et al., WNT and beta-catenin signalling: diseases and therapies. Nat. Rev. Genet 2004; 5: 691–701.

[102] Liu, T., et al., G protein signaling from activated rat frizzled-1 to the beta-catenin-Lef-Tcf pathway. Science 2001; 292: 1718–1722.

[103] Mann, B., M. Gelos, et al., Target genes of beta-catenin-T cell-factor/lymphoid-enhancer-factor signaling in human colorectal carcinomas. Proc Natl Acad Sci USA 1999, 96:1603–1608.

[104] Behrens, J., et al., Functional interaction of beta-catenin with the transcription factor LEF-1. Nature 1996; 382: 638–642.

[105] Kudo, J., et al., Aberrant nuclear localization of β-catenin without genetic alterations in β-catenin or Axin genes in esophageal cancer. World Journal of Surgical Oncology 2007; 5(21).
[106] Aberle, H., H. Schwartz, and R. Kemler, Cadherin-catenin complex: protein interactions and their implications for cadherin function. J Cell Biochem 1996; 61: 514–23.
[107] Barth, A.I., I.S. Nathke, and W.J. Nelson., Cadherins catenins and APC protein: interplay between cytoskeletal complexes and signaling pathways. Curr Opin Cell Biol 1997; 9: 683–90.
[108] Swami, S., S. Kumble, and G. Triadafilopoulos., E-cadherin expression in gastroesophageal reflux disease, Barrett's esophagus, and esophageal adenocarcinoma: an immunohistochemical and immunoblot study. Am J Gastroenterol 1995; 90: 1808–13.
[109] Washington, K., et al., Expression of beta-catenin, alpha-catenin, and E-cadherin in Barrett's esophagus and esophageal adenocarcinomas. Mod Pathol 1998; 11: 805–13.
[110] Seery, J.P., et al., Abnormal expression of the E-cadherin-catenin complex in dysplastic Barrett's oesophagus. Acta Oncol 1999; 38: 945–8.
[111] Dolan, K., J. Garde, et al., Allelotype analysis of oesophageal adenocarcinoma: loss of heterozygosity occurs at multiple sites. Br J Cancer 1998; 78: 950–7.
[112] Boynton, R.F., et al. Loss of heterozygosity involving the APC and MCC genetic loci occurs in the majority of human esophageal cancers. Proc Natl Acad Sci 1992; 89:3385- 8.
[113] Bektas, N., et al., Allelic loss involving the tumor suppressor genes APC and MCC and expression of the APC protein in the development of dysplasia and carcinoma in Barrett esophagus. Am J Clin Pathol 2000; 114(6): 890–5.
[114] Choi, Y.W., et al., Mutations in beta-catenin and APC genes are uncommon in esophageal and esophagogastric junction adenocarcinomas. Mod Pathol 2000; 13(10): 1055–9.
[115] Ogasawara, S., et al., Lack of mutations of the adenomatous polyposis coli gene in oesophageal and gastric carcinomas. Virchows Arch 1994; 424(6): 607–11.
[116] Li, H. and S. Lu, [Mutation of tumor suppressor genes APC and MCC in human esophageal cancer]. Zhonghua Zhong Liu Za Zhi 1995; 17(1): 9–12.
[117] Powell, S.M., et al., APC gene mutations in the mutation cluster region are rare in esophageal cancers. Gastroenterology 1994; 107(6): 1759–63.
[118] Voskas, D., L.S. Ling, and J.R. Woodgett, Does GSK-3 provide a shortcut for PI3K activation of Wnt signalling? F1000 Biol Reports 2010; 2:82
[119] Clement, G., et al., Alterations of the Wnt signaling pathway during the neoplastic progression of Barrett's esophagus. Oncogene 2006; 25(21): 3084–92.
[120] Clément, G., D. Jablons, and J. Benhattar, Targeting the Wnt signaling pathway to treat Barrett's esophagus. Expert Opin Ther Targets 2007; 11(3):375–89.
[121] Eads, C.A., et al., Fields of aberrant CpG island hypermethylation in Barrett's esophagus and associated adenocarcinoma. Cancer Res 2000; 60(18): 5021–6.
[122] Kawakami, K., et al., Hypermethylated APC DNA in plasma and prognosis of patients with esophageal adenocarcinoma. J Natl Cancer Inst 2000; 92(22): 1805–11.

[123] Ishii, T., et al., Oesophageal squamous cell carcinoma may develop within a background of accumulating DNA methylation in normal and dysplastic mucosa. Gut 2007; 56(1): 13–9.

[124] Zare, M., et al., Qualitative analysis of Adenomatous Polyposis Coli promoter: hypermethylation, engagement and effects on survival of patients with esophageal cancer in a high risk region of the world, a potential molecular marker. BMC Cancer 2009; 9(24).

[125] Wang, W., et al., Aberrant Changes of Wnt2/β-Catenin Signaling Pathway Induced by Sodium Nitroprusside in Human Esophageal Squamous Cell Carcinoma Cell Lines. Cancer Investigation 2010; 28(3): 230–241

[126] Ma, C., et al., The role of glycogen synthase kinase 3beta in the transformation of epidermal cells. Cancer Res 2007; 67:7756–7764.

[127] Kang, T., Y. Wei, et al., GSK-3 beta targets Cdc25A for ubiquitin-mediated proteolysis, and GSK-3 beta inactivation correlates with Cdc25A overproduction in human cancers. Cancer Cell 2008;13: 36-47.

[128] Greengard, P., The neurobiology of slow synaptic transmission. Science. 2001;294:1024–1030.

[129] Varis, A., A. Zaika., et al., Coamplified and overexpressed genes at ERBB2 locus in gastric cancer. Int J Cancer 2004; 109: 548–553.

[130] Beckler, A., C.A. Moskaluk, et al., Overexpression of the 32-kilodalton dopamine and cyclic adenosine 3',5'-monophosphate-regulated phosphoprotein in common adenocarcinomas. Cancer 2003; 98: 1547–1551.

[131] Belkhiri, A., A. Zaika, et al., Darpp-32: a novel antiapoptotic gene in upper gastrointestinal carcinomas. Cancer Res. 2005; 65: 6583–6592.

[132] Vangamudi, B., et al., Regulation of β-catenin by t-DARPP in upper gastrointestinal cancer cells. Mol Cancer 2011; 10: 32.

[133] Vanhaesebroeck, B. and M.D. Waterfield, Signaling by distinct classes of phosphoinositide 3-kinases. Exp Cell Res 1999; 253: 239–54.

[134] Cantley, L.C., The phosphoinositide 3-kinase pathway, Science 2002; 296:655–1657.

[135] Brader, S., and S.A. Eccles, Phosphoinositide 3-kinase signalling pathways in tumor progression, invasion and angiogenesis. Tumori 2004; 90: 2–8.

[136] Yen, C.C., et al., Genotypic analysis of esophageal squamous cell carcinoma by molecular cytogenetics and real-time quantitative polymerase chain reaction. Int J Oncol 2003; 23: 871–81.

[137] Zhang, G., X. Zhou, et al., Accumulation of cytoplasmic beta-catenin correlates with reduced expression of E-cadherin, but not with phosphorylated Akt in esophageal squamous cell carcinoma: immunohistochemical study. Pathol Int 2005; 55: 310–7.

[138] Miller, C.T., et al., Gene amplification in esophageal adenocarcinomas and Barrett's with high-grade dysplasia. Clin Cancer Res 2003; 9: 4819–25.

[139] Phillips, W.A., et al., Mutation analysis of PIK3CA and PIK3CB in esophageal cancer and Barrett's esophagus. Int. J. Cancer 2006; 118: 2644–2646.

[140] Mori, R., H. Ishiguro, et al., PIK3CA mutation status in Japanese esophageal squamous cell carcinoma. J Surg Res 2008; 145: 320–6.

[141] Yoshioka, A., H. Miyata, et al., The activation of Akt during preoperative chemotherapy for esophageal cancer correlates with poor prognosis. Oncol Rep 2008;19:1099–107.

[142] Ingham, P.W., Hedgehog signalling. Curr Biol 2008; 18: R238–41.

[143] Hooper, J.E. and M.P. Scott, Communicating with hedgehogs. Nat Rev Mol Cell Biol 2005; 6: 306–17.

[144] Philipp, M. and M.G. Caron, Hedgehog signaling: is Smo a G protein-coupled receptor? Curr Biol 2009;19:R125–7.

[145] Karhadkar, S.S., G.S. Bova, et al., Hedgehog signalling in prostate regeneration, neoplasia and metastasis. Nature 2004; 431:707–12.

[146] Ma, X., T. Sheng, et al., Hedgehog signaling is activated in subsets of esophageal cancers. Int J Cancer 2006; 118: 139–48.

[147] Mori, Y., T. Okumura, et al., Gli-1 expression is associated with lymph node metastasis and tumor progression in esophageal squamous cell carcinoma. Oncology 2006; 70: 378–89.

[148] Pasca di Magliano, M. et al., Hedgehog/Ras interactions regulate early stages of pancreatic cancer. Genes Dev 2006; 20: 3161–73.

[149] Faried, A. L.S. Faried, et al., RhoA and RhoC proteins promote both cell proliferation and cell invasion of human oesophageal squamous cell carcinoma cell lines in vitro and in vivo. Eur J Cancer 2006; 42: 1455–65.

[150] Wei, L. and Z. Xu, Cross-signaling among phosphinositide-3 kinase, mitogenactivated protein kinase and sonic hedgehog pathways exists in esophageal cancer. Int J Cancer 2010; 129(2): 275–234.

[151] Hui, C.M., P.Y. Cheung, et al., Id-1 promotes proliferation of p53-deficient esophageal cancer cells. Int J Cancer 2006; 119: 508–14.

[152] Yuen, H.F., Y.P. Chan, et al., Id-1 and Id-2 are markers for metastasis and prognosis in oesophageal squamous cell carcinoma. Br J Cancer 2007; 97: 1409–15.

[153] Li, B., et al., Id-1 activation of PI3K/Akt/NFkappaB signaling pathway and its significance in promoting survival of esophageal cancer cells. Carcinogenesis 2007;28: 2313–20.

[154] Li, B., et al., Id-1 promotes tumorigenicity and metastasis of human esophageal cancer cells through activation of PI3K/AKT signaling pathway. Int. J. Cancer 2009; 125: 2576–2585

[155] Benezra, R., R.L. Davis, et al., The protein Id: a negative regulator of helix-loop-helix DNA binding proteins. Cell 1990; 61:49–59.

[156] McCabe, M.L. and Z. Dlamini, The molecular mechanisms of oesophageal cancer. Int Immunopharmacol 2005; 5(7-8): 1113–30.

[157] Hollstein, M., et al., p53 mutations in human cancers. Science 1991; 253: 49–53.

[158] Olivier, M. et al., The IARC TP53 database: new online mutation analysis and recommendations to users. Hum Mutat 2002;19:607–14.

[159] el-Deiry, W.S., T. Tokino, et al., WAF1, a potential mediator of p53 tumor suppression. Cell 1993; 75:817–25.

[160] Oltvai, Z.N., C.L. Milliman and S.J. Korsmeyer, Bcl-2 heterodimerizes in vivo with a conserved homolog, Bax, that accelerates programmed cell death. Cell 1993;74:609–19.

[161] Miyashita, T., et al., Tumor suppressor p53 is a regulator of bcl-2 and bax gene expression in vitro and in vivo. Oncogene 1994; 9: 1799–805.
[162] Lane, D.P. Cancer. p53, guardian of the genome. Nature 1992; 358: 15–6.
[163] Ikeguchi, M., H. Saito, et al., Clinicopathologic significance of the expression of mutated p53 protein and the proliferative activity of cancer cells in patients with esophageal squamous cell carcinoma. J Am Coll Surg 1997; 185: 398–403.
[164] Ikeda, G., S. Isaji, et al., Prognostic significance of biologic factors in squamous cell carcinoma of the esophagus. Cancer 1999; 86: 1396–405.
[165] Lam, K.Y., et al., The clinicopathological significance of p21 and p53 expression in esophageal squamous cell carcinoma: an analysis of 153 patients. Am J Gastroenterol 1999; 94: 2060–8.
[166] Kato, H., M. Yoshikawa, et al., An immunohistochemical study of p16, pRb, p21 and p53 proteins in human esophageal cancers. Anticancer Res 2000; 20: 345–9.
[167] von Brevern, M.C., M.C. Hollstein., et al. Circulating anti-p53 antibodies in esophageal cancer patients are found predominantly in individuals with p53 core domain mutations in their tumors Cancer Res 1996; 56: 4917–21.
[168] Shimada, H., Nabeya, Y., et al. Prognostic significance of serum p53 antibody in patients with esophageal squamous cell carcinoma. Surgery 2002; 132: 41–7.
[169] Shimada, H., K. Nakajima, et al., Detection of serum p53 antibodies in patients with esophageal squamous cell carcinoma: correlation with clinicopathologic features and tumor markers. Oncol Rep 1998; 5: 871–4.
[170] Slebos, R.J., M.H. Lee, et al., p53-dependent G1 arrest involves pRB-related proteins and is disrupted by the human papillomavirus 16 E7 oncoprotein. Proc Natl Acad Sci USA 1994; 91: 5320–4.
[171] Shiohara, M., W.S. el-Deiry, et al., Absence of WAF1 mutations in a variety of human malignancies. Blood 1994; 84: 3781–4.
[172] Bahl, R., S. Arora, et al., Novel polymorphism in p21 (waf1/cip1) cyclin dependent kinase inhibitor gene: association with human esophageal cancer. Oncogene 2000; 19: 323–8.
[173] Masuda, N., H. Kato, et al., Synergistic decline in expressions of p73 and p21 with invasion in esophageal cancers. Cancer Sci 2003; 94: 612–7.
[174] Jost, C.A., M.C., Marin, and W.G., Kaelin, p73 is a human p53-related protein that can induce apoptosis. Nature 1997; 389: 191–4.
[175] Nita, M.E., H. Nagawa, et al., p21Waf1/Cip1 expression is a prognostic marker in curatively resected esophageal squamous cell carcinoma, but not p27Kip1, p53, or Rb. Ann Surg Oncol 1999;6:481–8.
[176] Natsugoe, S., S, Nakashima. et al., Expression of p21WAF1/Cip1 in the p53-dependent pathway is related to prognosis in patients with advanced esophageal carcinoma. Clin Cancer Res 1999;5: 2445–9.
[177] Shimada, Y., M. Imamura, et al., Prognostic factors of oesophageal squamous cell carcinoma from the perspective of molecular biology Br J Cancer 1999; 80: 1281–8.
[178] Sarbia, M., et al., Expression of p21WAF1 predicts outcome of esophageal cancer patients treated by surgery alone or by combined therapy modalities. Clin Cancer Res 1998; 4: 2615–23.

[179] Serrano, M., G.J. Hannon, and D. Beach, A new regulatory motif in cell-cycle control causing specific inhibition of cyclin D/CDK4. Nature 1993; 366: 704 -7.
[180] Lukas, J., D. Parry., et al., Retinoblastoma protein-dependent cell cycle inhibition by the tumor suppressor p16. Nature 1995; 375: 503–6.
[181] Igaki, H, H. Sasaki, et al., Highly frequent homozygous deletion of the p16 gene in esophageal cancer cell lines. Biochem Biophys Res Commun 1994;203:1090–5.
[182] Liu, Q., Y.X. Yan., et al., MTS-1 (CDKN2) tumor suppressor gene deletions are a frequent event in esophagus squamous cancer and pancreatic adenocarcinoma cell lines. Oncogene 1995; 10: 619–22.
[183] Tanaka, H., et al., Multiple types of aberrations in the p16(INK4a) and the p15(INK4b) genes in 30 esophageal squamous-cell-carcinoma cell lines. Int J Cancer 1997; 70: 437–42.
[184] Mohammad Ganji, S., et al., Associations of risk factors obesity and occupational airborne exposures with CDKN2A/p16 aberrant DNA methylation in esophageal cancer patients. Dis Esophagus, 2010. 23(7): p. 597–602.
[185] Maesawa, C., G. Tamura, et al., Inactivation of the CDKN2 gene by homozygous deletion and de novo methylation is associated with advanced stage esophageal squamous cell carcinoma. Cancer Res 1996; 56: 3875–8.
[186] Fong, L.Y., Nguyen VT, Farber JL, Huebner K, Magee PN. Early deregulation of the p16ink4a-cyclin D1/cyclin-dependent kinase4-retinoblastoma pathway in cell proliferation-driven esophageal tumorigenesis in zinc-deficient rats. Cancer Res 2000; 60: 4589–95.
[187] Tokugawa, T., H. Sugihara, T. Tani, T. Hattori, Modes of silencing of p16 in development of esophageal squamous cell carcinoma. Cancer Res 2002; 62: 4938–44.
[188] Xing, E.P., Y. Nie, et al., Aberrant methylation of p16INK4a and deletion of p15INK4b are frequent events in human esophageal cancer in Linxian, China. Carcinogenesis 1999; 20: 77–84.
[189] Wong, D.J., et al., p16INK4a promoter is hypermethylated at a high frequency in esophageal adenocarcinomas. Cancer Res 1997; 57: 2619–22.
[190] Eads, C.A., et al., Epigenetic patterns in the progression of esophageal adenocarcinoma. Cancer Res 2001; 61(8): 3410–8.
[191] Takeuchi, H., S. Ozawa, et al., Altered p16/MTS1/CDKN2 and cyclin D1/PRAD-1 gene expression is associated with the prognosis of squamous cell carcinoma of the esophagus. Clin Cancer Res 1997; 3: 2229– 36.
[192] Nie, Y., J. Liao, et al., Detection of multiple gene hypermethylation in the development of esophageal squamous cell carcinoma. Carcinogenesis 2002; 23: 1713–20.
[193] Hibi, K., M. Taguchi, et al., Molecular detection of p16 promoter methylation in the serum of patients with esophageal squamous cell carcinoma. Clin Cancer Res 2001; 7: 3135–8.
[194] Abbaszadegan, M.R., H. R. Raziee, et al., Aberrant p16 methylation, a possible epigenetic risk factor in familial esophageal squamous cell carcinoma. Int J Gastrointest Cancer 2005; 36: 47–54.
[195] Hannon, G.J., and D. Beach, p15INK4b is a potential effector of TGFβ-induced cell cycle arrest. Nature 1994; 371: 257–61.

[196] Weinberg, R.A., The retinoblastoma protein and cell cycle control. Cell 1995; 81: 323-30.

[197] Taya, Y., RB kinases and RB-binding proteins: new points of view. Trends Biochem Sci 1997; 22: 14-17.

[198] Ezhevsky, S.A., H. Nagahara, et al., Hypo-phosphorylation of the retinoblastoma protein (pRb) by cyclin D : Cdk4/6 complexes results in active pRb. Proc Natl Acad Sci USA 1997; 94: 10699-704.

[199] Boynton, R.F., Y. Huang, et al. Frequent loss of heterozygosity at the retinoblastoma locus in human esophageal cancers. Cancer Res 1991; 51: 5766-9.

[200] Huang, Y., S J. Meltzer, et al., Altered messenger RNA and unique mutational profiles of p53 and Rb in human esophageal carcinomas. Cancer Res 1993; 53: 1889-94.

[201] Coppola, D., R.H. Schreiber, et al., Significance of Fas and retinoblastoma protein expression during the progression of Barrett's metaplasia to adenocarcinoma. Ann Surg Oncol 1999; 6: 298-304.

[202] Xing, E.P., G.Y. Yang, et al., Loss of heterozygosity of the Rb gene correlates with pRb protein expression and associates with p53 alteration in human esophageal cancer. Clin Cancer Res 1999; 5: 1231-40.

[203] Li, L.W., et al., Expression of esophageal cancer related gene 4 (ECRG4), a novel tumor suppressor gene, in esophageal cancer and its inhibitory effect on the tumor growth in vitro and in vivo. Int J Cancer 2009; 125(7): 1505-1513.

[204] Chen, L., N. Matsubara, et al., Genetic alterations of candidate tumor suppressor ING1 in human esophageal squamous cell cancer. Cancer Res 2001; 61(11): 4345-4349.

[205] Kong, K.L., et al., Characterization of a Candidate Tumor Suppressor Gene Uroplakin 1A in Esophageal Squamous Cell Carcinoma. Cancer Res 2010; 70(21): 8832-8841.

[206] Mimori, K., et al., MAL gene expression in esophageal cancer suppresses motility, invasion and tumorigenicity and enhances apoptosis through the Fas pathway. Oncogene 2003; 22: 3463-3471.

[207] Daigo, Y., et al. Molecular cloning of a candidate tumour suppressor gene, DLC1, from chromosome 3p21.3. Cancer Res 1999; 59: 1966- 72.

[208] Kuroki, T., et al., Genetic alterations of the tumor suppressor gene WWOX in esophageal squamous cell carcinoma. Cancer Res 2002. 62: 2258- 60.

[209] Xia, S.H., et al., Three isoforms of annexin I are preferentially expressed in normal esophageal epithelia but down-regulated in esophageal squamous cell carcinomas. Oncogene 2002; 21(43): 6641-8.

[210] Liu, Y., et al., Translocation of annexin I from cellular membrane to the nuclear membrane in human esophageal squamous cell carcinoma. World J Gastroenterol 2003; 9(4): 645-649.

[211] Park, H.L., et al., DCC promoter hypermethylation in esophageal squamous cell carcinoma. Int J Cancer 2008; 122(11): 2498-502.

[212] Miyake, S., et al., Point mutations and allelic deletion of tumor suppressor gene DCC in human esophageal squamous cell carcinomas and their relation to metastasis. Cancer Res 1994; 54(11): 3007-10.

[213] O'Neill, G.M., J. Stehn, and P.W. Gunning, Tropomyosins as interpreters of the signaling environment to regulate the local cytoskeleton. Semin Cancer Biol 2008; 18(1): 35-44.

[214] Jazii, F.R., et al., Identification of squamous cell carcinoma associated proteins by proteomics and loss of beta tropomyosin expression in esophageal cancer. World J Gastroenterol 2006; 12(44): 7104-12.

[215] Lee, E.J., et al., CpG island hypermethylation of E-cadherin (CDH1) and integrin 4 is associated with recurrence of early stage esophageal squamous cell carcinoma. International Journal of Cancer 2008; 123 (9): 2073-2079.

[216] Pećina-Šlaus, N., Tumor suppressor gene E-cadherin and its role in normal and malignant cells. Cancer Cell International 2003; 3:17.

[217] Nishimori, T., et al., Proteomic analysis of primary esophageal squamous cell carcinoma reveals downregulation of a cell adhesion protein, periplakin. Proteomics 2006; 6: 1011-1018.

[218] Zhang, L.Y., et al., Loss of clusterin both in serum and tissue correlates with the tumorigenesis of esophageal squamous cell carcinoma via proteomics approaches. World J Gastroenterol 2003; 9(4): 650-654.

3

Biomarkers, Stem Cells and Esophageal Cancer

Irene Vegh and Ana I. Flores
Instituto de Investigación Hospital 12 de Octubre, Madrid, Spain

1. Introduction

There are two main forms of esophagus cancer with different malignant behaviors: epidermal or squamous carcinoma (ESCC) and esophagus adenocarcinoma (EA). ESCC is associated with ethanol and tobacco consumption (tobacco-specific-N- nitroso compounds). ESCC is among the more aggressive cancers known. The high mortality rate associated with this type of cancer is directly related to a late diagnosis. Thus there is an important challenge to identify biomarkers for early diagnosis (Shimada et al., 2003; Sobin & Fleming, 1997).

EA starts from a metaplasia mucosa-dysplasia-carcinoma sequence in the distal esophagus (Barrett's esophagus (BE), as a result of local injury and is associated with risk of malignant transformation. Cellular proliferation takes place through the subsequent phases of the cell cycle. During the cell cycle, there are different check points and, the transition from G1 to S phase is the most studied in neoplastic progression of Barrett's cells and alterations in growth factor expression. Its receptors and/or the signal transduction pathways have been found at various stages during the progression of metaplasia to EA (Lao-Sirieix et al., 2007; Lord et al., 2000). BE is clinically important because the risk of progressing to adenocarcinoma under the chronically damaging effect of gastrointestinal reflux. EA of the upper esophagus is rare and in some cases develops from areas of gastric heterotopias. It has been hypothesized that intestinal metaplasia could have a change in their differentiation pattern. Indeed, a clonal selection model suggests that malignant transformation occurs by multiple allelic alterations (Nowell, 1976; Souza et al., 2008).

The incidence of EA has increased in the last 40 years. However, the biology of both, the normal esophageal epithelium and the pathogenesis involved in the development of esophageal cancer are not well understood. Epithelial changes are due to stimulation of esophageal stem cells of the epithelium. These changes in the activity of the esophagus stem cells and the up- or down-regulation of stem cell markers appear to be related in the pathogenesis of esophageal cancer and final clinical outcome. Over the last 5 years, important progress has been made in the identification and understanding of adult gastrointestinal stem cells. However, esophageal stem cells are not well characterized. Isolation and characterization of adult esophageal stem cells and the factors that contribute to the development of dysplasia and malignancy is a very important issue for the development of efficient therapies for esophageal cancer (Adams and Strasser, 2008; Croagh et al., 2008; Hormi-Carver and Souza, 2009). The clonal selection theory was thought to be responsible for the development of gastrointestinal cancers, based on the evidence that some cells acquire genetic alterations giving them the capacity of self-renewal (Adams and Strasser, 2008). Recently, the cancer stem cell (CSC) theory has gained more attention based on the idea that some cancers are initiated by stem cells with genetic alterations. Cellular and tissue regeneration is based on the characteristics of self-renewal and multipotency of stem cells. In recent years, progress in stem cell identification and characterization indicate their potential therapeutic applications in regenerative medicine for the treatment of several pathologies. The different types of stem cells, embryonic, induced pluripotent and adult stem cells are emerging as a potential approach to treat gastrointestinal disorders.

2. Biomarkers or bio-indicators

The so called tumor markers and biological markers are usually used in place of each other. Initially, tumor markers were developed and used to detect some mucin antigens on the cancer cell surface and/or in the serum of cancer patients. Those tumor markers on the cell surface that form glyco-conjugates are involved in adhesion, motility and metastasis. The tumor markers can induce the immune response early during malignant transformation, and later are shed by cancer cells into blood vessels and detected in serum or plasma. The ideal tumor marker have to be specific for malignant cells, detectable early in the carcinogenesis process, measurable by simple invasive methods and the concentrations measured have to be proportional to the stage of malignancy and/or a pharmacological response to therapeutic intervention. There are different tumor markers, each indicative of a particular disease process and used in oncology to detect the presence of a cancer. Tumor markers can be produced by the tumor cells or by the non-tumor cells as a response to the presence of a disease. This was used for identification, evaluation and follows up of treatment, either for patients based or population based and even experimental condition. Brief descriptions for it were focused on these tumor markers in different cancer types. The carcinoembrionary antigen CEA, is a glycoprotein involved in cell adhesion that was studied in lung carcinoma (Vegh et al., 2002) and colorectal carcinoma (Vegh et al., 2007). Cancer antigen 125 (CA 125) was used principally for screening ovarian cancer (Frederick et al., 2011). CA 19.9, also called carbohydrate antigen 19-9 was detected in colorectal carcinoma (Morales-Gutierrez et al., 1999; Vegh et al., 2003). Alpha fetoprotein (AFP) levels were increased in hepatocellular carcinoma and esophagus carcinoma (Bellet et al., 1984). Beta human chorionic gonadotropin (βHCC) was evaluated in different diseases (Burg-Kurland et al., 1989). Carbohydrate antigen 15.3 (CA 15.3) was mostly studied in breast carcinoma (Bearz et al., 2007). Some epidemiologic studies observed that the incidence for EA in all races had variations according to this histology, age and gender. There is a striking male predominance in esophageal cancer. Sex hormones have been suggested as a contributing factor and these are influenced by histology, age and race. The highest sex ratios were seen in esophagus EA in the age group between 50-59 years old, rendering plausibility to the hypothesis that female sex hormone exposure may play a protective role in the development of this type of cancer (Nordenstedt et al., 2011).

Nowadays, biomarkers or bio-indicators in cell biology are molecules that allow the detection and isolation of a particular cell type. In genetics, a biomarker is a DNA sequence that causes or is associated with the development of diseases. Biomarkers are used to indicate the variation in the expression of a characteristic protein that correlates with the risk of development of pathology. Currently, most biomarkers used in clinic are proteins, while based on genetics they might be DNA or RNA and they could also be subject of determination or application in clinic, specially in case of viral infected or DNA or RNA which are shed from individual tumor tissue stream. The expression of several biomarkers in plasma and tissue from patients with esophagus cancer were analyzed, and looked for the biomarkers whose over-expression could be associated with a different behavior in esophagus cancer and could have potential prognostic implications.

In this chapter our aim was to discuss each specific biomarker in separate sections in the context of esophageal cancer, as some of these markers are also important in the development and evolution of other types of tumors.

2.1 Metalloproteinase

The extracellular matrix (ECM) is the extracellular part of a tissue which provides support to cells and is known as connective tissue (Bosman and Stamenkovic, 2003). ECM includes the interstitial matrix and the basement membrane. EMC is composed of a variety of proteins and glycoaminoglicans. Numerous families of enzymes (proteinases) are responsible for the degradation of ECM. The family of enzymes called matrix metalloproteinases (MMPs) are the major enzymes implicated in extracellular degradation and are essential for embryonic development, morphogenesis, remodeling and tissue repair. MMPs are classified into five classes: collagenases (MMP-1,-8 and -13), gelatinases (MMP-2 and -9), stromelysins (MMP-3 and -10), membrane type matrilysins (MMP-7 and -26) and others. The MMPs are zinc-dependent endo-peptidases and are inhibited by specific endogenous inhibitors, the tissue inhibitor of metalloproteinases (TIMP). This MMPs family currently includes more than 26 members. Proteases not only have cell-matrix interaction, but also can control the progression of angiogenesis by activating growth factors such as hepatocyte growth factor (HGF), basic fibroblast growth factor (bFGF) and vascular endothelial growth factor (VEGF) and can influence cellular behavior. MMPs can act also as an inhibitor of angiogenesis. The data indicate that proteases can acts either as positive or negative regulators of angiogenesis (Brooks et al., 1998). MMP-1 is an interstitial collagenase secreted from fibroblasts, macrophages and keratocytes. MMP-1 is related to cancer aggressiveness and its expression is associated with a multistep carcinogenesis from BE to EA according to the clonal selection model (Etoh et al., 2000; Grimm et al., 2010). MMP-7 (matrilysin) is the smallest molecule of the MMPs, whose function is to degrade elastin, proteoglycans, fibronectin and type IV collagen. It has been found that MMP-7 was over-expressed in a variety of epithelial and mesenchymal tumors such as esophagus, colon, liver, renal, and pancreas. Increased circulating levels of MMP-7 proteins were correlated with the presence of metastatic disease and poor patient survival in colorectal and renal cell cancer (Maurel et al., 2007; Szarvas et al., 2010; Yamamoto et al., 1999; Yamashita et al., 2000). Some authors concluded that the autoantibody levels of MMP-7 in serum may be a good biomarker for ESCC (J.H. Zhou et al., 2011). Some pharmacologic studies designed various MMP inhibitors with poor effect probably due to their high toxicity as has been demonstrated in clinical trials.

TIMPs (tissue inhibitor of metalloproteinases) comprise a family of four protease inhibitors: TIMP-1 (chromosome Xp11.3-p11.23); TIMP-2 (chromosome 17q25); TIMP-3 (chromosome

22q12.3); TIMP4 (chromosome 3q25). The first TIMP was described in 1975 as a protein which was able to inhibit collagenase activity (Bauer et al., 1975; Bosman and Stamenkovic, 2003). TIMPs and MMPs are found in all fluids, such as serum, plasma, urine, etc. All MMPs are inhibited by TIMPs once they are activated. The balance between MMPs and TIMPs plays a necessary role in maintaining the integrity of healthy tissue. An alteration of this balance is observed in different diseases. In cancer and rheumatoid arthritis, the imbalance is generally in favor of MMPs. By contrast to inhibition of MMPs by TIMPs, some studies founded that TIMP-2 was implicated in the activation of pro-MMP-2. This mechanism stimulates cell migration and progression to tumor metastasis and invasion (Yoshizuki et al., 2001). TIMPs are co-expressed with MMPs which depend on endogenously expressed growth factors and cytokines (Gomez et al., 1997).

The balance between MMPs and TIMPs is variable in both, in physiological processes such as growth and development, and in some diseases such as cancer. In esophagus cancer, we studied MMP-1 concentration in tumor and in non-tumor areas from the same patient with EA and observed a higher concentration in tumor areas (Vegh et al., 2007). Moreover, MMP-1 was associated with poor clinical outcome in esophageal cancer in different studies (Etoh et al., 2000; Murray et al., 1998; Yamashita et al., 2001). We found similar results in the concentration of MMP-1 in tumor vs. non-tumor areas in patients who had ESCC, but without being associated with the clinicopathological outcome (Vegh et al., 2007). On the other hand, we have observed that TIMP-1 expression in esophagus cancer showed higher values in tumor areas (Vegh et al., 2007). Interestingly, the same patients with lymph node negative showed higher values on TIMP-1 expression, whereas patients with more than three positive lymph nodes had lower values. This profile could indicate an inhibitory function for TIMP-1 on tumor growth and its possible dissemination. Numerous researchers considered that TIMP-1 has mitogenic activity on different cell types, whereas its over-expression reduced tumor growth in gastric carcinoma (Mimori et al., 1997). Furthermore, studies focusing on nitric oxide (NO) showed enhanced expression of MMP-1,-3,-7 and TIMP-1 in the progression from non-dysplasic BE to adenocarcinoma. This could indicate that NO play a role in Barrett's carcinogenesis through deregulating of MMP and TIMP expression to enhance invasive potential in dysplasic cells (Clemons et al., 2010). MMP-7 was cloned from ESCC tissues and higher levels were observed in serum in patients with ESCC than in their matched-control samples, therefore it was considered that MMP-7 may be a good diagnostic biomarker for ESCC (J.H. Zhou et al., 2011).

2.2 Polymorphisms and mutations

It has been well established that cancer is a genetic disease and carcinogenesis takes place in somatic mutations of the oncogenes or tumor suppressor genes. There have been several studies showing that BE and EA can occur within families indicating an inherent genetic risk (Eng et al., 1993; Romero et al., 1997). A pivotal role corresponds to phosphatidylinositol 3-kinase (PIK3CA) signaling pathway. In vitro ESCC proliferation was reduced by a PIK3CA inhibitor. This inhibition has more effects on the cells that contain a PIK3CA gene mutation than those without such mutation (Mori et al., 2008). It has also been speculated that some polymorphisms affecting the inflammatory response might be important in esophageal carcinoma. Such approaches may allow the identification of subsets of individuals within a population who are predisposed to EA. Accumulation of genetic alterations follows the dysplasia-adenocarcinoma sequence in the esophagus and identifies the patients with poor prognosis (Wu et al., 1998). The human genome receives exogenous and endogenous attacks that could promote genetic mutations, chromosomal rearrangements and finally development of cancer. Cells have an anti-DNA-damaging system to blockade both metabolic and external sources of DNA damaging agents. Activation of cell cycle checkpoints and DNA repair system are complex processes which help cellular responses to DNA damage. These checkpoints generally stop cell-cycle progression at the G1, S, and G2 phases. Gamma-radiation can induce single and double strand breaks. Some chemical carcinogenetic compounds, such as benzo(a) pyrene-diol-epoxide a tobacco procarcinogen benzo(a) pyrene, form bulky adducts and need nucleotide excision pathways to remove the adducts. Deficiencies in cell cycle checkpoint pathways are more frequently observed in esophagus cancer than in healthy donors. Shao et al, 2006 compared the mutagen-induced damage level among individuals with different S or G2-M phase cell accumulation and observed an increase of esophageal cancer risk.

2.3 Oncogen *p53*

Oncogen p*53* is a major regulator of the cell response to stress and acts as a tumor suppressor by inducing cell cycle arrest or apoptosis. Inactivation of the p53 signaling pathway has been seen in different human cancers. Previously, polymorphisms of p53 have been reported to be a possible risk factor for some types of tumors (Hrstka et al., 2009; Levine et al., 2004; Wu et al., 1998). The most common polymorphism on *p53* is at the 72nd amino acid residue with an arginine (Arg) to proline (Pro) change because of a G→C transverse. Differences in the biochemical or biological characteristics of the wild type *p53* variants have been reported. Some authors considered that the Arg72 variant can better induce apoptosis than the Pro72, indicating that the two polymorphic variants of *p53* (also so called *TP53*) are functionally distinct, which may influence cancer risk and treatment (Matlashewski et al., 1987; Thomas et al., 1999; Whibley et al., 2009). Numerous studies have reported this *p53* polymorphism in several cancers such as cervical, lung, breast, and gastric cancer (Dai et al., 2009; Dumont et al., 2003; Z. Zhang et al., 2011; Zhou et al., 2007), but its association with esophagus cancer remains elusive. Several specific molecular alterations play crucial roles in esophagus cancer, with tumor cell aneuploidy and p53 mutations being major hallmarks of both ESCC and EA (Blant et al., 2001; Fang et al., 2004; Jiang et al., 2010; Kuwano et al., 2005; Minu et al., 1994; Montesano et al., 1996; Souza, 2010; Whibley et al., 2009; Yu et al., 2007). Levine et al., 1991 considered that alteration or inactivation of p53 by mutations or interaction with oncogene products of DNA tumor viruses can lead to cancer. However, some researchers found no association between the immunomarkers p53, cyclin D1 and bcl-2 with the clinicopathological data and outcome in a selected population of esophagogastric junction adenocarcinoma patients (Lehrbach et al., 2009). The 17p is the chromosomial locus for *p53* oncogene. Studies of allelic alterations on chromosome 17p.13 and in 17p11.2-22 (microsatellite region adjacent to the *p53* locus) were performed by polymerase chain reaction (PCR) using two different primers (D17S513 and D17S514), (Table 1). An allelic alteration was observed in both tumor and non-tumor areas of esophagus cancer patients. Moreover, this dinucleotide repeat polymorphism was observed in both EA and ESCC. In addition, our studies showed statistically significant high levels of MMP-1 associated with this allelic alteration in the EA group. In the ESCC group, the allelic alteration was found associated with positive lymph nodes (Vegh et al., 2007).

Biomarker	Patients (n)	Values expressed	P	Overall survival time	References
CNR-1 *gene* (controls)	40	G/G: 60.0 % G/A: 40.0 % A/A: 0.0 %		ND	
CNR-1 *gene*; (EC)	29	G/G: 10.8 % G/A: 61.2 % A/A: 7.9 % No a. 20.1 %		G/G: 56.3 months versus A/A: 3.5 months P=0.04	Bedoya et al. 2009a
P53 (D17S513) A/A type, EA	23	a.a.: 69.9%		ND	
P53 (D17S514) A/A type, EA	23	a.a.: 82.6 %		ND	Vegh et al. 2007
P53 (D17S513) A/A type, ESCC	14	a.a.: 50.0%		ND	
P53 (D17S514) A/A type, ESCC	14	a.a.: 78.6%		ND	Vegh et al. 2007
VEGF tumor	39	300.6±99.7pg/mg			
VEGF no tumor	100	80.8±19.7 pg/mg	< 0.025	P= 0.11	Bedoya et al. 2009a
MMP1 (EA)	23	45.6±7.6 ng/mg			
TIMP1 (EA)	23	28.7±7.0 ng/mg	< 0.05	ND	Vegh et al. 2007
MMP1 (ESCC)	14	37.0±6.9 ng/mg			
TIMP1 (ESCC)	14	38.9±7.5 ng/mg	= 0.44	ND	Vegh et al. 2007

EC: esophageal cancer; VEGF: vascular endothelial growth factor; CNR1 *gene*: cannabinoid receptor 1 gene; G/G wild type, G/A heterozygous mutation; A/A homozygous mutation; P53: oncogene p53; D17S513 and D17S514: primers used; a.a.: with allelic alterations; MMP1: Matrix metalloproteinase, TIMP: Tissue inhibitor metalloproteinase; ND: no data; No a.: with no amplification; EA: esophagus adenocarcinoma; ESCC: esophagus squamous cell carcinoma; vs.: versus; P minor than 0.05 was considered statistically significant.

Table 1. *Biomarkers in esophagus cancer:* Analysis data of different markers in tissue of esophagus cancer patients, according our some experiences.

DNA repair inhibitors are used by the cells to protect or reverse themselves against mutagens and different carcinogens. Some authors considered the small cyclin dependent kinase-inhibiting protein p21 as a critical mediator of *p53* function and required for *p53* –mediated growth suppression of tumor cells (Waldman T et al., 1995).

2.4 Cannabinoids receptors and esophagus cancer

The CB1 receptor (or CNR1) is encoded by the *CNR1* gene and located in chromosome 6q14-q15 (size 26,056 bases). CNR1 molecular function corresponds to a receptor activity and their biological processes such as signal transduction and G-protein signaling-coupled with a cyclic nucleotide second messenger (cyclic AMP). CNR1 is expressed most widely in the brain. Endocannabinoids (anandamine and 2-arachidonylglycerol) released from the neurons bind to CBN1 receptors in the pre-synaptic neurons and produce a reduction in the release of the inhibitory neurotransmitter gamma-aminobutiric acid (GABA). Cannabinoid receptors are expressed on several cell types and have functions in liver, endocrine glands, on gastrointestinal and cardiovascular activity and on pain transmission. Endocannabinoids are agonists of cannabinoid receptors and have been shown to participate in the inhibition of malignant cells, in the proliferation of cancer tissues and have been associated with different stages of the disease (Pertwee, 1997). After the receptor is engaged, multiple intracellular signal transduction pathways are activated implicating potassium ion channels, calcium channels, protein kinase A and C, Raf-1, ERK, JNK, p38, c-fos, c-jun, etc. Previously, one simple nucleotide polymorphism (SNP) was detected at nucleotide positive 1359 G→A. Due to the high polymorphism information content, this SNP is considered as a useful intragenic marker which may be related to cannabinoid system alterations. The artificial creation of an *Mspl* restriction site in amplified wild type (G-allele) which is destroyed by the mutation (A-allele) has been useful to detect a silent mutation (Gadzicki et al., 1999). We have observed in *CNR-1gene* 10.8 % of wild type in esophagus tissue samples of esophagus cancer patients as compared to 60.0% in *CNR-1gene* in control patients (Figure 1). We

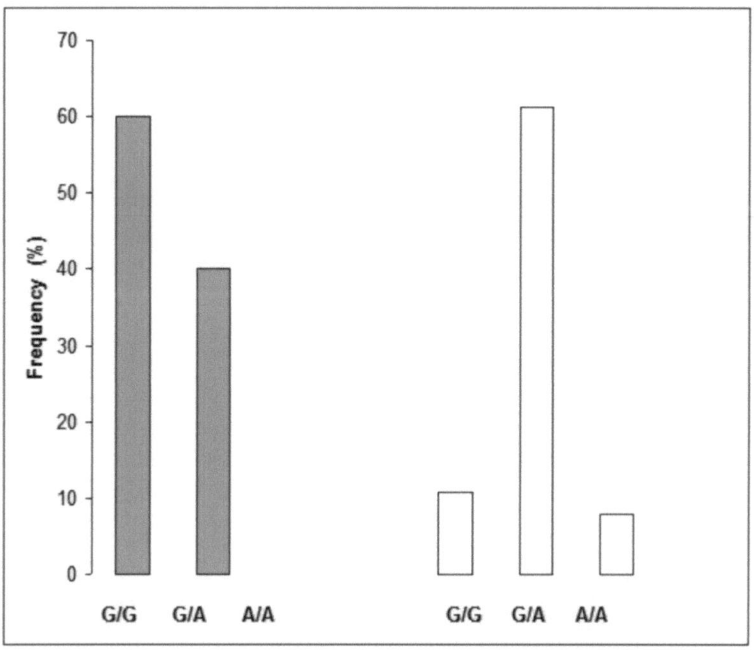

Fig. 1. *Frequency of CNR1 gene expression in esophageal tissue.* Grey bars, corresponding to control healthy patients (n=40) esophagus tissue, no A/A mutation was observed. White bars, corresponding to CNR1*gene* expression in tumor of esophagus cancer patients (n=29).

concluded that this alteration may be considered as a mutation and hypothesized that this mutation is an acquired somatic mutation. Moreover, we also found that the mean survival time in wild type G/G group was longer than A/A homozygous group, (P=0.04, chi-square: 4.26) (Table 1). However, we did not find any association of *CNR-1* with the angiogenic growth factor VEGF levels. However, VEGF expression was higher in tumor than in no-tumor (P< 0.025), but VEGF expression did not correlate with survival time. (Bedoya et al., 2009a). So, we can consider that CNR1 gene could be considered an independent marker for survival. In addition, in colorectal cancer patients we have also found that CNR1 gene genotype G/A plus A/A group of patients has a shorter overall survival time than G/G wild type patients (Bedoya et al., 2009b).

2.5 Vascular endothelial growth factor

In carcinogenesis, genetic and epigenetic changes are important for malignant transformation. The growth of solid tumors which is regulated partly by the angiogenesis process and vascular endothelial growth factor (VEGF) has been identified as the principal regulator of angiogenesis in both, physiological and pathological conditions (Ferrara, et al., 1997; Folkman, 1990). VEGF's function is to create new blood vessels during embryonic development. Binding of VEGF and other ligands to the VEGF-receptor (VEGFR) of endothelial cells activates the angiogenic pathways. VEGF is strongly expressed in many human cancers, including esophageal carcinomas (Inoue et al., 1997) and intestinal cancers (Bendardaf et al., 2008). High levels of VEGF have been associated with a poor prognosis in cancer patients. Our studies did not observe any statistically significant differences in plasma VEGF concentration in esophageal cancer patients at different clinical stages neither did in samples corresponding to different tumor and not tumor areas (Figure 2). In this study we assayed in plasma VEGF concentration of control healthy and esophagus cancer patients and the difference was not statistically significant. Analyses of VEGF expression in tumor homogenate of these patients using a cut-off level of 120 pg/mg of total protein did not appear to correlate with the overall survival time (Bedoya et al., 2009a). However, high hypoxia-inducible transcription factor-1 (HIF-1) is an important inducer of angiogenesis and VEGF expression is important as a prognostic factor and related to survival in ESCC patients (Kimura et al., 2004). Moreover, some authors considered that these factors could help to predict the response of the ESCC patients to several therapies (Shimada et al., 2002). The role of other angiogenic factors such as transforming growth factor-α (TGF-α) and basic fibroblast growth factor (bFGF) were studied by Li et al, 2000. They suggested that TGF-α as well as VEGF, PD-ECGF and bFGF may be associated with angiogenesis, and progression to metastases of ESCC patients. The diagnostic of lymph node status in esophagus cancer is a very important prognostic factor. VEGF-C is a potential angiogenic factor in lymph-nodes and selectively induces vasculature in the lymphatic glands. The expression of VEGF-C has a high correlation with the lymph node metastasis in patients with stage T*is* and T1 of esophagus cancer patients (Tanaka et al., 2010).

2.6 Epidermal growth factor receptor

Epidermal growth factor (EGF) plays an important role in the cell cycle and may regulate the production of MMPs via over-expression of the epidermal growth factor receptor (EGFR). EGF protein was discovered by Stanley Cohen and Rita Levi-Montachini and both won the Nobel Prize in 1986. EGF is a low molecular -weight polypeptide of 6045-Da protein. EGF includes different biological processes such as the activation of MAPKK activity, DNA replication, chromosome organization, EGFR signaling pathway and interaction with phosphatidylinosidol 3-kinase complex (PIK3R2). EGFR are on the cell surface and are activated by binding with its specific ligands (EGF, TGFα and others). Upon activation, EGFR undergoes a transition from an inactive to an active form. The EGFR dimerization stimulates its intrinsic intracellular protein-tyrosine kinase activity. Mutations that induce EGFR over-expression have been associated with cancer. These mutations have been the target of several treatments allowing the development of anticancer therapies such as gefitinib and erlotinib for lung cancer, cetuximab and panitumumab for colorectal cancer, as examples of a monoclonal antibody acting as inhibitors of tyrosine kinase proteins. Indeed, without kinase activity, EGFR is inactive and does not initiate the signaling cascade

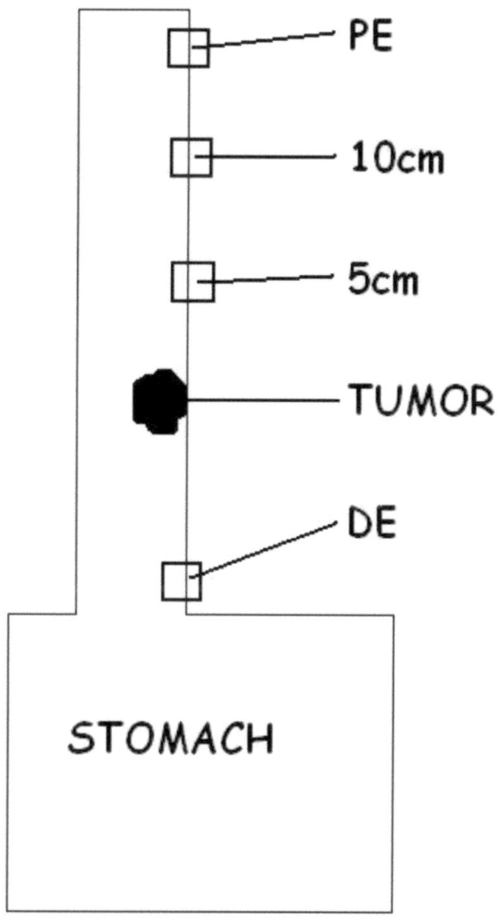

Fig. 2. *Diagram of esophagus areas studied.* PE: proximal edge of sample exceresis, 10 cm: sample from around tumor area; 5 com: sample around tumor area; T: tumor (EA or ESCC according to histopathologic diagnosis), DE: distal edge, sample obtained near to stomach.

pathway for growth in the cells (Lynch et al., 2004). Several studies have demonstrated that EGFR is over-expressed in tumors and ESCC cell lines. However, immunohistochemical evaluation of EGFR did not provide prognostic information for ESCC patients (Torzewski et a.l, 1997). The fact that EGFR correlated with age, depth of invasion, lymph node metastasis and poor prognosis was observed (Inada et al., 1999). Our results have found the over-expression of EGFR in membrane of tumor homogenate in a group of esophageal cancer patients with more than three positive lymph nodes. Nevertheless, we did not find any significant differences between mean levels of EGFR in both tumor and non-tumor areas of the esophagus (Vegh et al., 2007). EGFR over-expression and mutant *p53* tumor suppressor genes help the enrichment of a cellular subpopulation involved in epithelial to mesenchymal transition among telomerase- immortalized human esophageal epithelial cells during carcinogenesis (Ohashi et al., 2010).

2.7 Human chorionic gonadotropin-beta

The human chorionic gonadotropin (βHCG) is a glycoprotein synthesized by normal placenta and released by the trophoblastic cells and different neoplastic cells. In esophageal tumors, by immunostaining procedures Burg-Kurland et al., 1989 observed a variation in the staining intensity of the tumor cells. Cells were weakly stained in well differentiated squamous cell carcinomas, although the poorly differentiated cells showed a more generalized pattern of staining. Moreover, these studies considered that βHCG is associated with ESCC as well as EA and to pre-neoplastic lesions (Burg-Kurland et al., 1989). The characteristics of this tumor marker permit the monitoring and evaluation of the treatments.

2.8 Carcinoembryonic antigen

In 1965 Gold and coworkers demonstrated tumor-associated antigens in adenocarcinoma of the digestive tract in humans. The oncofetal carcinoembryonic antigen (CEA) is a glycoprotein with a molecular weight of 200,000 kDa originally isolated in colon carcinoma cells and is located on the luminal surface of the tumor cell membrane of endodermal as well as non-endodermal origin. CEA expression in serum of esophagus cancer patients is not well recognized as a biomarker. Nevertheless, correlation between CEA levels in serum and tissue was observed in patients with esophagus cancer (Sanders et al., 1994); and elevated serum CEA levels were useful for early detection of relapse in patients with EA (Kim et al., 1995). We have reported that in tissue homogenate of EA patients there were not statistically significant differences in mean levels of CEA in tumor areas when compared with non-tumor (Vegh et al., 2007). However, in ESCC tumors, CEA concentration showed statistically significant higher values in tumor samples from patients with negative lymph nodes. These results were similar to those observed in non-small–cell lung cancer patients (Vegh et al., 2002). Kosugi et al., 2004 determined the role of preoperative serum levels of CEA, CA19-9 and SSC in patients with esophagus cancer. They found that only preoperative high levels of serum SCC antigen indicate an adverse outcome after esophagectomy and the appearance of distant metastases (Kijima et al., 2000; Kosugi et al., 2004). In summary, the CEA marker is very useful for monitoring previously diagnosed cancer.

2.9 Interleukins

Interleukins (IL-1 through IL-17) are a group of cytokines that participate in stimulating the immune response in inflammation and in hematopoiesis. Interleukins are a group of cellular messenger molecules, so called cytokines, which act as modulators of cellular behavior and are secreted rapidly by cells in response to several stimuli such as an infectious agent. The first interleukin was identified in the 1970s (Gillis et al., 1978). Different types of interleukins have become known since then and are designated numerically. IL1 and IL2 are responsible for activating T and B lymphocytes. IL-1, along with IL-6, is also a mediator of inflammation. IL-6 expression at local tumor sites or in systemic circulation has been associated with disease progression and poor prognosis of esophageal cancer and may act as a resistance factor against cisplatin-based treatments (Suchi et al., 2011). The clinicopathological significance of IL-6 and other cytokine levels in esophageal cancer was associated with a poor outcome (Motoyama et al., 2011; Xin et al., 2010; H.Y. Zhang et al., 2011).

2.10 microRNAs

The expression of the miR-17-92 cluster was first shown in ESCC and is over-expressed in 75% of esophageal cancer patients (Liu et al., 2011). In addition, its over-expression could promote cellular growth in vivo and in vitro. Furthermore, antisense oligonucleotides (ONs) inhibited miR-19a and induced apoptosis while miR-17-5p, miR-18a, miR-20a and miR-92-1 were not affected. It was found that antagomir-19a treatment could impair tumor growth in vivo. In fact, using Human Apoptosis RT2 Profiler PCR Array 384HT was observed that tumor necrosis factor-α (TNF-α) was 12-fold up-regulated in cells transfected with miR-19a antisense ONs compared to the cells treated with the control scramble ONs. miR-19a was predicted to target the 3' untranslated region of TNF-α mRNA and this was confirmed by luciferase reporter assay. Taken together, they conclude that the miR-17-92 cluster is over-expressed in ESCC and that TNF-α could be a novel target of miR-19a (Liu et al., 2011).

2.11 c-erbB-2 or HER2 gene

HER-2/neu (c-erbB-2, HER2) gene amplification and protein over-expression have been associated with poor prognosis in several solid tumors, including breast and gastric cancer. However, its incidence and significance in EA is unknown (Thompson et al, 2011). Expression of erb-B2 in esophageal cancer patients was associated with longer survival and may be a good marker to monitoring the treatment sensitivity (D'Amico and Harpole, 2000).

2.12 TGF-alpha

Transforming growth factor-alpha (TGF-α) is produced by several human carcinomas. TGF-α maps to human chromosome 2p11-2p13. TGF-α is a small protein of 50 amino acids. This growth factor is found in plasma and urine and is produced by some non-transformed cells during the development such as, keratocytes, macrophages, platelets and hepatocytes. Their synthesis is induced by estrogens and is related to EGF. The biological activities of both growth factors are very similar and both bind to the same membrane receptor encoded by the cellular *erb* oncogene. Experimental studies in Wistar rats observed that TGF-α and EGFR play crucial roles in chronic reflux esophagitis (Fujiwara et al., 2004). The integrity of esophageal mucosa, acts upon the equilibrium between cellular protective mechanisms and different aggressive factors. It has been found that human esophageal submucosal glands elaborate protective biomarkers like TGF-α, EGF, prostaglandin E(2), bicarbonate and no-bicarbonate buffers (Sarosiek and McCallium, 2000). Nevertheless, an increased production of TGF-α is associated with malignant transformation in different cell types (Li et al., 2000). TGF-α can be assayed in plasma by a specific radioligant assay or the ELISA method and by colony formation assay. Aloia et al., 2001, analyzed the expression of the tumor markers P-gp, p53, and TGF-α in node-negative esophagus cancer patients. Their results showed that this type of analysis sustains the immunohistochemical prognostic value.

2.13 TGF-beta

Transforming growth factor beta (TGF-β) and Notch signaling pathways play important roles in regulating self-renewal of stem cells and cell-fate determination. Both pathways are frequently implicated in gastrointestinal carcinogenesis. TGF-β1 mediated the mesenchymal-epithelial transition and may be relevant in esophageal carcinogenesis (Rees et al., 2006; Thiery, 2002). However, others showed that the contribution of TGF-beta to esophageal adenocarcinoma remains associated with EGFR and *p53* (Ohashi et al, 2010). It is well known that the stromal compartment plays an important role in carcinogenesis. Genetic analysis showed a strong contribution of an inflammatory component and the key pathways included cytokine-cytokine receptor interactions and TGF-β in BE disease progression and how these can affect the outcome or progression (Saadi et al. 2010).

2.14 Alpha fetoprotein

Alpha fetoprotein (AFP) is a glycoprotein of 591 aminoacids and a carbohydrate moiety. AFP is highly expressed in human fetus but in adults, AFP levels are low with unknown function, although it can be used as a biomarker to detect tumors. It is indicative of germ-cell tumors, hepatocellular carcinoma and ectopic production of AFP has also been found in different tumors. In some tumors, the decrease of AFP levels indicates a good prognostic value. AFP expression is elevated in gastrointestinal malignancies and its expression is related to metastasis (Liu et al., 2010; Mizejewski, 2002). In summary, this tumor marker is very useful for monitoring previously diagnosed cancer.

2.15 CA 19-9

The carbohydrate antigen 19-9 (CA 19-9) tumor marker can be detected in blood serum and in the tumor homogenate of different cancer patients. Levels are often elevated in some gastrointestinal cancers, such as colorectal, pancreatic and esophagus cancer. As previously reported by our group, the level CA 19-9 was detected by ELISA in colorectal cancer patients and was considered as an independent prognostic factor for the relapse (Morales-Gutierrez et al, 1999). Studies performed in serum of human ESCC patients showed that CA19-9 is a link for E-selectin and this association may play an important role in tumor metastasis. Serum CA19-9 may be useful in the follow-up of recurrence and response to treatment (Mcknight et al, 1989; Oshiba et al, 2000). In EA patients, we observed a higher concentration of CA 19-9 in tumor areas than in non-tumor areas from the same patient, but these results did not correlate with their clinical characteristics (Vegh et al, 2007).

Nevertheless, CA 19-9 concentration was higher in patients with more than three positive lymph nodes than in patients with negative nodes. In ESCC patients, CA 19-9 concentration did not show any differences between tumor and non-tumor areas. In conclusion, patients who had advanced or metastatic cancer can be monitored by their CA 19-9 levels throughout the treatment.

2.16 Tumor Necrosis Factor –α

Tumor necrosis factor alpha (TNF-α) is a pro-inflammatory cytokine with conflicting effects in both, tumor growth and tumor regression. These paradoxical results seem to be related to differences in this cytokine concentration, as high therapeutic doses induced tumor regression while physiological levels of endogenous TNF-α promote tumor growth (Anderson et al., 2004). Clinical data related to TNF-α expression by esophageal cells are limited. Kilic et al. 2009, studied TNF-α and IL-2 expression in the distal esophageal muscle in patients with achalasia of the esophagus and observed that the proportion of inflammatory cells expressing TNF-α is inversely correlated with the duration of the clinical symptoms. Other studies have shown that TNF-α is up-regulated in the progression to Barret´s metaplasia suggesting a role of TNF-α in the transcription of gastrointestinal oncogenes (Tselepsis et al., 2002). In ESCC where the miR-17-92 cluster is over-expressed, TNF-α seems to be a novel target of miR-19a (Liu et al., 2011).

3. Esophageal cancer and stem cells

Despite the fact the incidence of EA has increased over the last 40 years, the biology of the normal esophageal epithelium and the pathogenesis of esophageal cancer is not well understood (Nguyen et al., 2011). Currently, it is still unknown if esophageal cancer initiation, growth and maintenance is caused: i) by the "clonal selection theory", i.e., through the accumulation of genetic alterations in some cells that acquire growth advantage over normal cells and leads to the selection of these clones; ii) by the "cancer stem cell (CSC) theory" based in the suggestion that only a small number of stem cells accumulate the genetic alterations and contribute to the esophageal tumor growth and maintenance; or iii) by a mixture of both models (Adams and Strasser, 2008; Hormi-Carver and Souza, 2009).

3.1 Cancer Stem Cell (CSC) theory and esophageal cancer

CSC theory is based on the idea that most cancers are initiated for stem cells with genetic alterations that are unable to undergo terminal differentiation, i.e., the proliferation capacity of stem cells can be difficult to control under certain circumstances and contribute to the tumor formation (Nguyen et al., 2011; Quante and Wang, 2009). In solid tumors including esophageal cancer, the CSCs have been correlated with resistance to chemotherapy and radiation, recurrence and metastasis (Zhang et al., 2005). It is interesting to highlight the lack of agreement on the best markers for CSCs in digestive tumors and doubts about the real phenotype and also the existence of the CSCs (Quante and Wang, 2009). There is little evidence for the existence of CSCs in esophageal cancer. Stimulation of esophageal stem cells of the epithelium contributes to both, esophageal epithelial regeneration and cancer. Changes in the activity of the esophagus stem cells and the up- or down-regulation of stem cell markers appear to be related to esophageal cancer development, tumor progression and final clinical outcome. Further understanding and characterization of adult esophageal stem cells and the factors that contribute to the development of dysplasia and malignancy it is a matter of critical importance (Croagh et al., 2008).

3.2 Stem cells in the esophagus

Stem cells are classified in two general groups as embryonic and adult stem cells. They have the ability to regenerate the tissue where they reside because of their characteristics of self-renewal and multipotency. Adult stem cells within the gastrointestinal tissue are classified as esophageal, gastric, intestinal, colonic, hepatic and pancreatic (Quante and Wang, 2009).

Stem cells in the human esophagus are present in the basal layer of the stratified squamous epithelium (Kalabis et al., 2008; Seery and Watt, 2000). Human esophagus is a complex tissue with a slow cell turnover (Croagh et al., 2008). A population of stem cells known as Side Population cells (SP cells) were isolated from mouse esophagus (Epperly et al., 2004; Kalabis et al., 2008). Esophageal SP cells have the ability to home in on and differentiate to esophagus cells as shown by in vitro and in vivo esophageal injury models. A rare stem cell population expressing high levels of α_6-integrin and low levels of CD71 was characterized in the basal layer of the mouse esophagus and whose final function is to form and/or regenerate the suprabasal layers (Croagh et al., 2007). A population of stem cells characterized by low expression of β1-integrin and high expression of β2-laminin chain was isolated from the human esophagus with the ability to reconstitute the esophageal epithelium in vitro (Seery and Watt, 2000). It has also shown that bone marrow stem cells may contribute to cell regeneration of normal and injured rat esophagus (Sarosi et al., 2008).

3.3 Stem cell markers involved in cancer development and evolution

It is a matter of crucial importance to known the markers characteristics of stem cells whose expression is significantly increased in the esophageal cancer cells and that would be involved in cancer development and associated with a poorer clinical outcome. However, there is little information about the phenotype and the biology of the stem cells and the cancer stem cells responsible of the low five-year survival rate in esophageal cancer (Kalabis et al., 2008; Nguyen et al., 2011).

The CD44, a glycoprotein involved in cell motility and migration, is one of the most used markers for the identification of CSCs in multiple tissues (Nguyen et al., 2011; Quante and Wang, 2009). CD44 is also a marker of esophageal CSCs and its expression is associated with metastasis and a poor prognosis (Takayama et al., 2003). However, CD133, another common CSC marker was not expressed in EA stem cells (Grotenhuis et al., 2010).

SP cells in the esophagus presented CSCs characteristics indicated by higher clone formation efficiency, up-regulation of stem-cell related genes such as Oct-4 and Sox-2, up-regulation of the ABC transporter genes, increased expression of the Notch and Wnt-related genes and a higher expression of beta-catenin protein (Epperly et al., 2004; Huang et al., 2009).

Analysis of tumors obtained from ESCC patients demonstrated a high expression of Oct-4 and Sox-2 genes and this expression was significantly associated with a higher histological grade and poorer clinical outcome (Bass et al., 2009; Wang et al., 2009; X. Zhou et al., 2011). The HIWI gene was identified in hematopoietic stem cells and germ cells and plays a role in stem cell pluripotency, self-renewal and differentiation. HIWI was also detected in human ESCC and its over-expression was associated with higher histological grade and poorer overall survival (He et al., 2009).

Musashi-1 is a RNA-biding protein identified as a marker of the intestinal stem cells and found in BE and significantly increased in EA, whereas it is absent in normal squamous epithelium indicating an important role in the development and maintenance of the esophagus diseases or even the cell of origin for esophagus cancer (Bobryshev et al., 2010).

Leucine-rich-repeat-containing G-protein-coupled receptor (LgR5) was first proposed as an intestinal stem cell marker and recently identified in EA but not in ESCC patients. LgR5 expression is related with the low survival rate in these patients (von Rahden et al., 2011). The neural stem cell marker low-affinity neurotrophin receptor p75NTR is expressed in esophageal keratinocyte stem cells with high proliferation properties (Okumura et al., 2003). This marker was present in an elevated number of ESCC and EA patients (Okumura et al., 2006; Sun et al., 2009). p75NTR could be a potential target for future specific esophageal therapies.

3.4 Adult stem cells as an approach for the treatment of gastrointestinal diseases

In recent years, the progress in stem cells identification and characterization indicate the potential therapeutic applications of stem cells in regenerative medicine for the treatment of several pathologies. The different types of stem cells, embryonic, induced pluripotent and adult stem cells are emerging as a potential approach to treat gastrointestinal disorders. Stem cells could be classified in two main groups, i.e., embryonic and adult stem cells. There is an increasing interest in the potential use of stem cells in regenerative medicine.

3.4.1 Embryonic stem cells

Embryonic stem cells (ESCs) have a high proliferation and differentiation capacity (pluripotency). However, there are several limitations to their use for therapeutic purposes including the ethical considerations, the elevated self-renewal properties that will induce tumors and the immune rejection as they are not patient-derived (Ao et al., 2011).

The induced pluripotent stem cells (iPSCs) are stem cells obtained from somatic stem cells by transfer of exogenous genes involved in the maintenance of ECSs. The iPSCs can be generated from the patients´ somatic cells preventing the immune rejection. However, like ESCs the risk of teratoma formation is an important problem to be overcome for future clinical application (Kooreman and Wu, 2010).

3.4.2 Adult stem cells

Adult stem cells are undifferentiated cells present a tissue or organ in very small amounts that can renew by themselves and differentiate into all of the specialized cell types of the tissue or organ. The principal role of adult stem cells is to maintain and repair the tissue in which they are found in case of any disease or injury. Adult stem cells have been found in almost all adult tissues, even in more tissues than was thought possible. Several adult stem cells such as adult hematopoietic stem cells from bone marrow or from umbilical cord blood have been used in transplants for 40 or 20 years, respectively.

Mesenchymal stem cells (MSCs) are adult stem cells also present in bone marrow. These non-hematopoietic stem cells are isolated from bone marrow by their adherence to the plastic plates after culture and characterized by the expression of a set of markers (CD105, CD73 and CD90) and the lack of expression of hematopoietic markers (CD45, CD34, CD14 or CD11b, CD79a or CD19) and the HLA class II surface molecules (Dominici et al., 2006). MSC are multipotent cells with the capacity of differentiation into bone, fat and cartilage (Horwitz et al., 2005). In addition to the mesodermal differentiation, MSC have been differentiated to cells of the endodermal and ectodermal embryonic layers. This differentiation capacity as well as their immunosuppressive and immunomodulatory properties makes MSCs a very attractive resource for tissue regeneration (Liu et al., 2009). Bone marrow MSC are the most used cells in both experimental and clinical settings, although MSCs have been isolated from numerous sources such as adipose tissue, umbilical cord blood, umbilical cord tissue, amniotic fluid and placenta (Broxmeyer et al., 2006; De Coppi et al., 2007; Igura et al., 2004; Macias et al., 2010; Miki et al., 2005; Sarugaser et al., 2005; Soncini et al., 2007; Tallone et al., 2011).

Human placenta is an especially complex organ composed of both fetal and maternal tissues. At the time of birth, placenta loses its function and is normally discarded. MSC obtained from human placenta are stem cells without ethical concerns, isolated without invasive procedures and present low risk of viral infection (Hemberger et al., 2008; Pappa and Anagnou, 2009; Parolini et al., 2008). Recently, we have described the isolation and characterization of a population of MSCs from the maternal part of human placenta, i.e. decidua parietalis (Macias et al., 2010). The cells named Decidua-derived Mesenchymal Stem Cells (DMSC) is a homogeneous population of MSCs that showed high proliferation and differentiation capacity into cell types from the three embryonic layers, genomic stability and until senescence and a decrease in telomerase activity indicating that DMSCs could be safely used in regenerative medicine. In addition, DMSCs are hypo-immunogenic cells suggesting that they could be used in both, autologous and allogenic transplantation for future clinical trials.

3.4.3 Mesenchymal stem cells for the treatment of gastrointestinal diseases

Recent studies have revealed that MSCs selectively migrate and home in on to damaged tissues and organs after systemic or local application (Kidd et al., 2009). This tropism for sites of injury, irrespective of the tissue or organ, indicates that MSCs can be useful as cellular vehicles as tumors are considered as "wounds that never heal" (Dvorak, 1986). Indeed, bone marrow stem cells migrate to esophageal epithelium and contribute to tissue regeneration under normal and/or pathological conditions (Sarosi et al., 2008). These migratory properties make MSCs a useful and efficient tool for the delivery of therapeutic anti-tumor genes to the tumor area (Hall et al., 2007). MSCs will later produce and release the anticancer agents in situ which would significantly increase the efficacy and decrease the side effects of these therapeutic agents (Nakamizo et al., 2005; Studeny et al., 2002; Studeny et al., 2004). Besides, these authors showed also evidences that MSCs can also be used as therapeutic agents themselves. The use of MSCs as cellular delivery vehicles offer several advantages such as MSCs from several sources are easy to isolate and culture; can be expanded in culture without losing their characteristics; and are hypoimmunogenic and show immunomodulatory properties to be well tolerated in allogeneic transplantation (Horwitz et al., 2005; Macias et al., 2010).

4. Conclusion

In EA and ESCC patients, standard treatments are similar although it is necessary to develop earlier diagnosis because of the poor prognosis of esophageal cancer compared to other digestive cancers. It is necessary to select the most appropriate predictive biomarkers - especially, those assayed in esophageal tissue- and determined in with the aim of designing specific treatments for each type of esophagus cancer patients and obtain a clear clinical benefit. The overall expression of a set of single markers together with the clinical data would be useful to predict the development and evolution of this type of tumors.

In the near future, integrated approaches to biomarkers discovery and development, analyses and simulations to predict and identify the most specific biomarkers in esophagus cancer, are necessary. In addition, will be important bioinformatics analyses and tissue array studies (genomic, proteomic and transcriptomic-based biomarkers) with high quality clinical samples.

The molecular and cellular events responsible for regulating both, the replacement of the normal esophageal epithelium and the development and maintenance of cancer are not well understood. It is important to understand how the stem cells fate is regulated and the factors that play a role in its de-regulation and will contribute to the formation of a tumor. MSCs contribute to the regeneration of several tissues and could be used as cellular vehicles of anti-cancer drugs increasing their efficacy and decreasing the side effects which would greatly improve the quality of life of esophagus cancer patients. In summary, understanding the biology of normal esophageal epithelium and the role of the biomarkers of tumor, non-tumor and esophageal stem cells it is crucial for designing more specific therapies in order to increase the reduced current clinical outcomes of esophagus cancer patients.

5. References

Adams, J.M. & Strasser, A. (2008). Is tumor growth sustained by rare cancer stem cells or dominant clones? *Cancer Research,* Vol. 68, No. 11, (June 2008), pp. 4018-4021, ISSN 0008-5472, EISSN 1538-7445

Aloia, T.A.; Harpole, D.H. Jr.; Reed, C.E.; Allegra, C.; Moore, M.B.; Herndon, J.E. 2nd & D'Amico, T.A. (2001). Tumor marker expression is predictive of survival in patients with esophageal cancer. *Annual Thoracic Surgery,* Vol. 72, No. 3, (September 2001), pp. 859-866, ISSN 0003-4975, EISSN 1552-6259

Anderson, G.M.; Nakada, M.T. & DeWitte, M. (2004). Tumor necrosis factor-α in the pathogenesis and treatment of cancer. *Current Opinion in Pharmacology,* Vol. 4, No. 4 (August 2004), pp.314-320, ISSN 1471-4892, EISSN 1471-4973

Ao, A.; Hao J. & Hong, C.C. (2011). Regenerative chemical biology: current challenges and future potential. *Chemistry & Biol*ogy, Vol.18, No. 4 (April 2011) pp. 413-424, ISSN 1472-6769

Bass, A.J.; Watanabe, H.; Mermel, C.H.; Yu, S.; Perner, S.; Verhaak, R.G.; Kim, S.Y.; Wardwell, L.; Tamayo, P.; Gat-Viks, I.; Ramos, A.H.; Woo, M.S.; Weir, B.A.; Getz,

G.; Beroukhim, R.; O'Kelly, M.; Dutt, A.; Rozenblatt-Rosen O.; Dziunycz, P.; Komisarof, J.; Chirieac, L.R.; LaFargue, C.J.; Scheble, V.; Wilbertz, T.; Ma, C.; Rao, S.; Nakagawa, H.; Stairs, D.B.; Lin, L.; Giordano, T.J.; Wagner, P.; Minna, J.D.; Gazdar, A.F.; Zhu, C.Q.; Brose, M.S.; Cecconello, I.; Ribeiro U. Jr.; Marie, S.K.; Dahl, O.; Shivdasani, R.A.; Tsao, M.S.; Rubin, M.A.; Wong, K.K.; Regev, A.; Hahn, W.C.; Beer, D.G.; Rustgi, A.K. & Meyerson, M.. (2009). SOX2 is an amplified lineage-survival oncogene in lung and esophageal squamous cell carcinomas. *Nature Genetics,* Vol. 41, No.11, (November 2009), pp.1238-1242, ISSN 1061-4036, EISSN 1546-1718

Bauer, E.A.; Strick, G.P.; Jeffry, J.J. & Eisen, A.Z. (1975). Collagenase production by human skin. *Biochemical and Biophysical Research Communications* Vol. 64, No. 1, (May 1975), pp. 232-240, ISSN 0006-291X

Bearz, A.; Talamini, R.; Vaccher, E.; Spina, M.; Simonelli, C.; Steffan, A.; Berretta, M.; Chimienti, E. & Tirelli, U. (2007). MUC-1 (CA 15-3 antigen) as a highly reliable predictor of response to EGFR inhibitors in patients with bronchioloalveolar carcinoma: an experience on 26 patients. *The International Journal of Biological Markers* Vol. 22, No. 4, (Oct-Dec), pp. 307–311, ISSN 1724-6008, EISSN 1724-6008

Bedoya, F.; Meneu, J.; Macias, M.I.; Moreno, A.; Enríquez de Salamanca, R.; Moreno-Gonzalez, E. & Vegh, I. (2009a). Mutation in CNR1 gene and VEGF expression in esophageal cancer. *Tumori,* Vol.95, No. 1, (January-February 2009), pp.68-75; ISSN 0300-8916, EISSN 2038-2529

Bedoya, F.; Rubio, J.C.; Morales-Gutierrez, C.; Abad-Badahona, A.; Lora Pablos, D.; Meneu, J.C.; Moreno-Gonzalez, E.; Enriquez de Salamanca, R. & Vegh, I. (2009b) Single nucleotide change in the cannabinoid receptor-1 (CNR1) gene in colorectal cancer outcome. *Oncology (Basel*), Vol. 76, No. 6, (May 5), pp. 435-441; ISSN 0030-2414, EISSN 1423-0232

Bellet, D.H.; Wands, J.R.; Isselbacher, K.J. & Bohuon, C. (1984). Serum alpha fetoprotein levels in human disease: perspective from a highly specific monoclonal radioimmunoassay. *Proceedings of the National Academy of Sciences USA* Vol. 81, No. 12, (June 1984), pp. 3869-3873; ISSN 0027-8424, EISSN 1091-6490

Bendardaf, R.; Bumeida, A.; Hilska, M.; Laato, M.; Syrjänen, K.; Collan, Y. & Pyrhönen, S. (2008) VEGF-1 expression in colorectal cancer is associated with disease localization, stage, and log-term disease specific survival. *Anticancer Research,* Vol. 28, No. 6B, (November-December 2008), pp. 3865-3870, ISSN0250-7005, EISSN 1791-7530

Blant, S.A.; Ballini, J.P.; Caron, C.T.; Fontolliet, C.; Monnier, P. & Laurini, N.R. (2001). Evolution of DNA ploidy during squamous cell carcinogenesis in the esophagus. *Diseases of Esophagus,* Vol. 14, No. 3-4 (October 2001), 178-184, ISSN 1120-8694, EISSN 1442-2050

Bobryshev, Y.V., Freeman A.K., Botelho N.K., Tran D., Levert-Mignon A.J. & Lord R.V.(2010). Expression of the putative stem cell marker Musashi-1 in Barrett's esophagus and esophageal adenocarcinoma. *Diseases of Esophagus,* Vol. 23, No. 7, (September 2010), pp. 580-58, ISSN 1120-8694, EISSN 1442-2050

Bosman, F.T. & Stamenkovic, I. (2003) Funtional structure and composition of the extracellular matrix. *Journal of Pathology,* Vol. 200, No. 4, (July 2003), pp. 423-428, ISSN 0022-3417, EISSN 1600-0714

Brooks, P.C.; Silletti, S.; von Schalscha, T.L.; Friedlander, M. & Cheresh, D.A. (1998). Disruption of angiogenesis by PEX, a noncatalytic metalloproteinase fragment with integrin binding activity. *Cell,* Vol. 92, No.3, (February 1998), pp. 391-400, ISSN 0092-8674, EISSN 1097-4172

Broxmeyer, H.E.; Srour, E.; Orschell, C.; Ingram, D.A.; Cooper, S.; Plett, P.A.; Mead, L.E. & Yoder, M.C. (2006). Cord blood stem and progenitor cells, In: *Methods in Enzymology*, Edited by Irina Klimanskaya and Robert Lanza, Vol. 419, pp.439-473, Elsevier, ISBN 978-0-12-373650-5

Burg-Kurland, C.L.; Purmell, D.M.; Combs, J.W.; Hillman, E.A.; Harris, C.C. & Trump, B.F. (1989). Immunocytochemical evaluation of human esophageal neoplasms and preneoplastic lesions for beta-chorionic gonadotropin, placental lactogen, alpha-fetoprotein, carcinoembryonic antigen, and nonspecific cross-reacting antigen. *Cancer Research,* Vol. 46, No. 11 (November 1986), pp. 2936-2943, ISSN 0008-5472, EISSN 1538-7445

Clemons, N.J.; Shannon, N.B.; Abeyratne, L.R.; Walker, C.E.; Saadi, A.; O'Donovan, M.L.; Lao-Sirieix, P.P. & Fitzgerald, R.C. (2010). Nitric oxide-mediated invasion in Barrett's high-grade dysplasia and adenocarcinoma. *Carcinogenesis,* Vol. 31, No. 9, (September 2010), pp. 1669-1675, ISSN 0143-3334, EISSN 1460-2180

Croagh, D., Phillips, W.A.; Redvers, R.; Thomas, R.J. & Kaur, P. (2007). Identification of candidate murine esophageal stem cells using a combination of cell kinetic studies and cell surface markers. *Stem Cells,* Vol. 25, No. 2, (February 2007), pp. 313-318, EISSN 1549-4918

Croagh, D.; Thomas, R.J.; Phillips, W.A. & Kaur, P. (2008). Esophageal stem cells-a review of their identification and characterization. *Stem Cell Reviews*, Vol. 4, No. 4, (December 2008), pp. 261-268, ISSN 1550-8943

Dai, S.; Mao, C.; Jiang, L.; Wang, G. & Cheng H. (2009). P53 polymorphism and lung cancer susceptibility: a pooled analysis of 32 case-control studies. *Human Genetics,* Vol. 125, No, 5-6, (June 2009), pp. 633-638, ISSN 0340-6717, EISSN 1432-1203

D'Amico, T.A. & Harpole, D.H. Jr. (2000). Molecular biology of esophageal cancer. *Chest surgery clinics of North America,* Vol. 10, No. 3, (August 2000), pp. 451-469, ISSN 1052-3359

De Coppi, P.; Bartsch, G. Jr.; Siddiqui, M.M.; Xu, T.; Santos, C.C.; Perin, L.; Mostoslavsky, G.; Serre, A.C.; Snyder, E.Y.; Yoo, J.J.; Furth, M.E.; Soker, S. & Atala, A. (2007). Isolation of amniotic stem cell lines with potential for therapy. *Nature Biotechnology*, Vol. 25, No.1, (January 2007), pp. 100-106, ISSN1087-0156, EISSN 1546-1696

Dominici, M.; Le Blanc, K.; Mueller, I.; Slaper-Cortenbach, I.; Marini, F.; Krause, D.; Deans, R.; Keating, A.; Prockop, D. & Horwitz, E. (2006). Minimal criteria for defining multipotent mesenchymal stromal cells. The International Society for Cellular Therapy position statement. *Cytotherapy,* Vol. 8, No. 4, (August 2006), pp. 315-317, ISSN 1465-3249, EISSN 1477-2566

Dumont, P.; Leu, J.I.; Della Pietra, A.C. 3rd; George, D.L. & Murphy, M. (2003) The codon 72 polymorphic variants of p53 have markedly different apoptotic potential. *Nature Genetics,* Vol. 33, No. 3, (March 2003), pp. 357-365, ISSN 1061-4036, EISSN1546-1718

Dvorak, H.F. (1986). Tumors: wounds that do not heal. Similarities between tumor stroma generation and wound healing. *New England Journal of Medicine,* Vol. 315, No.26 (December 1986), pp.1650-1659, ISSN 0028-4793, EISSN1533-4406

Eng, C.; Spechler, S. J.; Ruben, R. & Li, F.P. (1993). Familial Barrett esophagus and adenocarcinoma of the gastroesophageal junction. *Cancer Epidemiology Biomarkers & Prevention,* Vol. 2, No. 4, (July-August 1993), pp. 397–399, ISSN 1055-9965, EISSN1538-7755

Epperly, M.W.; Shen, H.; Jefferson, M. & Greenberger, J.S. (2004). In vitro differentiation capacity of esophageal progenitor cells with capacity for homing and repopulation of the ionizing irradiation-damaged esophagus. *In Vivo,* Vol.18 No. 6, (November-December 2004), pp. 675-85, ISSN 0258-851X

Etoh, T.; Inoue, H.; Yoshikawa, Y.; Barnard, G.F.; Kitano, S. & Mori, M. (2000). Increased expression of collagenase-3 (MMP-13) and MT1-MMP in esophageal cancer is related to cancer aggressiveness. *Gut,* Vol. 47, No. 1, (July 2000), pp. 50-56, ISSN 0017-5749, EISSN 1468-3288

Fang, M.; Lew, E.; Klein, M.; Sebo, T.; Su, Y. & Goyal, R. (2004). DNA abnormalities as marker of risk for progression of Barrett's esophagus to adenocarcinoma: image cytometric DNA analysis in formalin-fixed tissues. *The American Journal of Gastroenterology,* Vol. 99, No. 10, (October 2004), pp. 1887-1894, ISSN 0002-9270, EISSN1572-0241

Ferrara, N. & Davis-Smyth, T. (1997). The biology of vascular endothelial growth factor. *Endocrine Reviews,* Vol. 18, No. 1, (February 1997), pp. 4-15, ISSN 0163-769X, EISSN1945-7189

Folkman, J. (1990). What is the evidence that tumours are angiogenesis dependent? *Journal of the National Cancer Institute,* Vol. 82, No. 1, (January 3, 1990), pp. 68-75, ISSN 0027-8874, EISSN1460-2105

Frederick, P.J.; Ramirez, P.T.; McQuinn, L.; Milam, M.R.; Weber, D.M.; Coleman, R.L.; Gershenson, D.M. & Landen, C.N. Jr. (2011). Preoperative factors predicting survival after secondary cytoreduction for recurrent ovarian cancer. *International Journal of Gynecological Cancer,* Vol. 21, No.5, (July 2011), pp. 831-836, EISSN 1525-1438

Fujiwara, Y.; Higuchi, K.; Hamaguchi, M.; Takashima, T.; Watanabe, T.; Tominaga, K.; Oshitani, N.; Matsumoto, T.& Arakawa, T. (2004). Increased expression of transforming growth factor-alpha and epidermal growth factor receptors in rat chronic reflux esophagitis. *Journal of Gastroenterology and Hepatology,* Vol. 19, No. 5, (May 2004), pp.521-527, ISSN 0815-9319, EISSN1440-1746

Gadzicki, D.; Müller-Vahl, K. & Stuhrmann, M. (1999). A Frequent polymorphism in the coding exon of the human cannabinoid receptor (CNR1) gen. *Molecular and Cellular Probes,* Vol. 13, No. 4, (August 1999), pp. 321-323, ISSN 0890-8508, EISSN1096-1194

Gillis, S.; Ferm, M.; Ou, W. & Smith, K.A. (1978). T cell growth factor: parameters of production and a quantitative microassay for activity. *The Journal of Immunology,* Vol. 120, No. 6, (June 1978), pp. 2017-2032, ISSN 0022-1767, EISSN1550-6606

Gold, P. & Freedman, S.D. (1965). Demonstration of tumor-specific antigens in human colonic carcinomata by immunological tolerance and absortion techniques. *The Journal of Experimental Medicine,* Vol. 121, No. 3, (March 1965), pp. 439-462, ISSN 0022-1007, EISSN1540-9538

Gomez, D.E.; Alonso, D.F.; Yoshiji, H. & Thorgeirsson, U.P. (1997). Tissue inhibitors of metalloproteinases: structure, regulation and biological function. *The European Journal of Cell Biology,* Vol. 74, No. 2 (October 1997), pp. 111-122, ISSN 0171-9335

Grimm, M.; Lazariotou M.; Kircher, S.; Stuermer, L.; Reiber, C.; Höfelmayr, A.; Gattenlöhner, S.; Otto, C.; Germer, C.T. & von Rahden, B.H.A. (2010). MMP-1 is a pre-invasive factor in Barrett- associated esophageal adenocarcinomas and is associated with positive lymph node status. *Journal of Translational Medicine,* Vol. 8, (October 2010), pp. 99, ISSN 1479-5876

Grotenhuis, B.A.; Dinjens, W.N.; Wijnhoven, B.P; Sonneveld, P.; Sacchetti, A.; Franken, P.F.; van Dekken, H.; Tilanus, H.W.; van Lanschot, J.J. & Fodde, R.(2010). Barrett's oesophageal adenocarcinoma encompasses tumour-initiating cells that do not express common cancer stem cell markers. *The Journal of Pathology,* Vol. 221, No. 4, (August 2010), pp. 379-389, ISSN 0022-3417, EISSN 1096-9896

Hall, B.; Dembinski, J.; Sasser, A.K.; Studeny, M.; Andreeff, M. & Marini, F. (2007). Mesenchymal stem cells in cancer: tumor-associated fibroblasts and cell-based delivery vehicles. *International Journal of Hematology,* Vol. 86, No. 1, (July 2007), pp. 8-16, ISSN 0925-5710, EISSN1865-3774

He, W.; Wang, Z.; Wang, Q.; Fan, Q.; Shou, C.; Wang, J.; Giercksky, K.E.; Nesland, J.M. & Suo, Z. (2009). Expression of HIWI in human esophageal squamous cell carcinoma is significantly associated with poorer prognosis. *BMC Cancer,* Vol. 9, No. (December 2009), pp. 426-436, ISSN 1471-2407

Hemberger, M.; Yang, W.; Natale, D.; Brown, T.L.; Dunk, C.; Gargett, C.E. & Tanaka, S. (2008). Stem cells from fetal membranes - a workshop report. *Placenta,* Vol. 29, Suppl. A, (March 2008), pp. S17-19, ISSN 0143-4004

Hormi-Carver, K. & Souza, R.F. (2009). Molecular markers and genetics in cancer development. *Surgical oncology clinics of North America,* Vol. 18, No. 3, (July 2009), pp. 453-467, ISSN 1055-3207, EISSN 1558-5042

Horwitz, E.M.; Le Blanc, K.; Dominici, M. I.; Mueller, I.; Slaper-Cortenbach, F.; Marini, C.; Deans, R.J.; Krause, D.S. & Keating, A. (2005). Clarification of the nomenclature for MSC: The International Society for Cellular Therapy position statement. *Cytotherapy,* Vol. 7, No. 5, (January 2005), pp. 393-395, ISSN 1465-3249, EISSN1477-2566

Hrstka, R.; Coates, P.J. & Vojtesek, B. (2009) Polymorphisms in p53 and the p53 pathway: roles in cancer susceptibility and response to treatment. *Journal of Cellular and Molecular Medicine, Vol.* 13, No. 3, (March 2009), pp. 440-453 ISSN 1582-1838, EISSN 1582-4934

Huang, D.; Gao, Q.; Guo, L.; Zhang, C.; Jiang, W.; Li, H.; Wang, J.; Han, X.; Shi, Y. & Lu, S.H. (2009). Isolation and identification of cancer stem-like cells in esophageal carcinoma cell lines. *Stem Cells and Development,* Vol. 18, No. 3, (April 2009), pp. 465-473, ISSN 1547-3287, EISSN 1557-8534

Igura, K.; Zhang, X.; Takahashi, K.; Mitsuru, A.; Yamaguchi, S. & Takashi, T.A. (2004). Isolation and characterization of mesenchymal progenitor cells from chorionic villi of human placenta. *Cytotherapy,* Vol. 6, No. 6, (January 2004), pp. 543-53, ISSN 1465-3249, EISSN1477-2566

Inada, S.; Koto, T.; Futami, K.; Arima, S. & Iwashita, A. (1999) Evaluation of malignancy and prognosis of esophageal cancer based on an immunohistochemical growth factor receptor. *Surgery Today,* Vol. 29 No. 6, (June 1999), pp. 493-503, ISSN 0941-1291, EISSN 1436-2813

Inoue, K.; Ozeki, Y.; Suganuma, Y.; Sugiura, Y. & Tanaka, S. (1997). Vascular endotelial growth factor expression in primary oesophageal squamous cell carcinoma: association with angiogenesis and tumor progression. *Cancer,* Vol. 79, No. 2, (January 1997), pp. 206-213. ISSN 0008-543X, EISSN1097-0142

Jiang, D.K.; Yao, L.; Wang, W.Z.; Peng, B.; Ren, W.H.; Yang, X.M. & Yu, L. (2010) TP53 Arg72Pro polymorphism and esophageal cancer. *World Journal of Gastroenterology,* Vol. 17, No. 9, (March 2010) pp. 1227-1233, ISSN 1007-9327

Kalabis, J.; Oyama, K.; Okawa, T.; Nakagawa, H.; Michaylira, C.Z.; Stairs, D.B.; Figueiredo, J.L.; Mahmood, U.; Diehl, J.A.; Herlyn, M. & Rustgi, A.K. (2008). A subpopulation of mouse esophageal basal cells has properties of stem cells with the capacity for self-renewal and lineage specification. *The Journal of Clinical Investigation,* Vol. 118, No. 12 (December 2008), pp. 3860-3869, ISSN 0036-5513, EISSN 1502-7686

Kidd, S.; Spaeth, E.; Dembinski, J.L.; Dietrich, M.; Watson, K.; Klopp, A.; Battula, V.L.; Weil, M.; Andreeff, M. & Marini, F.C. (2009). Direct evidence of mesenchymal stem cell tropism for tumor and wounding microenvironments using in vivo bioluminescent imaging. *Stem Cells,* Vol. 27, No. 10, (October 2009), pp. 2614-2623, EISSN 1549-4918

Kijima, H.; Oshiba, G.; Kenmochi, T.; Kise, Y.; Tanaka, H.; Chino, O.; Shimada, H.; Ueyama, Y. & Makuuchi, H. (2000). Stromal CEA activity is correlated with lymphatic invasion of esophageal carcinoma. *The International Journal of Oncology,* Vol. 16, No. 4, (April 2000), pp. 677-682, ISSN 1341-9625, EISSN1437-7772

Kilic, A.; Owens, S.R.; Pennathur, A.; Luketich, J.D.; Landreneau, R.J. & Schuchert, M.J. (2009). An increased proportion of inflammatory cells express tumor necrosis factor alpha in idiopathic achalasia of the esophagus. *Diseases of Esophagus,* Vol. 22, No. 5, (August 2009), pp. 382-385, ISSN 1120-8694, EISSN1442-2050

Kim, Y.H.; Ajani, J.A.; Ota, D.M.; Lynch, P. & Roth, J.A. (1995) Value of serial carcinoembryonic antigen levels in patients with resectable adenocarcinoma of esophagus and stomach. *Cancer,* Vol. 75, No. 2, (January 1995), pp. 451-456, ISSN 0008-543X, EISSN1097-0142

Kimura, S.; Kitadai, Y.; Tanaka, S.; Kuwai, T.; Hihara, J.; Yoshida, K.; Toge, T. & Chayama, K. (2004) Expression of hypoxia-inducible factor (HIF)-1a expression and tumour angiogenesis in human oesophageal squamous cell carcinoma. *The European Journal of Cancer,* Vol. 40, No. 12, (August 2004), pp. 1904-1912, ISSN 0959-8049, EISSN1879-0852

Kooreman, N.G. & Wu, J.C. (2010). Tumorigenicity of pluripotent stem cells: biological insights from molecular imaging. *Journal of the Royal Society Interface,* Vol. 7, Suppl. 6, (December 2010), pp. S753-763, ISSN 1742-5689, EISSN 1742-5662

Kosugi, S.; Nishimaki, T.; Kanda, T.; Nagawa, S.; Ohashi, M. & Hatakeyama, K. (2004) Clinical significance of serum CEA, carbohydrate antigen 19-9, and squamous cell carcinoma levels in esophageal cancer patients. *World Journal of Surgery,* Vol. 28, No. 7, (July 2004), pp. 680-685, ISSN0364-2313, EISSN1432-2323

Kuwano, H.; Kato, H.; Miyazaki, T.; Fukuchi, M.; Masuda, N.; Nakajima, M.; Fukai, Y.; Sohda, M.; Kimura, H. & Faried, A. (2005). Genetic alterations in esophageal cancer. *Surgery Today,* Vol. 35, No. 1 (January 2005), pp. 7-18, ISSN0941-1291, EISSN 1436-2813

Lao-Sirieix, P.; Lovat, L. & Fitzgerald, R.C. (2007). Cyclin A immunocytology as a risk stratification tool for Barrett's esophagus: association with increased risk of adenocarcinoma. *Clinical Cancer Research,* Vol. 13, No. 2 Pt 1, (January 2007), pp. 659-665, ISSN 0008-5472, EISSN1538-7445

Lehrbach, D.M.; Cecconello, I.; Ribeiro, Jr. U.; Capelozzi, V.L.; Ab'saber, A.M. & Alves, V.A. (2009). Adenocarcinoma of the esophagastric junction: relationship between clinicopathological data and p53, cyclin D1 and Bcl-2 immunoexpressions. *Arquivos de Gastroenterologia,* Vol. 46, No. 4, (October-December 2009), pp. 315-320, ISSN 0004-2803, EISSN1678-4219

Levine, A.J.; Momand, J. & Finlay, C.A. (1991). The p53 tumor suppressor gene. *Nature,* Vol. 351, No. 6326, (June 1991), pp. 453-456, ISSN 0028-0836, EISSN1476-4687

Levine, A.J.; Finlay, C.A. & Hinds, P.W. (2004) P53 is a tumor suppressor gene. *Cell,* Vol. 116, No. 2 Supplement, (January 2004), pp. S67-S69, ISSN 0092-8674, EISSN1097-4172

Li, Z.; Shimada, Y.; Uchida, S.; Maeda, M.; Kawabw, A.; Mori, A.; Kano, M.; Watanabe, G & Immamura, M. (2000). TGF-alpha as well as VEGF, PD-ECGF and b FGF contribute to angiogenesis of esophageal squamous carcinoma. *The International Journal of Oncology,* Vol. 17, No. 3, (September 2000), pp. 453-460, ISSN 1341-9625, EISSN1437-7772

Liu, Z.J.; Zhuge, Y. & Velazquez, O.C. (2009). Trafficking and differentiation of mesenchymal stem cells. *Journal of Cellular Biochemistry,* Vol. 106, No. 6, (April 2009), pp. 984-991, ISSN 0730-2312, EISSN 1097-4644

Liu, X.; Cheng, Y.; Sheng, W.; Lu, H.; Xu, Y.; Long, Z.; Zhu, H. & Wang, Y. (2010). Clinicopathologic features and prognostic factors in alpha-fetoprotein-producing gastric cancers: analysis of 104 cases. *Journal of Surgical Oncology,* Vol. 102, No. 3, (September 2010), pp. 249-255, ISSN 0022-4790, EISSN1096-9098

Liu M, Wang Z, Yang S, Zhang W, He S, Hu C, Zhu H, Quan L, Bai J, Xu N. (2011). TNF-α is a novel target of miR-19a. *The International Journal of Oncology,* Vol. 38, No. 4, (April 2011), pp. 1013-1022, ISSN 1341-9625, EISSN1437-7772

Lord, R.V.; O'Grady, R.; Sheehan, C.; Field, A.F. & Ward, R.L. (2000). K-ras codon 12 mutations in Barrett's oesophagus and adenocarcinomas of the oesophagus and oesophagogastric junction. *Journal of Gastroenterology and Hepatology,* Vol. 15, No. 7, (July 2000), pp. 730-736, ISSN 0815-9319, EISSN1440-1746

Lynch, T.J.; Bell, D.W.; Sordella, R.; Gurubhagavatula, S. & Okimoto, R.A. (2004) Activating mutations in the epidermal growth factor receptor underlying responsiveness of non-small-cell lung cancer of gefitinib. *The New England Journal of Medicine,* Vol. 350, No. 21, (May 2004), pp. 2129-2139, ISSN 0028-4793, EISSN1533-4406

Macias, M.I.; Grande, J.; Moreno, A.; Dominguez, I.; Bornstein, R. & Flores, A.I. (2010). Isolation and characterization of true mesenchymal stem cells derived from human term decidua capable of multilineage differentiation into all 3 embryonic layers. *American Journal of Obstetrics and Gynecology,* Vol. 203, No.5, (November 2010), pp. 495.e9-495.e23, ISSN 0002-9378, EISSN1097-6868

McKnight, A.; Marnell, A. & Shperling, J. (1989). The role of carbohydrate antigen 19-9 as a tumour marker of oesophagus cancer, *British Journal of Cancer,* Vol. 60, No. 2, (August 1989), pp. 249-251, ISSN 0007-0920, EISSN1532-1827

Matlashewski, G.J.; Tuck, S.; Pim, D.; Lamb, P.; Schneider, J. & Crawford, L.V. (1987). Primary structure polymorphism at amino acid residue 72 of human p53. *Molecular and Cell Biology,* Vol. 7, No. 2, (February 1987), pp. 961-963, ISSN 0270-7306, EISSN1098-5549

Maurel, J.; Nadal, C.; Garcia-Albeniz, X.; Gallego, R.; Carcereny, E.; Almendro, V.; Mármol, M.; Gallardo, E.; Maria Augé, J.; Longarón, R.; Martínez-Fernandez, A.; Molina, R., Castells, A. & Gascón, P. (2007). Serum matrix metalloproteinase 7 levels identifies poor prognosis advanced colorectal cancer patients. *International Journal of Cancer,* Vol. 121, No. 5, (September 2007), pp. 1066-1071, ISSN 0020-7136, EISSN 1097-0215

Miki, T.; Lehmann, T.; Cai, H.; Stolz, D.B. & Strom, S.C. (2005). Stem cell characteristics of amniotic epithelial cells. *Stem Cells,* Vol. 23, No. 10, (November-December 2005), pp. 1549-1559, ISSN 1066-5099, EISSN 1549-4918

Mimori, K.; Mori, M.; Shiraishi, T.; Fujie, T.; Baba, K.; Haraguchi, M.; Abe, R.; Ueo, H. & Akiyoshi T. (1997). Clinical significance of tissue inhibitor of metalloproteinase expression in gastric carcinoma. *The British Journal of Cancer,* Vol. 76, No. 4, (August 1997), pp. 531-536, ISSN 0007-0920, EISSN 1532-1827

Minu, A.R.; Endo, M. & Sunagawa, M. (1994). Role of DNA ploidy patterns in esophageal squamous cell carcinoma. An ultraviolet microspectro-photometric study. *Cancer,* Vol. 74, No. 2, (July 1994), pp. 578-585, ISSN 0008-543X, EISSN1097-0142

Mizejewski, G.J. (2002). Biological role of alpha-fetoprotein in cancer: prospects for cancer therapy. *Expert Review of Anticancer Therapy,* Vol. 2, No. 6, (December 2002), pp. 709-735, ISSN 1473-7140

Montesano, R.; Hollstein, M, & Hainaut, P. (1996) Genetic alterations in esophageal cancer and their relevance to etiology and pathogenesis: a review. *International Journal of Cancer,* Vol. 69, No. 3, (June 1996), pp. 225-235. ISSN 0020-7136, EISSN1097-0215

Morales-Gutíerrez, C.; Vegh, I.; Colina, F.; Gomez-Cámara, A.; Landa, J.I.; Carreira, P.E. & Enríquez de Salamanca, R. (1999). Survival of patients with colorectal carcinoma: possible prognostic value of tissular carbohydrate antigen 19.9. *Cancer,* Vol. 86, No. 9, (November 1999), pp. 1675-1681. ISSN 0008-543X, EISSN 1097-0142

Mori, R.; Ishiguro, H.; Kimura, M.; Mitsui, A.; Sasaki, H.; Tomoda, K.; Mori, Y.; Ogawa, R.; Katada, T.; Kawano, O.; Harada, K.; Fujii, Y. & Kuwabara, Y. (2008). PIK3CA mutation status in Japanese esophageal squamous cell carcinoma. *Journal of Surgical Reseach,* Vol. 145, No. 2, (April 2008), pp. 320-326, ISSN 0022-4804

Motoyama, S.; Miura, M.; Hinai, Y.; Maruyama, K.; Usami, S.; Yoshino, K.; Nakatsu, T.; Saito, H.; Minamuya, Y. & Ogawa, J.I. (2011). Interleukin-2-330T>G genetic polymorphism associates with prognosis following surgery for thoracic esophageal squamous call cancer. *The Annals of Surgical Oncology,* Vol. 18, No. 7, (July 2011), pp. 1995-2002, ISSN 1068-9265, EISSN 1534-4681

Murray, G.I.; Duncan, M.E.; O'Neil, P.; McKay, J.A.; Melvin, W.T. & Fothergill, J.E. (1998). Matrix metalloproteinase-1 is associated with poor prognosis in oesophageal cancer. *The Journal of Pathology,* Vol. 185, No. 3, (July 1998), pp. 256-61, EISSN 1096-9896

Nakamizo, A.; Marini, F.; Amano, T.; Khan, A.; Studeny, M.; Gumin, J.; Chen, J.; Hentschel, S.; G. Vecil, J. Dembinski, M. Andreeff, and F.F. Lang. (2005). Human bone marrow-derived mesenchymal stem cells in the treatment of gliomas. *Cancer Research,* Vol. 65, No. 8, (April 2005), pp. 3307-3318. ISSN 0008-5472, EISSN 1538-7445

Nguyen, G.H.; Murph, M.M. & Chang, J.Y. (2011). Cancer Stem Cell Radioresistance and Enrichment: Where Frontline Radiation Therapy May Fail in Lung and Esophageal Cancers. *Cancers (Basel),* Vol. 3, No. 1, (March 2011), pp. 1232-1252, ISSN 2072-6694

Nordenstedt, H, & El-Srag, H. (2011). The influence of age, sex and race on the incidence of esophageal cancer in the United States (1992-2006) *Scandinavian Journal of Gastroenterology,* Vol. 46, No. 5, (May 2011), pp. 597-602, ISSN 0036-5521, EISSN 1502-7708

Nowell, P.C. (1976). The clonal evolution of tumor cell populations. *Science,* Vol. 194, No. 4260, (October 1976), pp. 23-28, ISSN 0036-8075, EISSN 1095-9203

Ohashi, S.; Natsuizaka, M.; Wong, G.S.; Michaylira, C.Z.; Grugan, K.D.; Stairs, D,B.; Kalabis, J.; Vega, M.E.; Kalman, R.A.; Nakagawa, M.; Klein-Szanto, A.J., Herlyn, M.; Diehl, A.; Rustgi, A.K. & Nakagawa, H. (2010). Epidermal growth factor and mutant p53 expand a esophageal subpopulation capable of epithelial-to mesenchymal transition through ZEB transcription factors. *Cancer Research,* Vol. 70, No. 10, (May 2010), pp. 4174-4184, ISSN 0008-5472, EISSN1538-7445

Okumura, T.; Shimada Y.; Imamura M. & Yasumoto S. (2003). Neurotrophin receptor p75(NTR) characterizes human esophageal keratinocyte stem cells in vitro. *Oncogene,* Vol. 22, No. 26, (June 2003), pp. 4017-4026, ISSN 0950-9232, EISSN1476-5594

Okumura, T.; Tsunoda S.; Mori Y.; Ito T.; Kikuchi K.; Wang T.C.; Yasumoto S.& Shimada Y. (2006). The biological role of the low-affinity p75 neurotrophin receptor in esophageal squamous cell carcinoma. *Clinical Cancer Research,* Vol. 12, No. 17, (September 2006), pp. 5096-5103, ISSN 1078-0432, EISSN1557-3265

Oshiba, G; Kijima, J.A.; Ota, D.M.; Lynch, P. & Roth, J.A. (2000). Frequent expression of sialkyl Lewis (a) in human squamous cell carcinoma. *The International Journal of*

Oncology, Vol. 17, No. 4, (October 2000), pp. 701-705, ISSN 1341-9625, EISSN 1437-7772

Pappa, K.I. & Anagnou, N.P. (2009). Novel sources of fetal stem cells: where do they fit on the developmental continuum? *Regenerative Medicine,* Vol. 4, No. 3, (May 2009), pp. 423-433, ISSN 1746-0751, EISSN1746-076X

Parolini, O.; Alviano, F.G.P.; Bagnara, G.; Bilic, H.J.; Buhring, M.; Evangelista, S.; Hennerbichler, B.; Liu, M.; Magatti, N.; Mao, T.; Miki, F.; Marongiu, H.; Nakajima, T.; Nikaido, C.B.; Portmann-Lanz, V.; Sankar, M.; Soncini, G.; Stadler, D.; Surbek, T.A.; Takahashi, H.; Redl, N.; Sakuragawa, S.; Wolbank, S.; Zeisberger, S.; Zisch, A. & Strom, S.C. (2008). Concise review: isolation and characterization of cells from human term placenta: outcome of the first international Workshop on Placenta Derived Stem Cells. *Stem Cells,* Vol. 26, No. 2, (February 2008), pp. 300-311, ISSN 1066-5099, EISSN 1549-4918

Pertwee, R.G. (1997). Pharmacology of cannabinoid CB1 and CB2 receptors. *Pharmacology & Therapeutics,* Vol. 74, No. 2, pp. 129-180, ISSN 0163-7258

Quante, M. & Wang, T.C. (2009). Stem cells in gastroenterology and hepatology. *Nature Reviews Gastroenterology & Hepatology,* Vol. 6, No. 12, (December 2009), pp. 724-737, ISSN 1759-5045

Rees, J.R.E.; Onwuegbusi, B.A.; Save, V.E.; Alderson, D. & Fitzgerald R.C. (2006). In vivo and in vitro evidence for transforming growth factor- β1-mediated epithelial to masenchymal transition in esophageal adenocarcinoma. *Cancer Research,* Vol. 66, No. 19, (October 2006), pp. 9583-9590, ISSN 0008-5472, EISSN1538-7445

Romero, Y.; Cameron, A. J.; Locke, G. R.; III, Schaid, D. J.; Slezak, J. M.; Branch, C. D. & Melton, L.J. (1997). Familial aggregation of gastroesophageal reflux in patients with Barrett's esophagus and esophageal adenocarcinoma. *Gastroenterology,* Vol. 113, No. 5, (November 1997), pp. 1449–1456, ISSN 0016-5085, EISSN1528-0012

Saadi, A.; Shanon, N.B.; Lao-Sirieix, P.; O'Donovan, M.; Walker, E.; Clemons, N.J.; Hardwick, J.S.; Zhang, C.; Das, M.; Save, V.; Novelli, M.; Balkwill, F. & Fitzgerald, R.C. (2010). Stromal genes discriminate pre-invasive from invasive disease, predict outcome and highlight inflammatory pathways in digestive cancers. *Proceedings of the National Academy of Sciences USA,* Vol. 107, No. 5, (February 2010), pp. 2177-2182, ISSN 0027-8424, EISSN1091-6490

Sanders, D.S.; Wilson, C.A.; Bryant, F.J.; Hopkins, J.; Johnson, G.D.; Milne, D.M. & Kerr, M.A. (1994). Classification and localization of carcinoembryonic antigen (CEA) related antigen expression in normal esophageal squamous mucosa and squamous carcinoma. *Gut,* Vol. 35, No. 8, (August 1994), pp. 1022-1025, ISSN 0017-5749, EISSN 1468-3288

Sarosi, G.; Brown, G.; Jaiswal, K.; Feagins, L.A.; Lee, E.; Crook, T.W.; Souza, R.F.; Zou, Y.S.; Shay J.W. & Spechler, S.J. (2008). Bone marrow progenitor cells contribute to esophageal regeneration and metaplasia in a rat model of Barrett's esophagus. *Diseases of Esophagus,* Vol. 21, No. 1, (February 2008), pp. 43-50, ISSN 1120-8694, EISSN1442-2050

Sarosiek, J. & McCallium, R.W. (2000). Mechanism of oesophageal mucosa defence. *Bailliere's Best Practice & Research Clinical Gastroenterology,* Vol. 14, No. 5, (October 2000), pp. 701-717, ISSN 1521-6918

Sarugaser, R.; Lickorish, D.; Baksh, D.; Hosseini, M.M. & Davies J.E. (2005). Human umbilical cord perivascular (HUCPV) cells: a source of mesenchymal progenitors. *Stem Cells,* Vol. 23, No. 2, (February 2005), pp. 220-229, ISSN 1066-5099, EISSN 1549-4918

Seery, J.P. & Watt, F.M. (2000). Asymmetric stem-cell divisions define the architecture of human oesophageal epithelium. *Current Biology,* Vol. 10, No. 22, (November 2000), pp. 1447-1450, ISSN 0960-9822, EISSN1879-0445

Shao, L.; Hottelman, W.N.; Lin, J.; Yang, H.; Ajani, J.A. & Wu, X. (2006). Deficiency of cell cycle checkpoints and ADN repair system predispose individuals to esophageal cancer. *Mutation Research,* Vol. 602, No. 1-2, (December 2006), pp. 143-150, ISSN 1383-5718

Shimada, H.; Hoshino, T.; Okazumi, S.; Matsubara, H.; Funami, Y.; Nabeya, Y.; Hayashi, H.; Takeda, A.; Shiratori, T.; Uno, T.; Ito, H. & Ochiai, T. (2002). Expression of angiogenic factors predicts response to chemoradiotherapy and prognosis of oesophageal squamous cell carcinoma. *British Journal of Cancer,* Vol. 86, No. 4, (February 2002), pp. 552-557, ISSN 0007-0920, EISSN 1532-1827

Shimada, H.; Nabeya, Y.; Okazumi, S.; Matsubara, H.; Shiratori, T.; Gunji, Y.; Kobayashi, H.; Hayashi, H & Ochiai, T. (2003). Prediction of survival with squamous cell carcinoma antigen in patients with resectable esophageal squamous cell carcinoma. *Surgery,* Vol. 133, No. 5, (May 2003), pp. 486-494, EISSN 1471-2482

Sobin, L.H. & Fleming, I.D. TNM Classification of Malignant Tumors, fifth edition (1997). Union Internationale Contre le Cancer and the American Joint Committee on Cancer. *Cancer,* Vol. 80, No. 9, (November 1997), pp. 1803-1804, ISSN 0008-543X, EISSN 1097-0142

Soncini, M.; Vertua, E.; Gibelli, L.; Zorzi, F.; Denegri, M.; Albertini, A.; Wengler, G.S. & Parolini, O. (2007). Isolation and characterization of mesenchymal cells from human fetal membranes. *Journal of Tissue Engineering and Regenerative Medicine,* Vol. 1. No. 4, (July-August 2007), pp. 296-305, ISSN 1932-6254, EISSN 1932-7005

Souza, R.F.; Krishnan, K. & Spechler, S.J. (2008). Acid bile, and CDX: the ABCs of making Barrett's metaplasia. *American Journal Physiology of Gastrointestinal and Liver Physiology,* Vol. 295, No. 2, (August 2008), pp. G211-G218, ISSN 0193-1857, EISSN 1522-1547

Souza, R.F. (2010) The molecular basis of carcinogenesis in Barrett's esophagus. *Journal of Gastrointestinal Surgery,* Vol. 14, No. 6, (June 2010), pp. 937-940, EISSN 1873-4626

Studeny, M.; Marini, F.C.; Dembinski, J.L.; Zompetta, C.; Cabreira-Hansen, M.; Bekele, B.N.; Champlin, R.E. & Andreeff, M. (2004). Mesenchymal stem cells: potential precursors for tumor stroma and targeted-delivery vehicles for anticancer agents. *The Journal of the National Cancer Institute,* Vol. 96, No. 21, (November 2004) pp. 1593-603, ISSN 0027-8874, EISSN 1460-2105

Suchi, K.; Fujuwara, H.; Okamura, H.; Umehara, S.; Todo, M.; Furutani, A.; Yoneda, M.; Shiozaki, A.; Kubota, T.; Ichikawa, D.; Okamoto, K. & Otsuji, E. (2011). Overexpression of interleukin-6 suppresses cisplatin-induced cytotoxicity in esophageal squamous cell carcinoma cells. *Anticancer Research,* Vol. 31, No. 1, (January 2011), pp. 67-75, ISSN 0250-7005, EISSN 1791-7530.

Sun, Z.G.; Huang, S.D.; Zhang, B.R.; Xu, Z.Y.; Liu, X.H.; Gong, D.J. & Yuan, Y. (2009). [Isolation and identification of cancer stem cells from human esophageal carcinoma]. *Zhonghua Yi Xue Za Zhi,* Vol. 89, No. 5, (February 2009), pp. 291-295, ISSN 03762491

Szarvas, T.; Becker, M.; von Dorp, F.; Gethmann, C.; Tötsch, M.; Bánkfalvi, A.; Schmid, K.W.; Romics, I.; Rübben, H. & Ergün, S. (2010). Matrix metalloproteinase-7 as a marker of metastasis and predictor of poor survival in bladder cancer. *Cancer Science,* Vol. 101, No. 5, (May 2010), pp- 1300-1308, ISSN 1347-9032, EISSN 1349-7006

Takayama, N.; Arima, S.; Haraoka, S.; Kotho, T.; Futami, K. & Iwashita, A. (2003). Relationship between the expression of adhesion molecules in primary esophageal squamous cell carcinoma and metastatic lymph nodes. *Anticancer Research,* Vol. 23, No. 6a, (November- December 2003), pp. 4435-4442, ISSN0250-7005, EISSN 1791-7530

Tallone, T.; Realini, C.; Bohmler, A.; Kornfeld, C.; Vassalli, G.; Moccetti, T.; Bardelli, S. & Soldati, G. (2011). Adult human adipose tissue contains several types of multipotent cells. *Journal of Cardiovascular Translational Research,* Vol. 4, No. 2, (April 2011), pp. 200-210, ISSN 1937-5387, EISSN 1937-5395

Tanaka, T.; Ishiguro, H.; Kuwabara, Y.; Kimura, M.; Mitsui, A.; Katada, T.; Shiozaki, M.; Naganawa, Y.; Fujii, T. & Takeyama, H. (2010). Vascular endothelial growth factor C (VEGF-C) in esophageal cancer correlates with lymph node metastasis and poor patient prognosis. *Journal of Experimental & Clinical Cancer Research,* Vol. 29, (June 2010), pp. 83, ISSN 1756- 9966

Tselepis, C.; Perry, I.; Dawson, C.; Hardy, R.; Darnton, S.J.; McConkey, C.; Stuart, R.C.; Wright, N.; Harrison, R. & Jankowski, J.A. (2002). Tumor necrosis factor-alpha in Barrett's oesophagus: a potential novel mechanism of action. *Oncogene,* Vol. 21, No. 39, (September 2002), pp. 6071-6081, ISSN 0950-9232, EISSN 1476-5594

Thiery, J.P. (2002). Epithermal-mesenchymal transition in tumor progression. *Nature Reviews Cancer,* Vol. 2, No. 6, (June 2002), pp. 442-454, ISSN 1474-175X, EISSN 1474-1768

Thomas, M.; Kalita, A.; Labrecque, S.; Pim, D.; Banks, L. & Matlashewski, G. (1999) Two polymorphic variants of wild-type p53 differ biochemically and biologically. *Molecular and Cellular Biology,* Vol. 19, No. 2, (February 1999), pp. 1092-1100, ISSN 0270-7306, EISSN 1098-5549

Thompson, S.K.; Sullivan, T.R.; Davies, R. & Ruszkiewicz, A.R. (2011). Her-2/neu gene amplification in esophageal adenocarcinoma and its influence on survival. *The Annals of Surgical Oncology,* Vol. 18, No. 7, (July 2011), pp. 2010-2017, ISSN 1068-9265 and EISSN 1543-4681

Torzewski, M.; Sarbia, M.; Verreet, P.; Bittinger, F.; Dutkowski, P.; Heep, H.; Willers, R. & Gabbert, H.E. (1997). The prognostic significance of epidermal growth factor receptor in squamous cell carcinomas of the esophagus. *Anticancer Research,* Vol. 17, No. 5B, (September-October 1997), pp. 3915-3919, ISSN 0250-7005, EISSN 1791-7530

Vegh, I.; Sotelo, T.; Estenoz, J.; Fontanellas, A.; Navarro, S.; Millán, I. & Enriquez de Salamanca, R. (2002). Tumor cytosol carcinoembryonic antigen as prognostic parameter in non-small-lung cancer. *Tumori,* Vol. 88, No. 2, (March-April 2002), pp. 142-146, ISSN 0300-8916

Vegh, I.; De La Cruz, J.; Navarro, S.; Morales, C.; Colina, F.; Abad, A.; De La Calle, A.; Enríquez de Salamanca, R.; Moreno-González, E. (2003). Colorectal cancer relapse: allelic alterations associated with tumour marker over-expression. *Oncology,* Vol. 65, No. 2, (August 2003), pp. 146-152, ISSN 0030-2414, EISSN 1423-0232

Vegh, I.; De-La-Calle Santiuste, A.; Colina, F.; Bor, L.; Bermejo, C.; Aragón, A.; Morán-Jimenez, M.J., Gomez-Cámara, A.; Enríquez de Salamanca, R. & Moreno-González, E. (2007). Relationship between biomarker expression and allelic alteration in esophageal carcinoma. *Journal of Gastroenterology and Hepatology,* Vol. 22, No. 12, (December 2007), pp. 2303-2309, ISSN 0815-9319, EISSN 1440-1746

von Rahden, B.H.; Kircher, S.; Lazariotou, M.; Reiber, C.; Stuermer, L.; Otto, C.; Germer, C.T. & Grimm, M. (2011). LgR5 expression and cancer stem cell hypothesis: clue to define the true origin of esophageal adenocarcinomas with and without Barrett's esophagus? *Journal of Experimental & Clinical Cancer Research,* Vol. 30, (February 2011), p. 23, ISSN 1756-9966

Waldman, T.; Kinzler, K.W. & Volgelstein, B. (1995) p21 is necessary for the p53-mediated G1 arrest in human cancer cells. *Cancer Research,* Vol. 55, No. 22, (November 1995), pp. 5187-5190, ISSN 1538-7445, EISSN 0008-5472

Wang Q, He W, Lu C, Wang Z, Wang J, Giercksky KE, Nesland JM, Suo Z. (2009). Oct3/4 and Sox2 are significantly associated with an unfavorable clinical outcome in human esophageal squamous cell carcinoma. *Anticancer Research,* Vol. 29, No. 4, (April 2009), pp. 1233-1241, ISSN 0250-7005, EISSN 1791-7530

Whibley, C.; Pahroah, P.D. & Hollstein, M. (2009). P53 polymorphisms: cancer implications. *Nature Reviews Cancer,* Vol. 9, No. 2, (February 2009), pp. 95-107, ISSN 1474-175X, EISSN1474-1768

Wu, T.T.; Watanabe, T.; Heimiller, R.; Zahurak, M.; Forastiere, A.A. & Hamilton, S.R. (1998). Genetic alterations in Barrett esophagus and adenocarcinoma of the esophagus and esophagogastric junction region. *The American Journal of Pathology,* Vol. 153, No. 1, (July 1998), pp. 287-294, ISSN 002-9440

Xin, Z.; Wenyu, F. & Shenhua, X. (2010). Clinicopathologic significance of cytokine levels in esophageal squamous cell carcinoma. *Hepatogastroenterology,* Vol. 57, No. 104, (November- December 2010), pp. 1416-1422, ISSN 0172-6390

Yamamoto, H.; Adachi, Y.; Itoh, F.; Iku, S.; Kusano, K.; Arimura, Y.; Endo, T.; Hinoda, Y.; Hosokawa, M. & Imai, K. (1999). Association of matrilysin expression with recurrence and poor prognosis in human esophageal squamous cell carcinoma. *Cancer Research,* Vol. 59, No. 14, (July 1999), pp. 3313-3316, ISSN 1538-7445 EISSN 0008-5472

Yamashita, K.; Mori, M.; Shiraishi, T.; Shibuta, K. & Sugimachi, K. (2000). Clinical significance of matrix metalloproteinase-7 expression in esophageal carcinoma. *Clinical Cancer Research,* Vol. 6, No. 3, (March 2000), pp. 1169-1174, ISSN 1557-3265, EISSN 1078 0432

Yamashita, K.; Mori, M.; Kataoka, A.; Inoue, H. & Sugimachi, K. (2001). The clinical significance of MMP-1 in oesophageal cancinoma. *British Journal of Cancer,* Vol. 84, No. 2, (January 2001), pp. 276-282, ISSN 0007-0920, EISSN 1532-1827

Yoshizuki, T.; Maruyama, Y.; Sato, H. & Furukawa, M. (2001). Expression of tissue inhibitor of matrix metalloproteinase-2 and predicts poor prognosis in the tongue squamous cell carcinoma. *International Journal of Cancer,* Vol. 95, No. 1, (January 2001), pp. 44-50, ISSN 1097-0215

Yu, C.; Zhang, X.; Huang, Q.; Klein, M. & Goyal, R.K. (2007). High-fidelity DNA histograms in neoplastic progression in Barrett's esophagus. *Laboratory Investigation,* Vol. 87, No. 5, (May 2007), pp. 466-472, ISSN 0023-6837 and EISSN 1530-0307

Zhang, X.; Cheung, R.M.; Komaki, R.; Fang, B. & Chang, J.Y. (2005). Radiotherapy sensitization by tumor-specific TRAIL gene targeting improves survival of mice bearing human non-small cell lung cancer. *Clinical Cancer Research,* Vol. 11, No. 18, (September 2005), pp. 6657-6668, ISSN 1557-3265, EISSN 1078-0432

Zhang, H.Y.; Zhang, Q.; Zhang, X.; Yu, C.; Huo, X.; Cheng, E.; Wang, D.H.; Spechler, S.J. & Souza, R.F. (2011). Cancer- Related inflammation and Barrett's carcinogenesis: interleukin-6 and Stat3 mediate apoptotic resistance in transformed Barrett's cells. *American Journal Physiology of Gastrointestinal and Liver Physiology,* Vol. 300, No. 3, (March 2011), pp. G454-G460, ISSN 0193-1857, EISSN 1522-1547

Zhang, Z.; Wang, M.; Wu, D.; Wang, M.; Tong, N.; Tian, Y. & Zhang, Z. (2011). P53 codon 72 polymorphism contributes to breast cancer. *World Journal of Gastroenterology,* Vol. 120, No. 2, (April 2010), pp. 509-517, ISSN 1007-9327

Zhou, Y.; Li, N.; Zhuang, W.; Liu, G.J.; Wu, T.X.; Yao, X.; Du, L.; Wei, M.L. & Wu, X.T. (2007). P53 codon 72 polymorphism and gastric cancer: a meta-analysis of the literature. *International Journal of Cancer,* Vol. 121, No. 7, (October 2007), pp. 1481-1486, ISSN 0020-7136, EISSN 1097-0215

Zhou, J.H.; Zhang, B.; Kmstine, K.H. & Zhong, L.O. (2011). Autoantibodies against MMP-7 as a novel diagnostic biomarker in esophageal squamous cell carcinoma. *World Journal of Gastroenterology,* Vol. 17, No. 10, (March 2011), pp. 1373-1378, ISSN 1007-9327

Zhou, X., G.R. Huang, and P. Hu. (2011). Over-expression of Oct4 in human esophageal squamous cell carcinoma. *Molecules and Cells,* [Epub ahead of print] May 2011, ISSN 1016-8478, EISSN 0219-1032

4

Proteomics and Esophageal Cancer

Mehdi Moghanibashi[1,2], Maryam Zare[1,3] and Ferdous Rastgar Jazii[1]
[1]*Department of Biochemistry, National Institute of Genetic Engineering and Biotechnology (NIGEB), Tehran,*
[2]*Islamic Azad University, Kazerun Branch, School of Medicine, Kazerun, Shiraz,*
[3]*Department of Biology, Payam-Noor University, Tehran,*
[4]*Department of Molecular Structure and Function, Research Institute, Hospital for Sick Children (Sickkids), Toronto, ON,*
[1,2,3]*Iran*
[4]*Canada*

1. Introduction

Following to completion of human genome project and accomplishment of the entire human genome sequence, it rose hopes that cure to many diseases would soon come true. This encouraged focusing efforts on the effect of gene expression and the mechanisms by which it could affect medicine, among which cancer. However, searches for the genes within genome (genome: the entire genes of an organism) whose alteration could be the cause of cancer has also been subject of hamper and complications by different mechanisms that genes might be transcribed (transcriptome: the entire transcripts of an organism or organelles within a specific condition) and subsequently into a variety of functional or structural unite known as proteins which can by themselves undergo essential changes [1]. As a powerful approach proteomics entails analysis of gene expression at protein (translation) and protein related levels such as posttranslational modifications, which complement the nucleic acid based level of gene expression. Protein based gene expression analysis is done by analyzing the 'proteome'; the entire protein expressed by a genome in cells, their sub-cellular structures such as organelles and tissues at a given time and specific condition. As a result, proteome is subject of change with time and condition of the being although it is direct product of a genome [2].

The definition of proteomics has changed greatly over the time. While currently it denotes any type of technology that focuses analysis of proteins constituent ranging from a single protein to thousands in one experiment, however it was originally attributed to the large scale protein analysis, high- throughput separation, and subsequent identification of proteins resolved by 2-dimensional polyacrylamide gel electrophoresis (2DE). 2DE is still the method of choice for protein separation and identification [2]. In subsequent sections, we provided a brief description of 2DE, proteomics, and its application in cancer research, the proteins and molecular markers, which were identified in esophageal cancer using this methodology.

2. Two Dimensional Electrophoresis (2DE) and protein identification

The first successful two-dimensional electrophoresis dates to the early 1970s by coupling denaturing IEF (isoelectric focusing) with the SDS-PAGE. Due to awkward process of 2DE, it was relatively unpublicized in its early advent; however, the story has substantially reversed several years later when the astonishing paper that revolutionized application of 2DE was published by O'Farrell [3]. By developing technical aspects of 2DE, O'Farrell was able to resolve hundreds of polypeptides in a single gel and in the same experiment. Since then, analysis of complex protein entities by 2DE has significantly improved, as in the late 1980s, 2DE has reached to a fully developed technique [4]. Though there is always space for development, 2DE still is subject of ongoing advancements along with seeking alternative methods for combining or replacing 2DE in order to achieve higher protein resolution. Nevertheless, the main argument that has put forth application of 2DE is that at present other methods are no more powerful as 2DE is or are hard enough to handle protein complement of the entire genome.

2DE is composed of proteins or polypeptides separation in two orthogonally (right angle) dimension techniques such that in one dimension separation is done based on isoelectric pH point (pI) of protein (or polypeptides) by a process which is called isoelectric focusing (IEF) and the second dimension based on their molecular weight. As a result of IEF proteins are separated based on their charge. Subsequent to IEF, proteins are further resolved or separated in the second dimension based on their molecular weight using sodium dodecyl sulfate polyacrylamide gel electrophoresis (SDS-PAGE).

From its early advent a requirement for 2DE was separation and comparison of complex protein mixtures with high resolution and reproducibility. The development of immobilized pH gradients (IPGs) on strips for IEF has fundamentally improved and solved this requirement, allowing intra- and inter-laboratory comparison of the separated protein profiles possible. The separated proteins can be detected by staining with dyes or metal ions. Silver staining is the most commonly used method for detection of proteins. The method is 100 folds more sensitive than other dye based staining methods such as Coomassie blue, however radiolabeling is still the most sensitive method, which can be used for autoradiography or fluorography of proteins (figure1).

Following to separation of proteins it is required to identify them in downstream process. While different methods of protein identification were established during past decades, nonetheless, peptide mass fingerprinting in combination with mass spectrometry based methods such as MALDI/TOF, MALDI/TOF/TOF, LC/MS/MS mass spectrometry as well as other methods which all are based on the mass of amino acids and peptides are commonly used for protein identification.

In addition; nowadays 2DE databases are available and could be used as a replacement or as a mean of preliminary analysis of the experimentally obtained 2DE separated and scanned polypeptides against such 2DE protein profile provided by databases for a specific cell type, organelle, body fluids, or tissues. While such supplementary sources of information are useful for primary analysis, however mass spectrometry based methods are still the best mean of protein identification with high confidence. The complexity and quantity of data available from 2DE gel patterns can be handled by image analysis techniques using automated computer analysis systems, which can provide both qualitative and quantitative information for polypeptides resolved in an individual gel and provide pattern matching between gels [2].

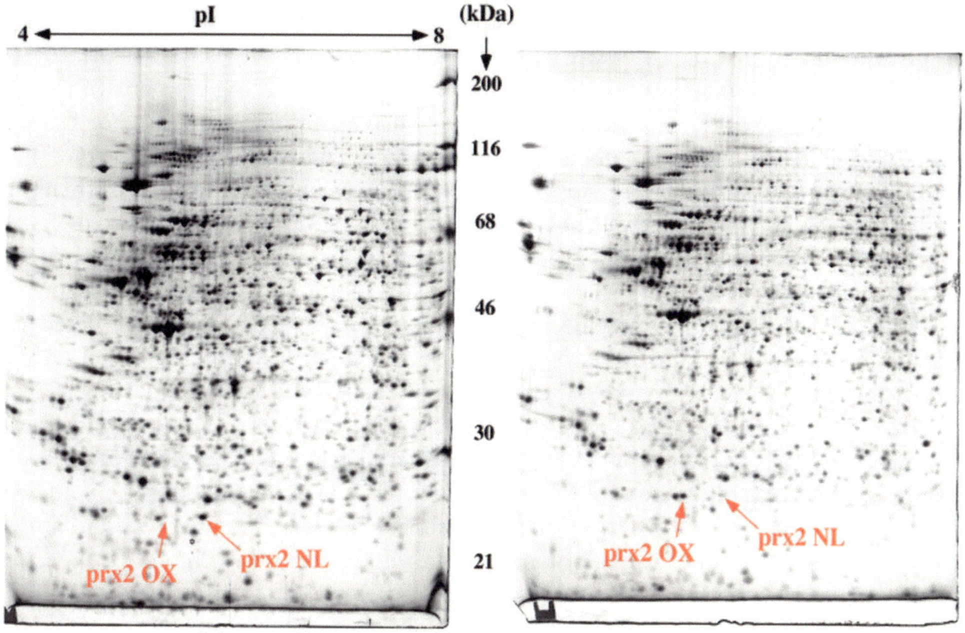

Fig. 1. Detection of proteins as well as modification of which by combining 2DE protein separation and mass spectrometry based identification. The figure represents peroxiredoxin and its modified form in Jurkat cells in normal cell culture conditions (panel A) or stressed with t-Butylhydroperoxide. Cells were lysed, and extracts were separated by two-dimensional electrophoresis: Linear pH gradient 4 – 8 was used for IEF first dimension and SDSPAGE was used for second dimension. Gels were subsequently stained with silver-nitrate. Arrows indicate the position of the normal (prx2NL) and the oxidized (prxOX) forms of peroxiredoxin 2. The change in pI (0.25 pH units) is due to the sole oxidation of the -SH group in peroxiredoxin 2 (adapted from Rabilloud, et al [4]).

3. Low abundance proteins and organelle proteomics

Although large-scale proteome analysis provides valuable information regarding cultured cells, tissues, or body fluids; nevertheless, analysis of the whole proteome might be too complex even at cellular level [5]. There are many proteins with low copy number, which might be far from resolution of the current methods when the whole tissue or cell is used as the source of proteins. Such proteins require enrichment before analysis. Considering the large variation in the expression level of proteins within a cell or tissue, the low abundance proteins become inevitably masked by high abundance proteins [6]. It should be noted that most regulatory proteins such as kinases, GTPases, certain membrane receptors, polymerases as well as transcription factors are present in low copy number. As a result an important layer of information would be lost [7]. This becomes even more important when there is only limited amount of material available for analysis (e.g. medical biopsies). Although genomic approaches have benefited from amplification methods such as polymerase chain reaction, protein based methods are poor in this regard as there is not currently any method available for their amplification. This drawback was solved in part by availability and application of accurate methods of identification such as mass spectrometry that require infinitesimal amount of proteins and to some extent using enrichment methods of low abundance proteins of interest by methods such as chromatography. For example, the total protein content of cells can be enriched by fractionation methods based on affinity procedures to isolate groups of proteins displaying similar features (lectin based isolation of glycoproteins, charge and hydrophobicity based protein separation or application of specific antibodies for isolation of phosphoproteins, etc.). This procedure has the advantage of simplifying the complexity of crude cell or tissue extracts, thereby maximizing the probability of detecting low abundance proteins. However, it should be noted that information with regard to the location of the protein of interest in the cell, organ or tissue remains to be elucidated. Organizing eukaryotic cells into sub-compartments with specialized features and functions; the organelles, provides a unique opportunity to link proteomics data with functional units. In addition identification of a specific protein within a specific organelle not only would be a step forward in our understanding of the function of the protein of interest and the molecular mechanisms in which it is involved but also the functional features of the related organelle as well. So far protein profile of several organelles have been elucidated by proteomic [5,7].

4. Proteomics in cancer research

Cancer is well known for its complex nature, which results from accumulation of numerous molecular alterations altogether lead to genetic instability, cellular proliferation, and acquisition of invasive phenotype and metastasis. While it has long been known that cancer to be a genetic disorder, but at functional level, it is rather a protein and proteomics related disease, since tumor progression, invasion and metastasis all depend on functional identity of cells or proteins such as growth factors, transcription factors, enzymes, signal transducers, proteases, etc. As a result different kinds of drugs that target different cellular components either protein [8] or nucleic acid constituent of the cells have so far been designed for treating the disease. Nonetheless such a broad range of drug could not lead to a satisfactory progress in complete treatment of the disease.

Despite our deeper understanding of the alterations and aberrations that happens in cancer cells along with advances in characterizing diversity of cancer transcriptomics, proteomics has the potential to complement further expansion the wealth of present information generated by genomics in cancers from different aspects. These aspects include; (i) there is generally not a direct correlation between level of transcription of specific genes and relative abundances of their corresponding proteins, since the resultant transcript might be subject of degradation, inactivation, or being kept in silent and inactive form until the time it is required (RNA granules) [9] (ii) due to the differential splicing and translation, each gene may encode several different protein variants with different properties; (iii) the key proteins driving malignant behavior of cancer cells can undergo post-translational modifications including phosphorylation, acylation, and glycosylation; and (iv) proteome reflects dynamic changes, it could be a suitable indicator of the disease progression and could be used for monitoring and following up the course and response of the disease to the therapy. And finally proteins represent the more accessible and relevant therapeutic targets [10,11].

Despite efforts and successes in prevention of cancers through applying screening programs along with public awareness, changes in habits, and application of better treatment strategies as well as postoperative programs, nevertheless, there wasn't so far prospect for a long life in case of many patients and cancer still remains the major cause of patients' death. The major cause of cancer death is metastasis. In most cases diagnosis of cancer and treatment of which is done when tumor has been developed well, metastasis has happened, and tumor has spread into distant organs. Proteomics could play important role not only in the study of molecular mechanism of carcinogenesis but also discovery of new cancer markers for early diagnosis of the disease, staging in addition to evaluating prognosis, prediction and monitoring of patients' response to a particular therapy. Such markers could directly be released from cancer cells or may represent as part of host's response to malignancy. They might be released into body fluids, which make their detection easy. Cells most often shed proteins into extracellular fluids including interstitial fluids, lymph and blood plasma. Whilst tissue interstitial fluids are in direct contact with tissue/cells via transfer of molecules, the composition of blood plasma results from its interaction with tissue's interstitial fluids. Blood plasma is dynamic; it influences the composition of other body fluids and becomes influenced by body fluids as well. It is important to realize that relative concentration of biomarkers is highest in the tissue of origin and surrounding interstitial fluid. However during the course of drainage from interstitial tissues' fluid into the lymph and lymph vessels and then into blood vessels the concentration of biomarker may become subject of crucial reduction. As a result, the concentration of specific biomarker in blood would significantly be lower than its original concentration in the interstitial fluid. Nevertheless, various body fluids represent more or less rich source of different types of biomarkers [10,11].

5. Proteomics of esophageal carcinoma

With 386000 annual death, eophageal cancer is the sixth leading cause of cancer death worldwide [12] [13]. The incidence of esophageal cancer is geographically diverse as a large variation could be observed for different parts of the world. The high incidence of esophageal cancer in certain parts of the world indicates a role for environmental as well as habitual factors in addition to genetics.

While reports indicate the highest incidence rate of esophageal cancer for northern Iran and certain parts in China, however, there are other high incidence areas in the world most of which are located in the Asian esophageal cancer belt. The Asian esophageal cancer belt consists of the central and eastern Asian countries including; Turkmenistan, Uzbekistan, Karakalpakstan (an autonomous republic in the eastern part of Uzbekistan), Kazakhstan, and parts of Turkey. Together these high-risk geographic areas appear to extend from north-western Iran to China, along the path of ancient Silk Road collectively known as "Central Asian Esophageal Cancer Belt" (Figure 2) [14].

Despite recent increase in the rate of esophageal adenocarcinoma in Western world, esophageal squamous cell carcinoma (ESCC) still remains the most prevalent subtype of esophageal cancer [16]. With five-year survival rate as less than 10% prognosis of esophageal cancer still remains poor. A primary cause for such high mortality is the fact that in most cases ESCC could be detected very late when tumor has developed well, invaded

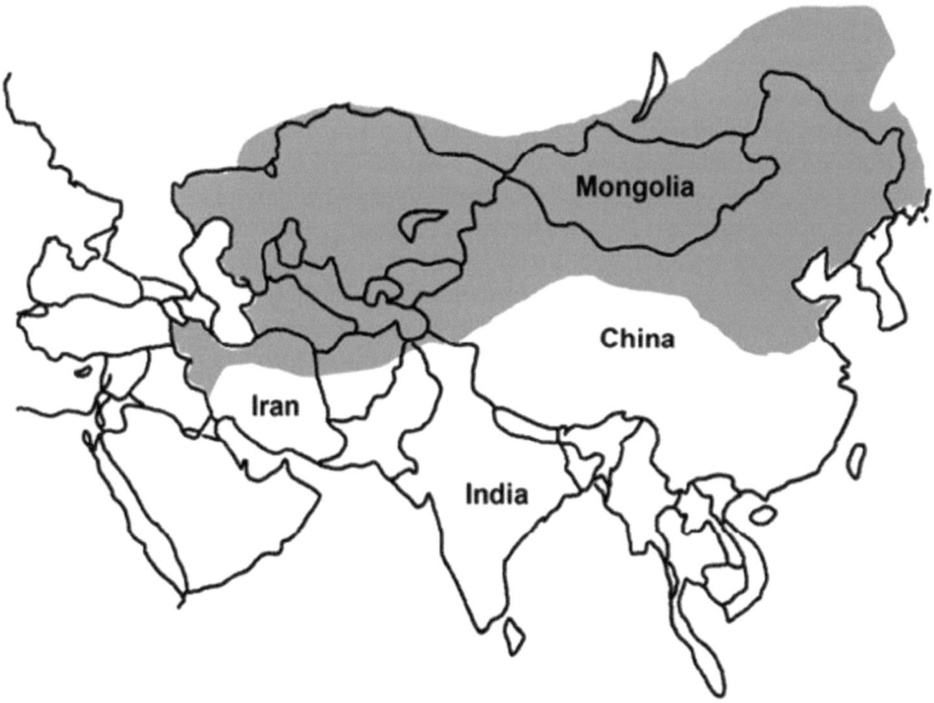

Fig. 2. The Asian esophageal cancer belt. The belt starts from eastern Anatolia in Turkey [15], extends through Iran to central Asian countries, China [14] and to the far east.

surrounding tissues and organs, and therefore at an advanced stage of the disease. Surgical resection has shown to be ineffective in 40%-60% of cases due to low resectability of the disease, the presence of distant metastases, in addition to high operation risk. Additionally, the conventional chemo and radiotherapies are relatively ineffective which further account for the poor long-term survival. The patient's survival becomes poor when the tumor spreads and extends through esophageal wall or when it is diagnosed with the widespread involvement of lymph nodes. Thus, early diagnosis and exact histological grading of the ESCC are critical for therapeutic management [17]. Over the past years, the molecular etiology of esophageal cancer was subject of extensive researches. Multiple genetic alterations, such as loss of tumor suppressor genes and activation of oncogenes were found to be associated with the development of esophageal cancer [18,19].

Although recent advancements such as microarray in addition to traditional molecular methods have been used for screening ESCC in order to find the important molecular alterations that ultimately result in ESCC [20-22], nevertheless, thus far target biomarkers applicable for the detection and therapeutic strategies and genes to act as molecular targets have not been well identified, indicating further limitations in the effective treatment of

ESCC. The high throughput and sensitive proteomic technology is hoped to open an effective venue for screening the novel cancer specific biomarkers for ESCC. Tissue and cell line based proteomics have widely been used in the study of ESCC and so far protein markers (biomarkers) have been identified as potential biomarkers for diagnosis of ESCC and possible follow-up of the treatment. Most of such identified protein molecular markers are those that are involved in cytoskeleton organization, metabolism, differentiation, apoptosis, cell growth, and metastasis as well as redox reactions. In subsequent sections, we present a summary of the recent achievements applying proteomics.

6. Cytoskeleton

Actin network is essential for several important cellular functions such as pseudopodia formation, motility, division, cell surface receptor movement, anchorage, and contact inhibition. During malignant transformation, alteration in the expression of actin microfilament network as well as other actin-associated proteins which are involved in the morphological changes and cytoskeletal organization could be seen. Among such proteins are tropomyosins (TPMs). As a major structural component of cytoskeletal microfilaments, multiple isoforms of TPMs were identified in the cultured non-muscle cells. At expression level different isoforms of TMP are regulated dissimilarly in tumors, implying that these isoforms may have different functions in cell transformation. TPM1 [23] and TPM2 [24] have shown to be subject of down-regulation while TPM4 [23] and TPM3 ([25], and as our unpublished result indicates (in a study on cell lines)) are significantly subject of up-regulation in ESCC tissues. In addition, fusion of TPM4-ALK was observed to happen in ESCC [24] which results in the up regulation of anaplastic leukemia kinase. Though as a cytoskeletal and housekeeping protein TPM4 promoter is constantly active, the fusion protein (TPM4-ALK) is constantly expressed in tumor cells which results in up regulation of fused anaplastic leukemia kinase in the cell and its oncogenic outcome. Deregulation of TPM isoforms may cause an imbalance in the normal phenotype of epithelial microfilaments, which leads to malignant phenotype of the aberrant cells. These alterations may provide clues for the early detection, diagnosis, and identification of therapeutic targets. In addition to TPMs altered expression of members of myosin family of proteins have also been reported in ESCC ([24] and our unpublished results).

Transgelin, a calponin related protein whose expression was observed to change in transformed cells is another member of cytoskeletal associated proteins that remarkably increases in ESCC. Distinct types of transgelin isoforms presents exclusively in cancer tissues [23]. Transgelin is an actin microfilament binding protein whose expression is regulated by deregulated Ras expression in a Raf independent pathway of transformation. Loss of transgelin in breast and colon tumors and in RIE-1 cells has also been reported [26].

Keratins are components of intermediate filaments of cytoskeleton functioning especially in epithelial cells. Keratin1 and keratin 8 ([24], as well as our unpublished results on ESCC cell lines, [27-29]) and keratin 13 were observed to be overexpressed in ESCC, while keratin 4 and keratin 14 are down regulated [30] in.

Desmin is another member of intermediate filaments that subjects to down regulation in ESCC [16]. As a 52 kDa protein, desmin is a subunit of intermediate filaments in the tissues of skeletal, smooth, and cardiac muscle [31] cells. While it is a muscle cell marker and important in muscle cell's development, nevertheless its exact role is not yet known for other cell types and demands further studies to unravel its true function.

Another actin binding protein is fascin that overexpression of which was observed in ESCC. Since overexpression of fascin was found to be associated with significant increase in the motility and dynamics of cell lines [16]; it could be concluded that the same consequences which are; the increased invasion and metastatic potential to happen for ESCC too.

α-actinins are actin binding and cross-linking proteins. Expression of alpha actinin 4 (ACTN4) was shown to increase progressively from stage I to stage III. Clinico-pathological correlation using TMA (tissue microarray) revealed that overexpression of ACTN4 is significantly associated with the advanced tumor stage and lymph node metastasis [25] in ESCC.

In addition gamma actin, tubulin alpha-1 chain, and tubulin beta-5 chain were also reported to be subject of change in expression in ESCC. Overexpression of these proteins was reported in ESCC [23].

7. Differentiation

Data obtained from models of carcinogenesis suggest that alteration in the normal differentiation process is associated with neoplastic transformation [16]. As a result, altered expression of proteins, which are related to differentiation, is expected to play role in carcinogenesis through dedifferentiation, resistance to terminal differentiation, or alteration of differentiation.

S100A8 ([32], and our unpublished data) and S100A9 [16] are the two other calcium binding proteins which are associated with the myeloid cell differentiation. These two proteins are subject of down regulation in ESCC. Recently, S100 family of proteins have received increasing attention as their possible involvement in several human diseases, including cancer.

Annexins [33,34] were shown to play important role in esophageal carcinogenesis. Annexin I down regulation has reportedly been observed in ESCC ([16, 35, 36], as well as our unpublished results). Loss of annexin AI correlates with the early onset of tumorigenesis in esophageal carcinoma. It was found that expression of annexin AI to be correlated with the differentiation status of esophageal carcinomas as high expression of annexin AI was reported to occur in the poor differentiated ESCC [35,36]. In addition to annexin AI, down-regulation of annexin A II and overexpression of annexin AIX were also observed in our studies on ESCC (unpublished results) and others [37-39].

Transglutaminases (TGases) are calcium dependent enzymes that catalyze formation of isopeptide bonds between amide group of glutamine and the Ɛ-amino group of lysine during the process of terminal differentiation in stratified squamous epithelia. It was shown TGases to be subject of down regulation in ESCC [16,25]. Among TGasese, the protein-glutamine gamma-glutamyltransferase E (TGM3) plays key role in epidermal terminal differentiation through cross-linking structural proteins such as involucrin, loricrin, and small proline-rich proteins. Although the role of TGM3 in the differentiation of skin keratinocytes has been well established, however, little information is available regarding its involvement in esophageal epithelium. TGM3 stabilizes the cornified envelope of the cells, a process that precedes the transition of keratinocytes to corneocytes by apoptosis [40, 41, 42]. It is among important molecules involved in the adhesion which is expressed by epithelial cells and regarded as inhibitor of invasion. As a result downregulation or loss of TGM3 correlates with dedifferentiation, increased invasion and high incidence of lymph node metastasis [43]. Although the role of TGM3 has well been established in the differentiation of skin keratinocytes, nonetheless, little information is available regarding its involvement in esophageal epithelium transformation. In addition to esophageal carcinoma, downregulation of TGM3 was also reported in laryngeal carcinoma [44], as well as head and neck squamous cell carcinoma [45].

The other protein that reports have indicated its low expression in ESCC is galectin7, a member of the galectin family. The low expression of this protein in ESCC is consistent with a differentiation defect in keratinocytes [16]. The major functions of galectin7 include regulation of cell to cell and cell to matrix interactions, apoptosis and immunity. It should be noted that both downregulation (above) as well as upregulation of galectin7 was reported with regard to ESCC. Upregulation of galectin7 was reported by Zhu et al (2010) in ESCC tissues [17].

Epidermal-type fatty acid-binding protein (E-FABP) is a member of the FABP family that mediates transport and utilization of fatty acids. FABPs are small cytosolic non-enzymic proteins that have tissue specific expression. They are involved in fatty acid signaling, cellular growth and differentiation. It was proposed that they play a role in cellular lipid uptake and transport, metabolic pathway, and regulation of protein metabolism. Downregulation of E-FABP in has been reported for ESCC [46].

8. Metabolism

Several proteins that are involved in cellular metabolism undergo overexpression in ESCC, for example, AKR (aldo-keto reductase) family 1, reflecting an increased metabolic and biosynthetic requirement of tumor cells and their possible involvement in carcinogens metabolism. AKR members have shown to be involved in carcinogen metabolism. As an example AKR can activate polycyclic aromatic hydrocarbons (PAHs) by oxidizing trans-dihydrodiol proximate carcinogens to reactive and redox active ortho-quinones. PAHs are ubiquitous environmental pollutants and human carcinogens. Overexpression of AKR might yield more active carcinogens and result in cellular transformation and tumor development in ESCC [16,47].

Glutathione transferases (GSTs) compose multigene family of dimeric enzymes of phase II detoxification that catalyze conjugation of glutathione to the lipophilic substrates in order to make them more water soluble or electrophile [48] essential for their excretion from the body. Since a large proportion of pro-mutagens and pro-carcinogens are lipophilic compounds, by conjugating them with the electrophilic glutathione they become more water soluble and easier targets for excretion into bile or urine. GSTs can be induced by many of their substrates and by some non-substrate compounds as well. For example, butyrate, an important luminal component produced from bacterial fermentation of dietary fibers, is an efficient inducer of GSTs in colonic carcinoma cell lines. M and P family of GSTs have a regulatory role in mitogen-activated protein (MAP) pathway and resistance to drugs.

In addition, overexpression of GSTs is associated with the increased resistance to apoptosis that could be initiated by various stimuli [49]. GSTM1, GSTP1 and GSTT2 are expressed in esophagus mucosa. Higher expression of GSTP1 has been observed in esophagus compared to other GSTs [50]. GSTM2 was found to be over-expressed in ESCC. The overexpression of this enzyme in ESCC might be a response to the increased GSTM substrates or to the bacterial metabolites in the esophagus. In addition to GSTM2, overexpression of GSTP was also reported in ESCC [16,51].

Alpha enolase is a multi-functional enzyme in the glycolytic pathway which catalyzes formation of phosphoenol pyruvate from 2-phosphoglycerate. The expression of alpha enolase was seen to be elevated in ESCC tissues [52] that might indicate a higher metabolic rate as well as switch to glycolytic pathway as possibly the main source of providing the required energy.

Another metabolism related protein whose expression is affected by cancer is glutamate dehydrogenase (mitochondrial) GLUD1. The enzyme is involved in glutaminolysis that is important in cancer metabolism [53]. Our observation in the cell lines prepared from ESCC also indicates that GLUD1 subjects to down regulation in ESCC.

9. Redox reaction

Accumulating evidences indicate that intracellular redox state plays important roles in cellular signal transduction and gene expression [54]. Reactive oxygen species (ROSs) which are produced during physiological processes in response to external stimuli, can affect intracellular redox state. At low levels, ROS modulate gene expression through modulating cellular redox state, however, at higher levels ROSs are extremely deleterious and potentially damage DNA, proteins, carbohydrates, and lipids. It has been suggested that ROSs play roles in all stages of carcinogenesis, including initiation, promotion, and progression [55,56]. In order to protect cells from oxidative radical stress, cells have developed defense systems that comprise proteins superoxide dismutases (SODs), catatalse, glutathione peroxidases, and peroxiredoxins (PRXs). The up-regulation of MnSOD and PRX1 in ESCC and their linear correlation with progression of disease from premalignant to invasive cancer reflect the cell defense effort in maintaining intracellular homeostasis. Interestingly, a minor down-regulation of PRX2 isoform was detected in ESCC [23,24] suggesting that different PRX isoforms may have slightly different functions unique to the esophageal neoplasms [23] . We observed PRDX5 overexpression in ESCC (unpublished observation). Thioredoxin peroxidase (TxP) uses thiol groups as reducing equivalent donors to scavenge oxidants. By reducing reactive oxygen species formation, TxP inhibits caspase activity and hence apoptosis. Overexpression of TxP in ESCC may increase the number of proliferating ESCC cells by inhibiting apoptosis [16].

10. Heat shock proteins

Heat shock proteins are the highly conserved cytoprotective proteins in all species. They play essential role in protein folding, transport, translocation, degradation, and assembly, even under unstressed conditions. GRP78 is an endoplasmic reticulum (ER) chaperone calcium binding protein. It is involved in many cellular processes including the translocation of newly synthesized polypeptides across the ER membrane, facilitation of the folding and assembly of newly synthesized proteins, degradation of misfolded proteins through proteasome, and regulation of calcium homeostasis. In addition to above functions GRP78 endows cancer cells ability to resist against anticancer drugs such as chemotherapy, antiangiogensis antibodies, and anti hormonal therapy. It was shown to be involved in tumor cell immune resistance, proliferation and metastasis added to its role against apoptosis. Thus, it is reasonable that its overexpression accompany with the increased rate of carcinogenesis. In accordance with these properties, elevated expression of GRP78 could be observed in ESCC. ESCC patients with higher expression of GRP78 show a shorter survival than those with low or no expression of GRP78 [52,57].

Calreticulin is another calcium binding endoplasmic reticulum specific protein whose up regulation was observed in ESCC [24,52]. It is involved in the regulation of intracellular calcium homeostasis and endoplasmic reticulum calcium storage capacity [52,58]. Calreticulin is a lectin that interacts with the nascent and newly synthesized glycoproteins. It functions as a molecular chaperon during folding of glycoprotein [59]. It cooperates with calnexin, glycoprotein glucosyltransferase and glucosidase in calnexin/calreticulin cycle of protein folding. Role of this cycle is engagement in selective folding of newly synthesized glycoproteins in the process of protein translation [60,61]. Approximately all glycoproteins transiently interact with one or both of these two proteins (i.e. calnexin or calreticulin) during maturation or degradadtion after misfolding [62,63].

AlphaB-Cryst is a member of the small heat shock proteins (HSPs), which are ubiquitous chaperone molecules related to stresses. They bind to partially denatured proteins, dissociating protein aggregates, modulating the correct folding, and cooperating in transporting newly synthesized polypeptides to the target organelles. AlphaB-Cryst is able to inhibit both mitochondrial and the death receptor apoptotic pathways through abolishing the autoproteolytic maturation of the partially processed caspase-3 intermediate. Intriguingly, while other HSPs were usually up-regulated in tumors, alphaB-Cryst was often down-regulated in various cancers including in ESCC tissues. These results point out that alphaB-Cryst plays a role distinct from other HSPs in the carcinogenesis and its underexpression might candidate it as a general tumor marker for various types of cancers [23].

gp96 and Hsp27 are the two other chaperones whose expression change have been reported in esophageal cancer. Reports indicate upregulation of gp96 and down regulation of Hsp27 in ESCC. Hsp27 and gp96 are stress-response proteins. gp96 also plays a role in tumor immunity [16]. In addition to gp96, overexpression of HSP70 has also been reported in ESCC [24].

11. Cell growth

Several cell growth related proteins' expression was seen to change in ESCC. PCNA is among such proteins whose overexoression could be observed in ESCC [16]. As a highly conserved protein in eukaryotes, it is essential factor for DNA replication and DNA repair. In addition to PCNA, upregulation of DNA directed RNA polymerase B has formerly been reported by our group in ESCC [24].

RNA binding motif proteins 8A (RBM8A), the other growth related protein is also overexpressed in ESCC [16]. RBMs play key role in post-transcriptional regulation of gene expression in eukaryotic cells and mediate mRNA processing including terminal processing of which; intron splicing, editing and deamination of nucleotides [64].

Clusterin, the so-called testosterone repressed prostate message, sulfated glycoprotein, complement associated protein SP-40, and complement cytolysis inhibitor, is an 80-kDa heterodimeric highly conserved secreted glycoprotein expressed in a wide variety of tissues and was found in all human fluids. It responses to a number of diverse stimuli, including hormone ablation and has been attributed to function in several diverse physiological processes such as sperm maturation, lipid transportation, complement inhibition, tissue remodeling, membrane recycling, cell adhesion and cell- substratum interactions, stabilization of stressed proteins in a folding competent state and is involved in promotion or inhibition of apoptosis. In addition, loss and downregulation of clusterin in ESCC, it was also lost or decreased in tumor cell lines and tissues [65].

Another potential tumor suppressor protein is prohibitin that was found to be differentially expressed in cancerous tissues compared to the adjacent normal epithelium. Interestingly, while expression of prohibitin is positively correlated with the progression of precancerous lesions, however, it is inversely correlated with the differentiation grade of squamous cell carcinoma of esophagus. The expression of prohibitin drops with dedifferentiation of ESCC. This pattern of expression implies that prohibitin may play different roles in different stages of esophageal tumorigenesis [23].

Eukaryotic translation initiation factor 1 a (eIF-1a), reticulocalbin and transmembrane protein 4 are three other proteins that overexpress in ESCC [16]. eIF-1a stabilizes Met-tRNA to the 40S ribosomal subunit, thus prevents pre-maturation association of 40S ribosomal subunit to 60S subunit of ribosome [66]. eIF-1a along with other eIFs stimulate decoding of AUG start codon in mRNA [67].

Reticulocalbin is a calcium binding protein located in the endoplasmic reticulum lumen. Overexpression of this protein plays a role in tumorogenesis, tumor invasion and resistance to drug [68,69].

12. Metastasis

Cancer cells escape the primary tumor mass and penetrate into the surrounding tissues or tissues at far distant through the process of invasion and metastasis, the two processes that require degradation of extracellular matrix and/or basement membranes. The key molecules involved in the degradation of these structures are cysteine, serine, and aspartic acid protease as well as matrix metalloproteinases (MMPs). MMPs contains collagenases (MMP-1, MMP-8, MMP-13, MMP-18), gelatinases (MMP-2, MMP-9), stromelysins (MMP-3, MMP-10, MMP-11) matrilysins (MMP-7, MMP-26) mating type (MMP-14, MMP-15, MMP-16, MMP-24, MMP-17, MMP-25) and non-classified (RASI-1, enamelysin) [70]. Generally, gelatinases are more often observed in tumor tissues. It seems that they are involved more in the invasion rather than other members of matrix metalloproteinases [71,72]. High expression of MMP-1 [73], MMP-7 [74], MMP-11 [75] is associated with the worse prognosis of tumors, while MMP-9 and MT1-MMP are involved in the depth of invasion [76,77]. MMP-2 and MMP-3 were found to be correlated with the lymph node metastasis in ESCC [78].

Down-regulation of neutrophil elastase inhibitor and SCCA1 (below) in ESCC was among other observation by proteomic studies. Neutrophil elastase is an inflammatory protein that is mainly produced by neutrophils. The protease degrades extracellular matrix thereby increases ability of neutrophils to infiltrate into the tissues. Neutrophil elastase might also be released by some cancer cells to serve a similar function. Low expression of elastase inhibitor in ESCC would result in an increased enzyme activity, facilitating tumor invasion and metastasis.

Squamous Cell Carcinoma Antigens (SCCAs), are members of serine protease inhibitors (serpins) [79] superfamily that strong expression of which could be observed in different epithelial cancers. Two different isoforms of SCCA are encoded by two highly homologous genes SCCA1 and SCCA2 [80]. Both the SCCA1 and SCCA2 proteins are physiologically present in the suprabasal layers of normal stratified squamous epithelium[81]. SCCA1 [23] was shown to inhibit papain like cysteine proteinases, cathepsin S, K, and L. Serpins are involved in the multiple cellular biological processes including tumor cell invasion, cellular differentiation, and apoptosis. SCCA1 may function intra as well as extracellularly, serving as a cytoprotective mediator [16,23].

APA-1, a zinc finger protein, was shown to be overexpressed in ESCC. APA-1 is a transcription factor which activates transcription of matrix remodeling genes such as matrix metalloproteinase 1 (MMP-1) during fibroblast senescence [52]. The same role for APA-1 overexpression could be envisaged for esophageal cancer.

13. Apoptosis

Apoptosis is a major barrier for cancer cells that they must have to overcome in order to survive. The modest increase observed in COX-2 and p53 protein expression with progression from normal to dysplasia suggests that these markers may be the most informative in the more advanced state of neoplasias [17,30]. Cyclooxygenases (Cox-1 and Cox-2) are enzymes which are involved in the formation of prostaglandins from arachidonic acid. While Cox-1 is constitutively expressed; Cox-2 is induced by cytokines, tumor promoters, growth factors and viral induced transformation. Cox-2 was found to be expressed in various malignant tumors [82]. Expression of Cox-2 could be induced by p53. In turn, Cox-2 negatively affects p53 activity through physical interaction with p53. Cox-2 is a positive regulator of growth while p53 is a negative regulator of growth thus increasing expression of Cox-2 by p53 seems to be a controlling event of growth by creating a balance between induction and inhibition of cellular division. It is suggested that p53-dependent induction of Cox-2 abate apoptotic and growth inhibitory effect of p53 [83].

14-3-3 protein sigma, also known as stratifin or HME-1, has recently reported to be down regulated in ESCC. It is transactivated by p53 in response to DNA damage and negatively regulates both G1/S and G2/M cell cycle progression. Overexpression of stratifin increases stabilization of p53 through blocking Mdm2 mediated p53 ubiquitination and enhanced oligomerization of p53, leading to the increased p53 transcriptional activity. Additionally, expression of stratifin inversely correlates with the differentiation grade of ESCC indicating that malignant cells arising from esophageal epithelium may lose stratifin in progressive dedifferentiation [23]. Stratifin is a checkpoint protein that causes G2 arrest following to DNA damage. Inactivation of this protein; mainly by methylation, was reported in some tumors. Likely loss of this protein impairs the function of G2/M checkpoint results in the accumulation of genetic defects and ultimately cancer [84].

Table 1 represents proteins that were identified using proteomic based methods in ESCC and we discussed here. These are not the only proteins identified with regard to ESCC, though other proteins could also be found in other literatures. Here we focused on some proteins as examples for documenting the applicability of proteomic based methodologies in the molecular etiology of cancers and among which esophageal cancer in particular. A long list of proteins for ESCC could be found in literatures that are far from scope of the present book chapter. We propose that in future studies attempts to be focused on narrowing down the list of proteins to as small number and to as tissue specific as possible till each of such proteins could be correlated with a specific type of cancer. Such a narrowing down is important from that respect that makes detection and prediction of specific type of cancer possible before the onset of the disease, especially by using such proteins as markers in body fluids, body secretions and excretions and other rout of discharge from the body. Fortunately, recent reports indicate the potential of proteomic based studies in correlating and establishing fine relationship between the expression patterns of several proteins with the stage of carcinogenesis as well as differentiation or grade of cancer. Among such reports are papers published by Qi and colleagues [23] and Nishimori, et al. [85] that showed well such a correlation. These proteins have significant clinical value since they could be used as molecular markers in order to evaluate the tumor per se and prognosis for evaluating the efficacy of the treatment as well as prediction of recurrence, etc. (figure 3).

Classification (cellular function)	Upregulated	Downregulated
Cytoskeleton	TPM4 TPM3 Transgelin Keratin 1 Keratin 8 Keratin 13 Tubulin alpha chain 1 Fascin Tubulin Beta-5 chain Alpha actinin 4	TPM1 TPM2 Keratin 4 Keratin 14 Desmin
Differentiation	Annexin A4 Galectin 7	S100A9 S100A8 Annexin A1 Annexin A2 TGM3 Galectin 7
Metabolism	AKR GSTM2 Alpha enolase	GLUD1
Redox reaction	MnsOD PRX1 PRX5 TxP	PRX2

Classification (cellular function)	Upregulated	Downregulated
Heat Shock Protein	GRP78 Calreticulin Gp96 Hsp70	αβ-Cryst Hsp27
Cell growth	PCNA DNA direct RNA Polymerase B RBM8A Prohibitin eIF-1A Reticulocalbin Transmembrane protein 4	Clusterin
Metastasis	MMP-1 MMP-7 MMP-11 MMP-9 MT1-MMP MMp-2 MMP-3 APA-1	SCCA1 Neutrophil elastase inhibitor
Apoptosis	Cox-2 P53	14-3-3 Protein Sigma

Table 1. Proteins identified by proteomics in ESCC and discussed in the text.

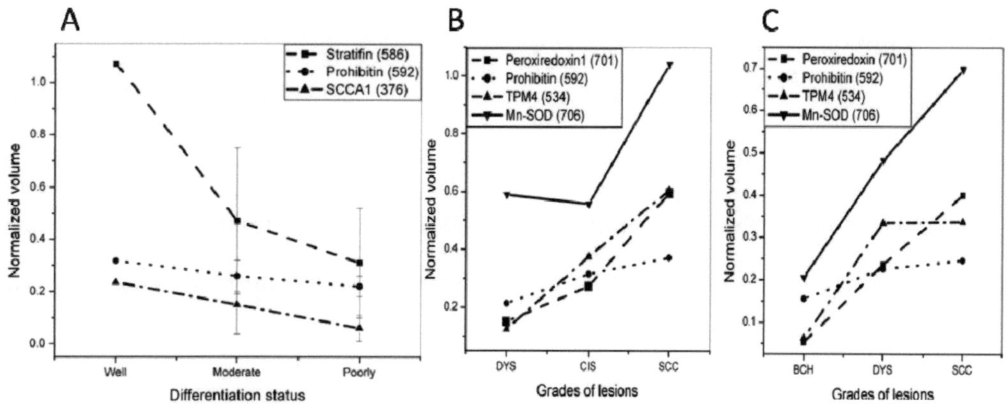

Fig. 3. Correlation between expression patterns of several proteins identified by 2DE and differentiation status (A), grade (B) or the degree of lesion (C) in ESCC. Numbers in the parenthesis indicate the spot number in 2DE gel pattern explained in the text by the authors. A well correlation could be established for stratifin, TPM4, peroxiredoxin and the other member of redox family of proteins; peroxiredoxin1, as well as Mn-SOD with the degree of

the disease progression. Other proteins show more or less the same pattern of expression change (adapted from Takanori Nishimori, et al [85]).

14. Conclusion

The complexity of the carcinogenesis in addition to the dynamics of the protein constituent of the cells demand new approaches for the analysis of the molecular etiology of cancers and among which ESCC for establishing appropriate strategies of their successful detection, treatment, and follow up. Proteomics is a powerful mean of gene expression analysis applicable both at translational as well as posttranslational level. In addition it could be used for studying protein-nucleic acid, or protein-drug interaction, along with vast other applications. As a result, proteomics could be an appropriate complement for the gene expression based analyses. It enables to put further steps of information ahead which is the entire genes being expressed in a cell or tissue at a given time and under specific condition. So far many proteins in different steps of carcinogenesis have been identified that found to be subject of alteration in carcinogenesis. Accumulating data indicate that proteomics could be an efficient approach for the identification of molecular alterations in ESCC carcinogenesis in addition to other cancers.

The data generated by proteomics in ESCC has so far lead us to the identification of a set of proteins, which are involved in the different stages of ESCC carcinogenesis. These proteins are not only related to the alterations in the structure but also to the function of ESCC among which cell growth and division along with apoptosis and invasion. Moreover, several of such identified proteins were also found to be as appropriate biomarkers of ESCC, which authenticates the efficacy of the proteomic based strategies in clinical investigations and practical application. It is expected that proteomic evaluation of tissues and body fluids could open a venue to the achievement of the proper approaches of the assessment of the overall status of health and prognosis of cancers including ESCC.

15. References

[1] Chuthapisith, S., Layfield, R., Kerr, I. and Eremin, O. (2007) Principles of proteomics and its applications in cancer. *The Surgeon*, 5, 14-22.

[2] Baak, J., Path, F., Hermsen, M., Meijer, G., Schmidt, J. and Janssen, E. (2003) Genomics and proteomics in cancer. *European Journal of Cancer*, 39, 1199-1215.

[3] O'Farrell, P.H. (1975) High resolution two-dimensional electrophoresis of proteins. *Journal of biological chemistry*, 250, 4007.

[4] Rabilloud, T., Chevallet, M., Luche, S. and Lelong, C. (2010) Two-dimensional gel electrophoresis in proteomics: past, present and future. *Journal of proteomics*, 73, 2064-2077.

[5] Yates Iii, J.R., Gilchrist, A., Howell, K.E. and Bergeron, J.J.M. (2005) Proteomics of organelles and large cellular structures. *Nature Reviews Molecular Cell Biology*, 6, 702-714.

[6] Patterson, S.D. and Aebersold, R.H. (2003) Proteomics: the first decade and beyond. *nature genetics*, 33, 311-323.

[7] Brunet, S., Thibault, P., Gagnon, E., Kearney, P., Bergeron, J.J.M. and Desjardins, M. (2003) Organelle proteomics: looking at less to see more. *Trends in cell biology*, 13, 629-638.

[8] Ebert, M., Yu, J., Lordick, F. and Röcken, C. (2006) Proteomics in gastrointestinal cancer. *Annals of Oncology*, 17, x253.
[9] Anderson, P. and Kedersha, N. (2009) RNA granules: post-transcriptional and epigenetic modulators of gene expression. *Nature Reviews Molecular Cell Biology*, 10, 430-436.
[10] Bertucci, F., Birnbaum, D. and Goncalves, A. (2006) Proteomics of breast cancer. *Molecular & Cellular Proteomics*, 5, 1772.
[11] Martinkova, J., Gadher, S.J., Hajduch, M. and Kovarova, H. (2009) Challenges in cancer research and multifaceted approaches for cancer biomarker quest. *FEBS letters*, 583, 1772-1784.
[12] Ohigashi, Y., Sho, M., Yamada, Y., Tsurui, Y., Hamada, K., Ikeda, N., Mizuno, T., Yoriki, R., Kashizuka, H. and Yane, K. (2005) Clinical significance of programmed death-1 ligand-1 and programmed death-1 ligand-2 expression in human esophageal cancer. *Clinical cancer research*, 11, 2947.
[13] Wu, M., Zhang, Z.F., Kampman, E., Zhou, J.Y., Han, R.Q., Yang, J., Zhang, X.F., Gu, X.P., Liu, A.M. and van't Veer, P. (2010) Does family history of cancer modify the effects of lifestyle risk factors on esophageal cancer? a population based case-control study in China. *International Journal of Cancer.*
[14] Kamangar, F., Malekzadeh, R., Dawsey, S.M. and Saidi, F. (2007) Esophageal cancer in Northeastern Iran: a review. *Arch Iran Med*, 10, 70-82.
[15] Türkdogan, M., Testereci, H., Akman, N., Kahraman, T., Kara, K. and Tuncer, I. (2003) Dietary nitrate and nitrite levels in an endemic upper gastrointestinal (esophageal and gastric) cancer region of Turkey. *Turk J Gastroenterol*, 14, 50-53.
[16] Zhou, G., Li, H., Gong, Y., Zhao, Y., Cheng, J. and Lee, P. (2005) Proteomic analysis of global alteration of protein expression in squamous cell carcinoma of the esophagus. *Proteomics*, 5, 3814-3821.
[17] Zhu, X., Ding, M., Yu, M.L., Feng, M.X., Tan, L.J. and Zhao, F.K. (2010) Identification of galectin-7 as a potential biomarker for esophageal squamous cell carcinoma by proteomic analysis. *BMC cancer*, 10, 290.
[18] Kwong, K.F. (2005) Molecular biology of esophageal cancer in the genomics era. *The Surgical clinics of North America*, 85.
[19] Enzinger, P.C. and Mayer, R.J. (2003) Esophageal cancer. *New England Journal of Medicine*, 349, 2241-2252.
[20] Imazawa, M., Hibi, K., Fujitake, S.I., Kodera, Y., Ito, K., Akiyama, S. and Nakao, A. (2005) S100A2 overexpression is frequently observed in esophageal squamous cell carcinoma. *Anticancer research*, 25, 1247.
[21] Xiong, X.D., Xu, L.Y., Shen, Z.Y., Cai, W.J., Luo, J.M., Han, Y.L. and Li, E.M. (2002) Identification of differentially expressed proteins between human esophageal immortalized and carcinomatous cell lines by two-dimensional electrophoresis and MALDI-TOF-mass spectrometry. *World Journal of Gastroenterology*, 8, 777-781.
[22] Yoshitake, Y., Nakatsura, T., Monji, M., Senju, S., Matsuyoshi, H., Tsukamoto, H., Hosaka, S., Komori, H., Fukuma, D. and Ikuta, Y. (2004) Proliferation potential-related protein, an ideal esophageal cancer antigen for immunotherapy, identified using complementary DNA microarray analysis. *Clinical cancer research*, 10, 6437.
[23] Qi, Y., Chiu, J., Wang, L., Kwong, D.L.W. and He, Q. (2005) Comparative proteomic analysis of esophageal squamous cell carcinoma.

[24] Jazii, F.R., Najafi, Z., Malekzadeh, R., Conrads, T.P., Ziaee, A.A., Abnet, C., Yazdznbod, M., Karkhane, A.A. and Salekdeh, G.H. (2006) Identification of squamous cell carcinoma associated proteins by proteomics and loss of beta tropomyosin expression in esophageal cancer. *WORLD JOURNAL OF GASTROENTEROLOGY*, 12, 7104.

[25] Fu, L., Qin, Y.R., Xie, D., Chow, H.Y., Ngai, S.M., Kwong, D.L.W., Li, Y. and Guan, X.Y. (2007) Identification of alpha actinin 4 and 67 kDa laminin receptor as stage specific markers in esophageal cancer via proteomic approaches. *Cancer*, 110, 2672-2681.

[26] Shields, J.M., Rogers-Graham, K. and Der, C.J. (2002) Loss of transgelin in breast and colon tumors and in RIE-1 cells by Ras deregulation of gene expression through Raf-independent pathways. *Journal of biological chemistry*, 277, 9790.

[27] Makino, T., Yamasaki, M., Takeno, A., Shirakawa, M., Miyata, H., Takiguchi, S., Nakajima, K., Fujiwara, Y., Nishida, T. and Matsuura, N. (2009) Cytokeratins 18 and 8 are poor prognostic markers in patients with squamous cell carcinoma of the oesophagus. *British journal of cancer*, 101, 1298-1306.

[28] Singh, A., Kapur, S., Chattopadhyay, I., Purkayastha, J., Sharma, J., Mishra, A., Hewitt, S.M. and Saxena, S. (2009) Cytokeratin immunoexpression in esophageal squamous cell carcinoma of high-risk population in Northeast India. *Applied immunohistochemistry & molecular morphology: AIMM/official publication of the Society for Applied Immunohistochemistry*, 17, 419.

[29] Cintorino, M., Tripod, S.A., Santopietro, R., Antonio, P., Lutfi, A., Chang, F., Syrjänen, S., Shen, Q., Tosi, P. and Syrjänen, K. (2001) Cytokeratin expression patterns as an indicator of tumour progression in oesophageal squamous cell carcinoma. *Anticancer research*, 21, 4195.

[30] Chung, J.Y., Braunschweig, T., Hu, N., Roth, M., Traicoff, J.L., Wang, Q.H., Knezevic, V., Taylor, P.R. and Hewitt, S.M. (2006) A multiplex tissue immunoblotting assay for proteomic profiling: a pilot study of the normal to tumor transition of esophageal squamous cell carcinoma. *Cancer Epidemiology Biomarkers & Prevention*, 15, 1403.

[31] Li, Z., Mericskay, M., Agbulut, O., Butler-Browne, G., Carlsson, L., Thornell, L.E., Babinet, C. and Paulin, D. (1997) Desmin is essential for the tensile strength and integrity of myofibrils but not for myogenic commitment, differentiation, and fusion of skeletal muscle. *The Journal of cell biology*, 139, 129.

[32] Kong, J.P., Ding, F., Zhou, C.N., Wang, X.Q., Miao, X.P., Wu, M. and Liu, Z.H. (2004) Loss of myeloid-related proteins 8 and myeloid-related proteins 14 expression in human esophageal squamous cell carcinoma correlates with poor differentiation. *World Journal of Gastroenterology*, 10, 1093-1097.

[33] Violette, S., King, I., Browning, J., Pepinsky, R., Wallner, B. and Sartorelli, A. (1990) Role of lipocortin I in the glucocorticoid induction of the terminal differentiation of a human squamous carcinoma. *Journal of cellular physiology*, 142, 70-77.

[34] Hu, N., Flaig, M.J., Su, H., Shou, J.Z., Roth, M.J., Li, W.J., Wang, C., Goldstein, A.M., Li, G. and Emmert-Buck, M.R. (2004) Comprehensive characterization of annexin I alterations in esophageal squamous cell carcinoma. *Clinical cancer research*, 10, 6013.

[35] Paweletz, C.P., Ornstein, D.K., Roth, M.J., Bichsel, V.E., Gillespie, J.W., Calvert, V.S., Vocke, C.D., Hewitt, S.M., Duray, P.H. and Herring, J. (2000) Loss of annexin 1

correlates with early onset of tumorigenesis in esophageal and prostate carcinoma. *Cancer research*, 60, 6293.

[36] Wang, K.L., Wu, T.T., Resetkova, E., Wang, H., Correa, A.M., Hofstetter, W.L., Swisher, S.G., Ajani, J.A., Rashid, A. and Hamilton, S.R. (2006) Expression of annexin A1 in esophageal and esophagogastric junction adenocarcinomas: association with poor outcome. *Clinical cancer research*, 12, 4598.

[37] Liu, Z., Feng, J., Tuersun, A., Liu, T., Liu, H., Liu, Q., Zheng, S., Huang, C., Lv, G. and Sheyhidin, I. (2011) Proteomic identification of differentially-expressed proteins in esophageal cancer in three ethnic groups in Xinjiang. *Molecular Biology Reports*, 1-9.

[38] Qi, Y.J., He, Q.Y., Ma, Y.F., Du, Y.W., Liu, G.C., Li, Y.J., Tsao, G.S.W., Ngai, S.M. and Chiu, J.F. (2008) Proteomic identification of malignant transformation related proteins in esophageal squamous cell carcinoma. *Journal of cellular biochemistry*, 104, 1625-1635.

[39] Qi, Y., Wang, L., Jiao, X., Feng, X., Fan, Z., Gao, S., He, X., Li, J. and Chang, F. (2007) Dysregulation of Annexin II expression in esophageal squamous cell cancer and adjacent tissues from a high-incidence area for esophageal cancer in Henan province]. *Ai zheng= Aizheng= Chinese journal of cancer*, 26, 730.

[40] Ahvazi, B., Boeshans, K.M., Idler, W., Baxa, U., Steinert, P.M. and Rastinejad, F. (2004) Structural basis for the coordinated regulation of transglutaminase 3 by guanine nucleotides and calcium/magnesium. *Journal of biological chemistry*, 279, 7180.

[41] Kim, I.G., Gorman, J., Park, S.C., Chung, S. and Steinert, P. (1993) The deduced sequence of the novel protransglutaminase E (TGase3) of human and mouse. *Journal of Biological Chemistry*, 268, 12682.

[42] Uemura, N., Nakanishi, Y., Kato, H., Saito, S., Nagino, M., Hirohashi, S. and Kondo, T. (2009) Transglutaminase 3 as a prognostic biomarker in esophageal cancer revealed by proteomics. *International Journal of Cancer*, 124, 2106-2115.

[43] Liu, W., Yu, Z.C., Cao, W.F., Ding, F. and Liu, Z.H. (2006) Functional studies of a novel oncogene TGM3 in human esophageal squamous cell carcinoma. *World Journal of Gastroenterology*, 12, 3929.

[44] He, G., Zhao, Z., Fu, W., Sun, X., Xu, Z. and Sun, K. (2002) Study on the loss of heterozygosity and expression of transglutaminase 3 gene in laryngeal carcinoma]. *Zhonghua yi xue yi chuan xue za zhi= Zhonghua yixue yichuanxue zazhi= Chinese journal of medical genetics*, 19, 120.

[45] Gonzalez, H.E., Gujrati, M., Frederick, M., Henderson, Y., Arumugam, J., Spring, P.W., Mitsudo, K., Kim, H.W. and Clayman, G.L. (2003) Identification of 9 genes differentially expressed in head and neck squamous cell carcinoma. *Archives of Otolaryngology- Head and Neck Surgery*, 129, 754.

[46] Gutiérrez-González, L.H., Ludwig, C., Hohoff, C., Rademacher, M., Hanhoff, T., Rüterjans, H., Spener, F. and Lücke, C. (2002) Solution structure and backbone dynamics of human epidermal-type fatty acid-binding protein (E-FABP). *Biochemical Journal*, 364, 725.

[47] Palackal, N.T., Lee, S.H., Harvey, R.G., Blair, I.A. and Penning, T.M. (2002) Activation of Polycyclic Aromatic Hydrocarbontrans-Dihydrodiol Proximate Carcinogens by Human Aldo-keto Reductase (AKR1C) Enzymes and Their Functional Overexpression in Human Lung Carcinoma (A549) Cells. *Journal of Biological Chemistry*, 277, 24799.

[48] Strange, R.C., Spiteri, M.A., Ramachandran, S. and Fryer, A.A. (2001) Glutathione-S-transferase family of enzymes. *Mutation Research/Fundamental and Molecular Mechanisms of Mutagenesis*, 482, 21-26.

[49] Townsend, D.M. and Tew, K.D. (2003) The role of glutathione-S-transferase in anti-cancer drug resistance. *Oncogene*, 22, 7369-7375.

[50] Abbas, A., Delvinquière, K., Lechevrel, M., Lebailly, P., Gauduchon, P., Launoy, G. and Sichel, F. (2004) GSTM1, GSTT1, GSTP1 and CYP1A1 genetic polymorphisms and susceptibility to esophageal cancer in a French population: different pattern of squamous cell carcinoma and adenocarcinoma. *World J Gastroenterol*, 10, 3389-93.

[51] Li, Z., Zhang, R. and Luo, X. (2001) Expression of glutathione S-transferase-pi in human esophageal squamous cell carcinoma]. *Zhonghua zhong liu za zhi [Chinese journal of oncology]*, 23, 39.

[52] Du, X.L., Hu, H., Lin, D.C., Xia, S.H., Shen, X.M., Zhang, Y., Luo, M.L., Feng, Y.B., Cai, Y. and Xu, X. (2007) Proteomic profiling of proteins dysregulted in Chinese esophageal squamous cell carcinoma. *Journal of Molecular Medicine*, 85, 863-875.

[53] Tennant, D.A., Durán, R.V., Boulahbel, H. and Gottlieb, E. (2009) Metabolic transformation in cancer. *Carcinogenesis*, 30, 1269.

[54] Kamata, H. and Hirata, H. (1999) Redox regulation of cellular signalling. *Cellular signalling*, 11, 1-14.

[55] Klaunig, J.E. and Kamendulis, L.M. (2004) The role of oxidative stress in carcinogenesis. *Annu. Rev. Pharmacol. Toxicol.*, 44, 239-267.

[56] Neumann, C.A. and Fang, Q. (2007) Are peroxiredoxins tumor suppressors? *Current opinion in pharmacology*, 7, 375-380.

[57] Lee, A.S. (2007) GRP78 induction in cancer: therapeutic and prognostic implications. *Cancer research*, 67, 3496.

[58] Gelebart, P., Opas, M. and Michalak, M. (2005) Calreticulin, a Ca2+-binding chaperone of the endoplasmic reticulum. *The international journal of biochemistry & cell biology*, 37, 260-266.

[59] Parodi, A.J. (2000) Protein glucosylation and its role in protein folding. *Annual review of biochemistry*, 69, 69-93.

[60] Hammond, C. and Helenius, A. (1993) A chaperone with a sweet tooth. *Current biology: CB*, 3, 884.

[61] Molinari, M., Calanca, V., Galli, C., Lucca, P. and Paganetti, P. (2003) Role of EDEM in the release of misfolded glycoproteins from the calnexin cycle. *Science*, 299, 1397.

[62] Schrag, J.D., Procopio, D.O., Cygler, M., Thomas, D.Y. and Bergeron, J.J.M. (2003) Lectin control of protein folding and sorting in the secretory pathway. *Trends in biochemical sciences*, 28, 49-57.

[63] Oda, Y., Hosokawa, N., Wada, I. and Nagata, K. (2003) EDEM as an acceptor of terminally misfolded glycoproteins released from calnexin. *Science*, 299, 1394.

[64] Salicioni, A.M., Xi, M., Vanderveer, L.A., Balsara, B., Testa, J.R. and Dunbrack, R.L. (2000) Identification and Structural Analysis of Human RBM8A and RBM8B: Two Highly Conserved RNA-Binding Motif Proteins That Interact with OVCA1, a Candidate Tumor Suppressor* 1. *Genomics*, 69, 54-62.

[65] Zhang, L.Y., Ying, W.T., Mao, Y.S., He, H.Z., Liu, Y., Wang, H.X., Liu, F., Wang, K., Zhang, D.C. and Wang, Y. (2003) Loss of clusterin both in serum and tissue

correlates with the tumorigenesis of esophageal squamous cell carcinoma via proteomics approaches. *World Journal of Gastroenterology*, 9, 650-654.

[66] Battiste, J.L., Pestova, T.V., Hellen, C.U.T. and Wagner, G. (2000) The eIF1A solution structure reveals a large RNA-binding surface important for scanning function. *Molecular Cell*, 5, 109-119.

[67] Fekete, C.A., Mitchell, S.F., Cherkasova, V.A., Applefield, D., Algire, M.A., Maag, D., Saini, A.K., Lorsch, J.R. and Hinnebusch, A.G. (2007) N-and C-terminal residues of eIF1A have opposing effects on the fidelity of start codon selection. *The EMBO Journal*, 26, 1602-1614.

[68] Ozawa, M. and Muramatsu, T. (1993) Reticulocalbin, a novel endoplasmic reticulum resident Ca (2+)-binding protein with multiple EF-hand motifs and a carboxyl-terminal HDEL sequence. *Journal of biological chemistry*, 268, 699.

[69] Fukuda, T., Oyamada, H., Isshiki, T., Maeda, M., Kusakabe, T., Hozumi, A., Yamaguchi, T., Igarashi, T., Hasegawa, H. and Seidoh, T. (2007) Distribution and variable expression of secretory pathway protein reticulocalbin in normal human organs and non-neoplastic pathological conditions. *Journal of Histochemistry & Cytochemistry*, 55, 335.

[70] Urlin, V., Ioana, M. and Ple EA, I. (2011) Genetic patterns of metalloproteinases and their tissular inhibitors–clinicopathologic and prognostic significance in colorectal cancer. *Rom J Morphol Embryol*, 52, 231-236.

[71] Wilson, C.L., Heppner, K.J., Labosky, P.A., Hogan, B.L.M. and Matrisian, L.M. (1997) Intestinal tumorigenesis is suppressed in mice lacking the metalloproteinase matrilysin. *Proceedings of the National Academy of Sciences*, 94, 1402.

[72] Fingleton, B.M., Goss, K.J.H., Crawford, H.C. and Matrisian, L.M. (1999) Matrilysin in early stage intestinal tumorigenesis. *Apmis*, 107, 102-110.

[73] Murray, G.I., Duncan, M.E., O'Neil, P., McKay, J.A., Melvin, W.T. and Fothergill, J.E. (1998) Matrix metalloproteinase 1 is associated with poor prognosis in oesophageal cancer. *The Journal of pathology*, 185, 256-261.

[74] Yamamoto, H., Adachi, Y., Itoh, F., Iku, S., Matsuno, K., Kusano, M., Arimura, Y., Endo, T., Hinoda, Y. and Hosokawa, M. (1999) Association of matrilysin expression with recurrence and poor prognosis in human esophageal squamous cell carcinoma. *Cancer research*, 59, 3313.

[75] Porte, H., Triboulet, J.P., Kotelevets, L., Carrat, F., Prevot, S., Nordlinger, B., DiGioia, Y., Wurtz, A., Comoglio, P. and Gespach, C. (1998) Overexpression of stromelysin-3, BM-40/SPARC, and MET genes in human esophageal carcinoma: implications for prognosis. *Clinical cancer research*, 4, 1375.

[76] Yamashita, K., Tanaka, Y., Mimori, K., Inoue, H. and Mori, M. (2004) Differential expression of MMP and uPA systems and prognostic relevance of their expression in esophageal squamous cell carcinoma. *International Journal of Cancer*, 110, 201-207.

[77] Ohashi, K., Nemoto, T., Nakamura, K. and Nemori, R. (2000) Increased expression of matrix metalloproteinase 7 and 9 and membrane type 1 matrix metalloproteinase in esophageal squamous cell carcinomas. *Cancer*, 88, 2201-2209.

[78] Fingleton, B. and Matrisian, L.M. (2001) Matrix metalloproteinases in cancer. *Matrix metalloproteinase inhibitors in cancer therapy*, 85–112.

[79] Suminami, Y., Kishi, F., Sekiguchi, K. and Kato, H. (1991) Squamous cell carcinoma antigen is a new member of the serine protease inhibitors. *Biochemical and biophysical research communications*, 181, 51-58.

[80] Schneider, S.S., Schick, C., Fish, K.E., Miller, E., Pena, J.C., Treter, S.D., Hui, S.M. and Silverman, G.A. (1995) A serine proteinase inhibitor locus at 18q21. 3 contains a tandem duplication of the human squamous cell carcinoma antigen gene. *Proceedings of the National Academy of Sciences*, 92, 3147.

[81] Kato, H., Suehiro, Y., Morioka, H., Torigoe, T., Myoga, A., Sekiguchi, K. and Ikeda, I. (1987) Heterogeneous distribution of acidic TA-4 in cervical squamous cell carcinoma: immunohistochemical demonstration with monoclonal antibodies. *Japanese journal of cancer research: Gann*, 78, 1246.

[82] Thun, M.J., Henley, S.J. and Patrono, C. (2002) Nonsteroidal anti-inflammatory drugs as anticancer agents: mechanistic, pharmacologic, and clinical issues. *Journal of the National Cancer Institute*, 94, 252.

[83] Corcoran, C.A., He, Q., Huang, Y. and Sheikh, M.S. (2004) Cyclooxygenase-2 interacts with p53 and interferes with p53-dependent transcription and apoptosis. *Oncogene*, 24, 1634-1640.

[84] Tanaka, K., Hatada, T., Kobayashi, M., Mohri, Y., Tonouchi, H., Miki, C., Nobori, T. and Kusunoki, M. (2004) The clinical implication of 14-3-3 sigma expression in primary gastrointestinal malignancy. *International journal of oncology*, 25, 1591-1597.

[85] Nishimori, T., Tomonaga, T., Matsushita, K., Oh Ishi, M., Kodera, Y., Maeda, T., Nomura, F., Matsubara, H., Shimada, H. and Ochiai, T. (2006) Proteomic analysis of primary esophageal squamous cell carcinoma reveals downregulation of a cell adhesion protein, periplakin. *Proteomics*, 6, 1011-1018.

5

The Interaction Between the Metabolism of Retinol and Ethanol in Esophageal Mucosa – A Possible Mechanism of Esophageal Cancer in Alcoholics

Hirokazu Yokoyama, Haruko-Shiraishi Yokoyama and Toshifumi Hibi
Department of Internal Medicine, Keio University
Japan

1. Introduction

It has been well established that excessive ethanol consumption is associated with an increased risk of cancers in various organs (Bann et al. 2007). It is estimated that alcohol consumption accounts for 3.6% of all cancer cases and 3.5% of cancer deaths in the world (Boffetta et al. 2006). However, the mechanisms by which ethanol causes cancer remains obscure.

Recently, aberrant statuses of retinoids, which are structurally and/or functionally related to vitamin A (retinol), have been implicated in the pathogenesis of some types of cancers. It is well established that, at least in natural conditions, retinoic acids (RAs) are mainly responsible for retinoid actions among various retinoids. A current consensus is that RAs are supplied via retinol metabolisms *in vivo.*

Both retinol and ethanol are types of alcohol. Thus, features of their metabolic pathways are similar to each other. The aim of this chaper is to summarize the latest knowledge on the supply pathway of RA *in vivo* and that on carcinogenesis due to short supply of RA. Moreover, we recently suggested that *in situ* RA supply was disturbed by ethanol metabolism in esophageal mucosa, and hypothesized that this could account for the pathogenesis of esophageal cancer seen in alcoholics. In this chapter, we also discussed how this hypothesis could be fit to the clinical characteristics of esophageal cancer seen in alcoholics. Since many of the views introduced in this chapter are obtained from animal models, we must interpret them carefully. However, we believe that most of these views are fully applicable for clinical cases.

2. Cancers in heavy drinkers and their characteristics

2.1 Organ specificities in cancers related to ethanol consumption

Many reports suggest that ethanol consumption could be a risk factor for malignancies of multiple organs (Alcohol and Cancer- Widipeda, http://en.wikipedia.org/wiki/ Alcohol_ and_ cancer). However, the current consensus, established by a meeting of the International Agency for Research on Cancer (IARC) in 2007, is as follows: Alcohol beverages are definitely carcinogenic to humans and they contribute to the development of human cancers in the oral cavity, pharynx, larynx, esophagus, liver, colorectum, and the female breast, but they are not related to the development of human renal cell cancer and non-Hodgkins lymphoma (Bann et al. 2007). Currently, it is acceptable to assume that alcoholic beverages could be carcinogenic but there are apparent organ specific susceptibilities to the carcinogenicity of ethanol, and the esophagus is one of these susceptive organs.

2.2 Genetic variations and cancers related to ethanol consumption

Imbibed ethanol is metabolized mainly by an NAD-dependent mechanism *in vivo*. In this pathway, ethanol is oxidized to acetaldehyde, which is further oxidized to acetate (Lieber 1984). This process is performed mainly in the liver where alcohol dehydrognease 1 (ADH1), comprising ADH1A, 1B, and 1C, is responsible for ethanol oxidation to acetaldehyde and aldehyde dehydrogenase 2 (ALDH2) is responsible for acetaldehyde oxidation to acetate. Among these enzymes, genetic variations of ADH1C and ALDH2 are known to affect ethanol metabolism. ADH1C includes two polymorphisms i.e., ADH1C*1 and ADH1C*2, encoding $\gamma 1$ and $\gamma 2$ subunits, respectively. The Kcat values for ethanol of $\gamma 1\gamma 1$ and $\gamma 2\gamma 2$ isoforms were shown to be 87 min^{-1} and 35 min^{-1}, respectively (Bosron and Li, 1987), indicating that the former catalyzes ethanol faster than the latter, such that the former produces larger amounts of acetaldehyde than the latter during a constant period when they encounter the same amount of ethanol. On the other hand, ALDH2 also includes two distinct polymorphisms i.e. ALDH2*1 and ALDH2*2, and the latter encodes a variant subunit of ALDH2 lacking catalytic activity for acetaldehyde. This variant is often seen in Asians but is rare in other races (Goedde, 1992). Most homozygous carriers of this allele are non-drinkers, since they can not oxidize acetaldehyde and can not complete ethanol metabolism *in vivo*. Thus, they are hardly exposed to the harmful effects associated with ethanol consumption including carcinogenesis. Heterozygous carriers of ALDH 2*1 / 2*2, who account for around 40% of the population in some Asian countries, including Japan, can consume alcohol beverages. However, since the catalytic activity for acetaldehyde in the heterozygous carriers is around 10% of that of homozygous carriers of ALDH2*1/2*1 (Thomasson et al. 1993), significant acetaldehyde accumulation, of which symptoms are represented by the flushing phenomenon, occurs after drinking. Importantly, the risks of several cancers, including esophageal cancer seen in alcoholics, have been reported to be higher in alcoholics having the variant ADH1C*1 (Homann et al. 2006) and ALDH2*2 (Yokoyama et al. 1996). However, contradictory findings have also been published for the ADH1C*1 variant (Brennan et al. 2004) and a consensus statement of a meeting of IARC in 2007 only accepted a higher risk of cancer in subjects with the ALDH2*2 variant (Bann et al. 2007). At any rate, genetic differences in ethanol-oxidizing enzymes, which alter *in vivo* acetaldehyde levels after drinking affect the inceidence of cancers in alcoholics.

2.3 Field cancerization in cancer related to ethanol consumption

The concept of field cancerization has been recognized. Namely, during the development of some cancers, such as that in aerodigestive organs, some genetic alterations which are peculiar to cancer cells occur not only in cancer cells, but also in non-cancer cells adjacent to the malignant tumor, or in advanced pre-malignant lesions in cancer-free patients (Hong et al. 1995). Alteration of the p53 gene and accumulation of its protein are typical observations seen in field cancerization (Shin et al. 1994). The fact that a mutated p53 protein has a longer half-life compared to that of wild-type p53 may account for its accumulation (Gao et al. 1994). The field cancerization has been confirmed in human esophageal mucosa (Gao et al. 1994), and furthermore, in that of alcoholics (Yokoyama et al. 2011). Namely, it is fully expected that esophageal cancer develops in a manner of field concerization in some alcoholcs..

2.4 Animal models of cancers related to ethanol consumption

There are several lines of animal models demonstrating the carcinogenicity of ethanol, however, in most models, cancers were produced by the combination of ethanol and other carcinogens. Notably, Sofferitti et al. demonstrated that the administration of 10% ethanol ad libitum for 104-152 weeks alone could produce cancers in Sprague-Dawley rats, including breeders and offspring. They demonstrated that ethanol consumption increased the risk of head and neck cancers. However, other cancers, which were induced by this model, were different from those seen in human alcoholics, for example, interstitial cell adenocarcinoma of the testis, Sertoli cell tumor in the ovary, uterus carcinoma, pheochromoblastoma, and head osteosarcoma (Soffritti et al. 2002). Moreover, at least in their model, ethanol administration did not affect the incidence of cancers of the esophagus, lung, colorectum, breast, and liver, which are now regarded as related to ethanol consumption in humans (Bann et al. 2007). These observations indicate that ethanol is also carcinogenic in the rat, however, the features are different from those in humans. There seems to be strain specific susceptibilities to the carcinogenicity of imbibed ethanol. On the other hand, one paper demosntrated that the administration of acetaldehyde vapour produced various lesions in the respiratory epithelium including squamous metaplasia and squamous cell carcinoma (Feron et al. 1986).

3. *In vivo* dynamics of vitamin A for the production of RA

Molecules which are structurally and/or functionally related to vitamin A (retinol) are called retinoids. Presently, over 4000 retinoids including natural and synthetic ones have been identified. They are biologically important since they participate in the regulation of various phenomenon of life. Since mammals can not synthesize retinoids *in vivo,* they must take them from foods. The current consensus is that the effects of retinoids are mainly attributable to retinoic acids (RAs). In spite of the large demands for RAs in tissues, its serum level has been reported to be just 2-3 ng/ml (Moulas et al., 2006). This level was too low to satisfy all *in vivo* demands, suggesting the existence of a compensatory supply system *in situ*. And, recently, it became clear as to how RAs were produced from retinol *in situ.* The following is a summary of recent knowledge as to *in vivo* retinoid dynamics.

3.1 Absorption, storage, and delivery of retinol to a target cell

Food contains retinol, retinyl ester, and β-carotene, which are absorbed in the small intestine. When intestinal epithelial cells absorb retinyl esters, they are converted into retinol via retinyl ester hydrolase (REH) *in situ*. β-carotene is cleaved to retinal via β–β–carotene-15,15′ monooxygenase and the retinal formed is converted into retinol via retinol dehydrogenase. Retinol, then, binds to celluar retinol binding protein (CRBP), which contributes to the stabilization of retinol and its solubilization in the aqueous phase. In turn, this complex is converted to retinyl esters via lecithin retinol acetyltransferase (LRAT). Retinyl esters formed are released into blood vessels and transported to the liver. In hepatocytes, retinyl esters are converted into retinol via REH, and the retinol forms a retinol-CRBP complex with CRBP. A part of this complex is transported to hepatic stellate cells, which are major storage sites of retinol *in vivo*. There, the retinol-CRBP complex is converted to retinyl esters again via LRAT for storage. Upon *in vivo* requests for retinol, they are converted back to the retinol-CRBP complex via REH, which is returned to the hepatocytes. Recently, Bcmo1, an enzyme, which participates in β-carotene metabolism, was shown to be highly expressed in hepatic stellate cells, suggesting that they also contribute to β-carotene metabolism (Shmarakov 2010). Further studies are necessary to clarify the significance of this enzyme in stellate cells. In hepatocytes, CRBP of the retinol-CRBP complex is converted to serum retinol-binding protein (sRBP or RBP4). The retinol-RBP4 complex is released from the liver into blood vessels, and is delivered to retinoid target cells. In blood vessels, transthyretin (TTR) binds to the retinol-RBP complex, preventing efflux of the complex from the kidney. These features are summarized in Figure 1.

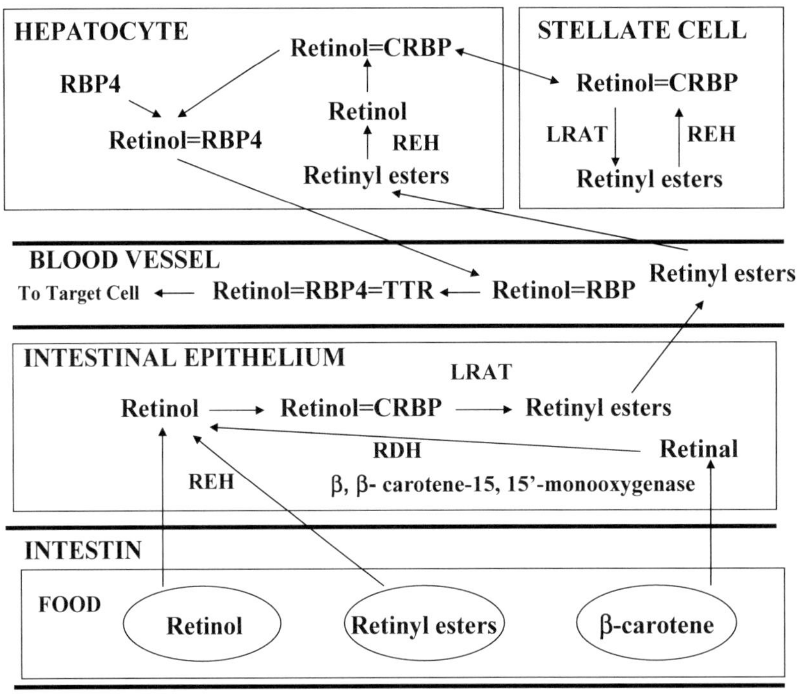

Retinol, retinyl esters, and β-carotene in food are absorbed mainly by the small intestine and stored in hepatic stellate cells. Retinol binds to retinol binding protein (RBP) -4 in the liver and transthyretin (TTR) in blood vessels and is delivered to target cells. [CRBP; cellular retinol binding protein, RDH; retinol dehydrogenase LRAT; lecithin retinol acetyltransferase, REH; retinyl ester hydrolase]

Fig. 1. Absorption, storage, and delivery to a target cell of retinol.

3.2 RA formation from retinol in RA target cell

A cell which requires RA, namely a RA target cell usually expresses a receptor for RBP4, named "stimulated by retinoic acid 6 (STRA6)", on its surface and their combination allows for the retinol-RBP4-TTR complex to bind to the cell curface. From the complex, the cell incorporates only retinol by the action of LRAT. A part of free retinol binds to CRBP, forming a retinol-CRBP complex in the cell. Since the CRBP-1 gene has a binding site for RAR-α at its promoter region, it may be up-regulated by RA, suggesting that the protein contributes to retinol storage when RA is over supplied in the cell. On the other hand, free retinol is converted to RA via a two step oxidation process in which retinol is first oxidized to retinal via retinol dehydrogenase (RDH), and is then oxidized to RA via retinal dehydrogenase (RalDH). The formed RA binds to a cellular RA binding protein (CRABP), which may contribute to RA storage in the cell. The formation of a RA-CRABP complex may also facilitate the migration of RA from the cytosol into the nucleus, and the formation of RA-RA receptor complex binding to RA target genes. Free RA is further catalyzed to 4-hydroxyl-retinoic acid (4-OH-RA), 18-hydroxy-retinoic acid (18-OHRA), 4-oxo-retinoic acid ((4-oxo-RA), and 5,6-epoxy-retinoic acid (5,6-epoxy-RA) in the cell via Cyp26A, B, and C, enzymes of a P450 familiy. Among these RA metabolites, 4-oxo-RA has been shown to have RA activity (Baron et al.). These features are summarized in Figure 2.

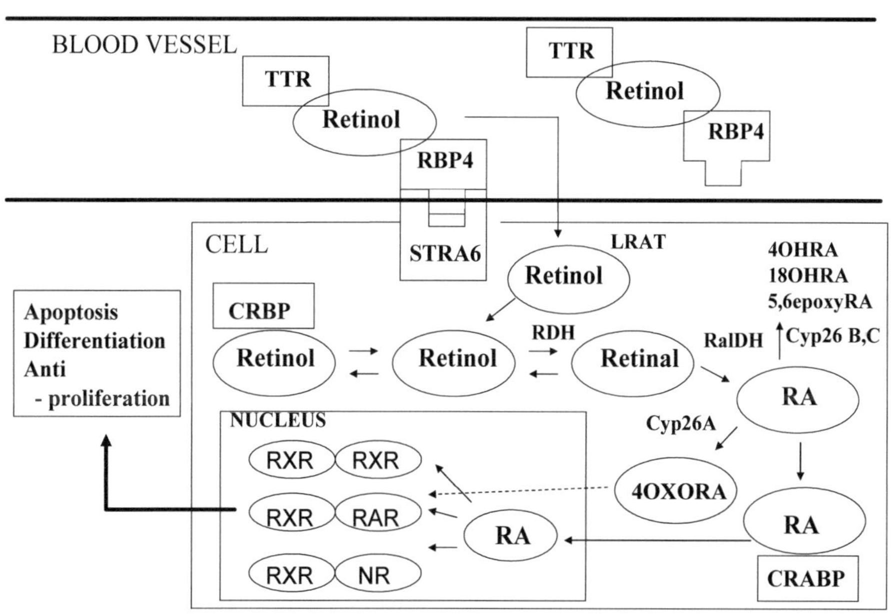

A cell incorporates retinol from a Retinol-RBP4-TTR complex in blood vessels via STRA6. Retinol is metabolized to retinoic acid (RA) via a two step oxidation process. RA binds to a cellular retinoic acid binding protein (CRABP), and is transferred into the nucleus, when it exhibits its action. 4-oxo-RA, a metabolite of RA, may also have a RA effect. [CRBP; cellular retinol binding protein, RDH; retinol dehydrogenase RalDH; retinal dehydrogenase, RBP4; retinol binding protein 4, TTR; transthyretin, LRAT; lecithin retinol acetyltransferase]

Fig. 2. Retinoic acid formation from retinol in a retinoic acid target cell.

4. RA and gene expression

4.1 RA receptors

When RA is transported into the nucleus, it binds to RA receptors which usually bind to the promoter regions of RA target genes. They comprise two classes, i.e. retinoic acid receptors (RAR) and retinoid X receptors (RXR), and each comprises three subtypes designated as α, β, γ, respectively. Furthermore, each subtype has several isoforms, namely two isoforms of RARα (α1, α2), five isoforms of RARβ (β1–β4 and β1′), two isoforms of RARγ (γ1, γ2), and two isoforms of RXRα (α1, α2), two isoforms of RXRβ (β1, β2), and two isoforms of RXRγ (γ1, γ2). RARs have affinity to *all-trans* and *9-cis* RA, and RXRs have affinity to *9-cis* RA. They show cDNA sequence homology with receptors of vitamin D, glucocorticoid, and estrogen. RXR can form homodimers with RXR and heterodimers with RAR. Furthermore, RXR can form heterodimers with peroxisomal proliferation activated receptors (PPAR), farnesoid X receptors (FXR), liver X receptors (LXR), pregnant X receptors (PXR), constitutive androstane receptors (CAR), and vitamin D receptors (VDR). In these cases, RA, especially *9-cis* RA, may regulate gene expression with the other regulators which are originally required by partner receptors, namely fatty acid, bile acid, oxysterol, some xenobiotics, vitamin D, and their analogs, except for the cases where RXR is non-functional. Notably, the RXR-RXR homodimer was shown to activate PPARs (Ijpenberg et al.2004)

4.2 Gene regulation by RA

RA regulates gene transcription via multiple mechanisms. The simplest way is that RA directly affects transcription of the target gene via RA receptors. The hetero- or homo- dimer of RA receptors, i.e., RXR-RXR, RAR-RAR, or RXR-RAR, binds to the RA DNA Response Element (the specific sequence of GGTTCA(N5)AGTTCA, RARE), usually located at the promoter region of the target gene. When RA and co-activators, such as the pCIP/p300 complex, binds to the dimer, gene transcription starts under the presence of RNA polymerase II. This condition is schematically illustrated in Figure 3.

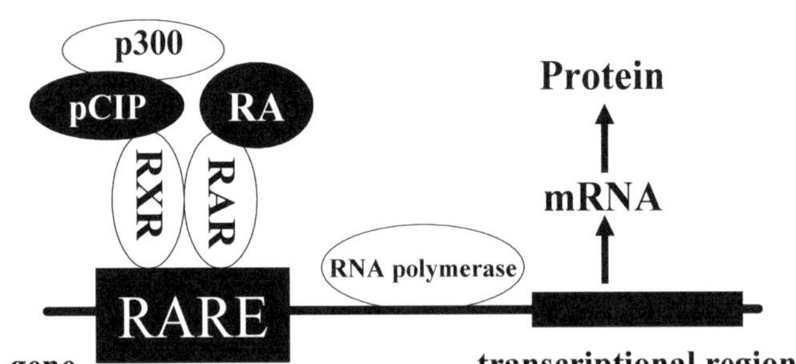

When RA binds to RARE, located at the 5′ region of a gene via RA receptors, gene transcription starts. For this event, co-activators, such as a pCIP/p300 complex and RNA polymerase II, are required.

Fig. 3. Regulation of gene transcription by RA (1).

There are several lines of evidence to suggest that the functions of RARs are also regulated by their phosphorylation statuses. The enzymes responsible for their phosporylation processes remain obscure. However, observations suggest that regulation of gene transcription by RA is not a simple event in such a simple model. The identification of enzymes responsible for this process will provide further information as to how RAs regulate gene expressions.

Sometimes, RA can regulate the expression of some genes lacking RARE. Namely, RA regulates the expression of a transcriptional factor, such as Hox1, which regulates that of another gene, as illustrated in Figure 4.

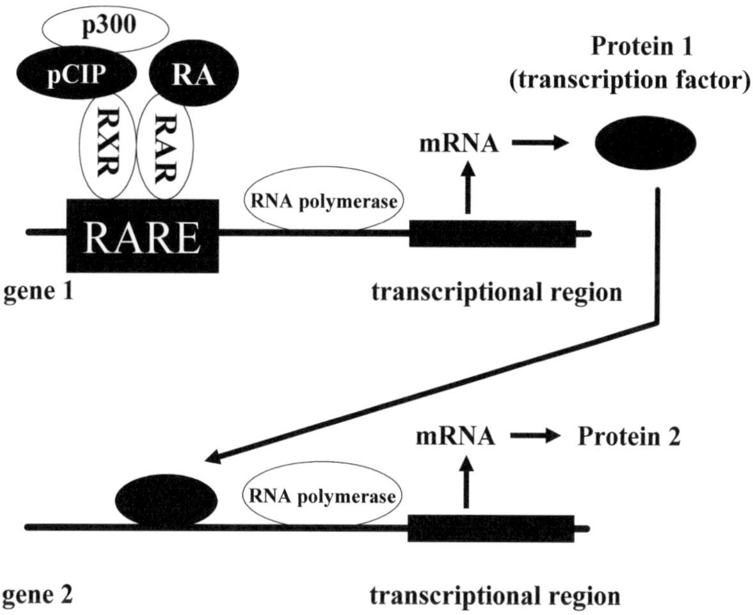

Some transcriptional factors are produced from some RA-regulated genes (gene 1). When the transcriptional factor binds to the binding site on another gene (gene 2), its transcription starts and protein 2 is produced. In this case, protein 2 is thought to be RA regulated.

Fig. 4. Regulation of gene transcription by RA (2).

The transcription of some genes is regulated by polycomb group proteins (PcG, Simon and Kingston 2009). Although it is still unclear how PcGs recognize their specific sites on DNA, they bind to some regions on their target gene. In this situation, co-activators, such as the pCIP/p300 protein, can not bind to retinoid receptors binding to the gene, and gene translation does not occur. Gillespie and Gudas demonstrated that RA regulates this PcGs-DNA binding. Namely, when RA binds to the RAR-RXR complex, which binds to RARE sometimes located at the 3′ region of the gene, PcGs are removed from the gene, facilitating the binding of the gene co-activator(s), starting gene transcription (Figure 5). They demonstrated that the RARγ–RXR-RA complex exclusively exhibits such an action, but not others. Expressions of Cyp26a1, and RARβ2 are known to be controlled in this way (Gillespie and Gudas 2007).

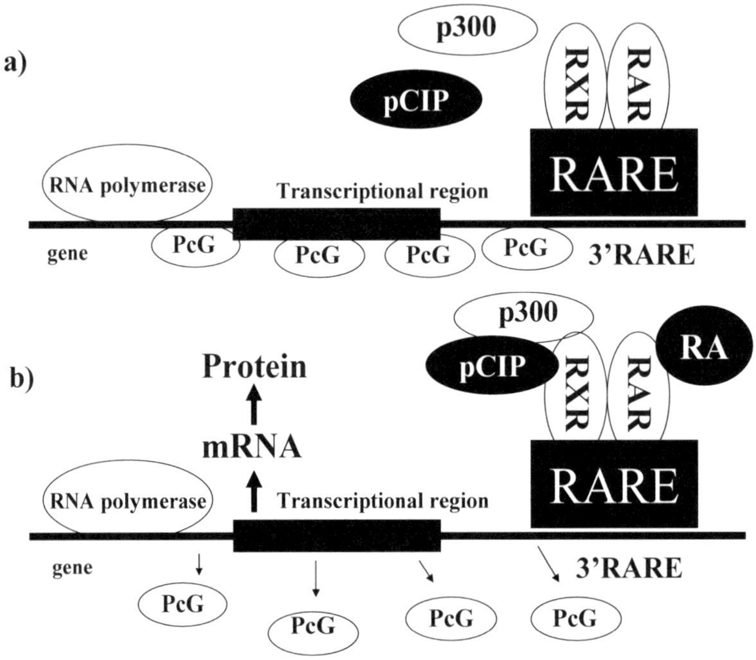

Transcription of some genes is regulated by RA via the polycomb group proteins (PcGs) status. In such a gene, transcription does not occur without RA since PcGs binding to the gene inhibit its transcription (a). However, when RA makes a complex with its receptor, and the complex binds to the RARE of the gene which is usually located at its 3′ region, PcGs are removed from the gene, allowing the binding of co-factors to the gene via the retinoid receptor, and its transcription starts (b). (modified from a figure from Gillespie and Gudas 2007)

Fig. 5. Regulation of gene transcription by RA via PcGs.

5. Retinoids and cancer

When vitamin A, a major source of RAs, is depleted, metaplasia of squamous cells occurs (Harris et al. 1972,Lotan et al. 1993). In clinical cases, vitamin A deficiency has been implicated in the development of esophageal cancer (Mellow et al. 1983). *In vitro* studies clearly demonstrated that retinoids inhibit cell proliferation of normal cells (Lee et al. 1995). The current consensus is that normal differentiation and proliferation of the cell are spoiled when intercellular homeostasis of retinoids is disturbed (Zou et al. 1994). Apparently, an abnormal retinoid status is related to carcinogenesis. Therefore, it is not surprising that the administration of retinoid prevents the development of squamous cell carcinoma in the skin, oral cavity, and lung in animal models (Moon et al. 1994). Notably, some synthetic retinoids were reported to be effective in preventing the development of esophageal cancer from severe esophageal squamous dysplasia (Han 1993).

Retinoids also act against malignant cells. They suppress the growth rate of various tumor cells including melanoma, neuroblastoma, glioma, retinoblastoma, embryonal carcinoma, lymphoma, leukemia, myeloma, various sarcoma, as well as cancers of the breast, prostate, bladder, colon, head and neck, and cervix. Most malignancies develop based on the complicated accumulation of various events including genetic alterations, dysregulation of cell growth, abnormal cell differentiation, and changes in the phenotype and cell function. Retinoids may be involved in all of these steps and usually exhibit anti-cancer effects.

5.1 Retinoids and apoptosis

It is well established that retinoids induce apoptosis and cell cycle arrest in some malignant cells. *All-trans* retinoic acid (ATRA) has been known to produce p53 dependent apoptosis in promyelocytic leukemia HL-60 cells (Noguchi et al. 1995). Moreover, a synthetic retinoid up-regulated the expression of p21 (WAF1/CP1), Bax, and Killer/DR5, resulting in cell-cycle arrest of the G1 phase and apoptosis in human non-small cell lung cancer cell. These phenomena were observed only in cell lines having a wild type of p53, but not in those with mutant p53, indicating that they were p53 dependent (Sun et al. 1999a). On the other hand, retinoids were shown to produce cell-cycle arrest of the G0/G1 phase and apoptosis in a p53 independent manner in human breast cancer cells (Shao et al. 1995). Apoptosis due to retinoids via the BCL2 pathway in orbital fibroblasts (Pasquali et al. 2003), via caspase-3 in esophageal squamous cells (Wan et al. 2001), and via CPP32-like caspase in lung non-small cell carcinoma (Sun et al. 1999b) have been also demonstrated. In addition, c-Myc and its downstream genes have been shown to be involved in apoptosis caused by a synthetic retinoid in human lung cancer cell (Sun et al. 1999c). The mitogen-activated protein kinase (MAPKs) pathway is now recognized as an important cascade regulating the expressions of various genes related to apoptosis and cell proliferation. RA also activates MEK-dependent ERK2, a member of the MAPK family, and subsequent RB hypophosphorylation, resulting in cell differentiation and G0 arrest in the myeloid leukemia cell line (Yen et al. 1998).

Obviously, retinoids have the potential to produce apoptosis in various cells, resulting in the reduction of cell growth. Thus, it is fully conceivable that an RA deficiency causes the reduction of cellular apoptosis, which may cause carcinogenesis. Although the mechanisms as to how retinoid causes apoptosis have not been unified, differences in experimental conditions, including characteristics of target cells, structures of retinoids used, and amounts of retinoids used, may account, at least in part, for this complexity.

5.2 Retinoids and cell differentiation

Retinoids maintain proper differentiation in normal cells at physiological doses as well as restore demolished regulation of differentiation and/or cell growth of certain malignant or pre-malignant cells at pharmacological doses. At any rate, they usually enhance cell differentiation (Gudas et al. 1994). RA signals via RAR-β2 seem to be responsible for the maintenance of normal cell differentiation in epithelial cells. RAR-β2 signals are known to suppress the expression of EGFR (or ErbB-1). Thus, its reduction causes over expression of EGFR and its downstream proteins comprising activating protein-1 (AP-1) and COX-2, resulting in the disturbance of normal cell differentiation. The RAR-β2 signals are also known to attenuate the phosphorylation of extracellular signal-regulated protein kinases 1 and 2 (Erk1/2), contributing to the down-regulation of AP-1 in esophageal cancer cells (Li et al. 2002). Recently, a new protein named retinoid receptor induced gene 1 (RRIG1), mediating the anticancer effects of RAR-β2, was cloned from esophageal cells. When its expression is maintained, the expression of RhoA and its downstream proteins including

Cyclin D1, the phosphorylation of Erk1/2, and COX-2 are suppressed. RhoA also causes f-actin formation which induces colony formation, invasion, and proliferation of cells. Suppression of RhoA is required to keep these malignant characteristics in stationary states. When RRGI1 expression is attenuated using its antisense mRNA, these malignant characteristics were induced in esophageal squamous cancer cell lines (Liang et al. 2006).

Preservation of cell-cell communication is an important characteristic for maintaining normal cell differentiation. Retinoids induce expression of connexin 43, a gap junction protein, contributing to the meintenance of cell-cell communication (Rogers et al. 1990). Retinoids also participate in the maintenance of gene expression of various extracellular matrix proteins, including integrins, lamminin (Ross et al. 1994), and hyaluronic acid (Kim et al. 2010) to prevent the transformation of normal cells. RA signals via RAR-β may participate in the expression of several cell adhesion proteins, such as LSAMP which has anti cancer effects, and PCDH11Y which guides normal development (Wallden et al. 2005).

5.3 Retinoids and anti cancer effect via immunity

Retinoids also exhibit anti tumor effects via immunological mechanisms. Treatment of tumors with ATRA resulted in increased sensitivity to CTL and NK-cell-mediated lysis via MHC class I (Santin et al. 1998, Thompson et al. 2006). ATRA administration was shown to enhance apoptosis induced by IFN-γ in human glioblastoma cells. IFN-γ causes expression of HLA class II and HLA-DM molecules, and expression levels become higher when cells are treated with ATRA. Apparently, ATRA contributes to the production of apoptosis via the class II-mediated immune system (Haque et al. 2007). Recently, upregulation of HER2 (or ErbB-2) is implicated in the carcinogenesis of some cancers. IFNγ is known to downregulate HER2 oncoprotein p185 and this may be an event explaining the anti cancer effect of IFNγ. Ou et al. demonstrated that IFNγ induces the expression of RRIG1, which is responsible for the downregulation of the HER2 oncoprotein p185 in ovarian cancer cells. Thus, retinoids, which are essential factors for maintaining RRIG1 expression, should be important in exhibiting the anti-cancer effect of IFNγ (Ou et al. 2008). Retinoids exhibit anti cancer effects not only via ErbB-1, as shonw in section 5.2, but also ErbB-2.

RA signals via RAR-β2 have been shown to increase the expression of tumor cell antigens, such as CTAG1, CTAG2, and those of RIG-1/DDX58, responsible for the innate immune response (Wallden et al. 2005). From this viewpoint, retinoids are also indispensable for the anti cancer effect via immunity.

5.4 Lack of RAR-β2 expression and carcinogenesis

There is no doubt that RA has anticancer effects, however, some cancers exhibit RA resistance (Lippman and Davis 1997). Although the mechanisms behind this phenomenon are still obscure, the role of RAR-β2, one of the RA receptor, is of major interest, recently. The importance of RAR-β2 signals for anti cancer effects are mentioned in section 5.2 and 5.3, and recently, the relationship between suppression of RAR-β2 expression and RA resistance was demonstrated in various cell lines established from cancers in the kidney, esophagus, lung, breast, and prostate. Importantly, when RAR-β2 cDNA is compulsorily expressed using an adequate vector in cancer cells lacking RAR-β2 expression and acquiring RA resistance, they regain RA sensitivities (Houle et al. 1993). Furthermore, when COX-2, a downstream protein of RAR-β2, was reduced in esophageal cancer cells exhibiting RA resistance, they recovered RA sensitivity (Song et al. 2005). On the other hand, when RAR-β2 expression was compulsorily suppressed by its antisense, lung cancer developed in mice (Berard et al.1996).

In clinical cases, the reduction of RAR-β2 was observed in cancers of head and neck, esophagus, lung, breast, pancreas, cervix, and prostate. Interestingly, a lack of RXR-β expression is also observed in pre-malignant lesions in the oral cavity (Lotan et al. 1995) and the bronchus (Xu et al. 1999), as well as in morphologically normal cells adjacent to cancer cells (Widschwendter et al. 1997). It can be assumed that the alteration of RAR-β expression status is involved in the neoplastic transformation from normal cells, and these aspects are consistent with the concept of field cancerization which was mentioned in section 2.3. As also mentioned in section 2.3, where one of characteristic features of field cancerization is the accumulation of mutant p53 not only in malignant cells, but also in pre-malignant lesions. The reduction of RAR-β2 has been also implicated in the accumulation of mutant p53 in some cancers. The accumulation of p53 in pre-malignant lesions in the oral cavity has been shown to be correlated with RA resistance, possibly due to a lack of RAR–β up-regulation (Lippman et al. 1997). Moreover, immortalized dysplastic cells of oral mucosa have been reported to be characterized by the accumulation of mutation p53, induction of hTERT mRNA, and a lack of RAR-β2 and p16 expression (McGregor et al.1997). Consequently, the same group concluded that the lack of RAR-β2 and p16 expression are the only essential factors for this transformation process among these events, at least for their model (Muntoni et al. 2003).

Clinically, the preservation of RAR-β2 expression is associated with a higher efficacy in RA treatment of premalignant lesions in oral mucosa (Lotan et al. 1995), and also with a better prognosis in neuroblastoma cases (Cheung et al. 1998).

The mechanisms which lie behind the reduction in RAR-β2 expression still remain obscure. In a lung cancer cell line lacking RAR-β2 expression, deletion of chromosome 3p, a site responsible for RAR-β2, was observed (Geradts et al. 1993). However, this seems to be a rare case. On the other hand, Lin et al. found that the orphan receptor COUP-TF was essential for RAR-β2 expression and the lack of COUP-TF caused a reduction in RAR-B2 expression in some cancers (Lin et al 2000). A recently prevailing view is that the lack of RAR-β2 is attributed to epigenetic mechanisms, namely the unusual methylation status of the RAR-β2 gene, and the aberrant acetylation or phosphorylation of the histone wrapping the gene (Widschwendter et al. 2000, Lewis et al. 2005, Bean et al. 2005). In addition, Lefebvre et al. have demonstrated that an alteration of the PI3K/Akt signaling pathway is involved in the abnormal phosphorylation of the RAR-β2 histone, resulting in the loss of RAR-β2 expression in the cell (Lefebvre et al. 2006).

Importantly, the genes of RAR-β2 and RRIG1 constituting the RAR-β2 pathway, are RA inducible genes. The fact that the expression of RAR-β2 is regulated by RA via PcGs is mentioned in section 4.2. This suggests that cellular RA levels affect the expression of RAR-β2 levels and the status of its downstream proteins. The reduction in RAR-β2 expression has been demonstrated in some tissues of rats fed with vitamin A deficient diet (Verma et al. 1992). Moreover, Xu et al. found that intercellular RA levels were lower in premalignant lesions of human oral mucosa compared to normal ones (Xu et al. 1995). These observations support the view that an RA deficiency causes the reduction in RAR-β2 expression, which is closely related to carcinogenesis. (This section (5.4) was written referring to the review of Xu et al., 2007).

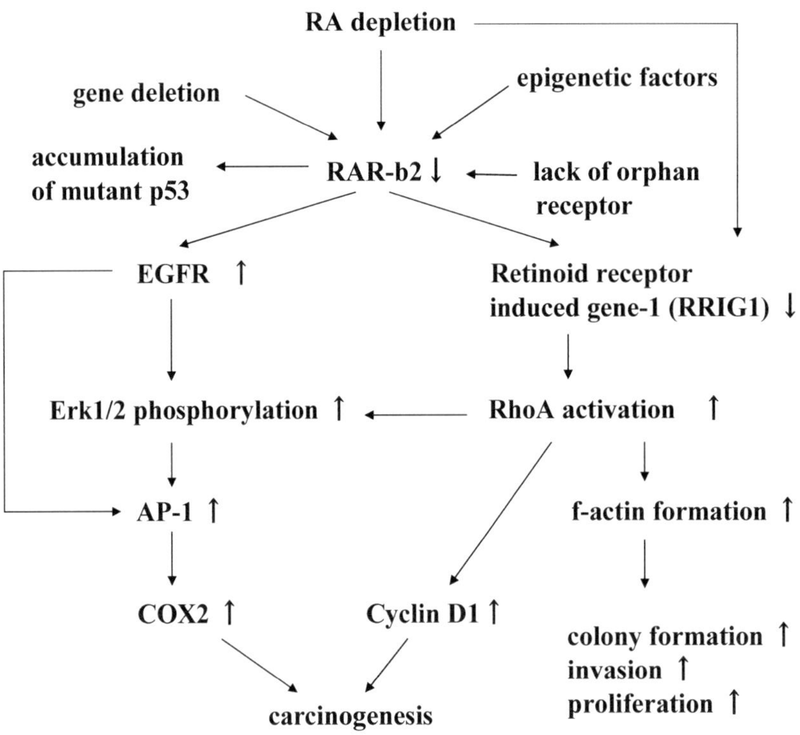

Reduction in RAR-β2 is now assumed to be closely related to carcinogenesis in some organs. In addition, the reduction of RAR-β2 is also implicated in the accumulation of mutant P53, which is often observed in some cancer cells and their premalignant regions. Multiple factors may affect RAR-β2 expression. Since RAR-β2 and RRIG1 are RA inducible genes, RA depletion is expected to reduce their expression, changing the features of their downstream proteins. A decrease in the RAR–β2 signal increases expression of EGFR, and phosporylation of Erk1/2, resulting in an increase in the expressions of AP-1 and COX-2. It also decreases the expressions of RRIG1, resulting in increases in RhoA and Cyclin D1. An increase in RohA also causes Erk1/2 phosphorylation and COX2 activation. These changes cause carcinogenesis. In addition, RhoA is implicated in the activation of f-actin formation, resulting in colony formation, proliferation, and invasion of cells. (modified from a figure from Xu et al. 2007)

Fig. 6. Possible mechanisms for the development of cancer by RA depletion via a reduction in RAR-β2 expression.

6. Structural and functional features of *the in situ* RA supply system in esophageal mucosa and its implication with the clinical aspects of esophageal cancer in alcoholics

As mentioned above, RAs are produced from vitamin A (retinol) in RA target cells *in situ* via a two step oxidation process, namely retinol is oxidized to retinal, a type of aldehyde, then retinal is oxidized to RA, a type of acid. The structural feature of this pathway is fundamentally the same as that of ethanol metabolism, in which ethanol is oxidized to acetaldehyde, a type of aldehyde, then acetaldehyde is oxidized to acetate, a type of acid. It is well established that the former pathway comprises retinol dehydrogenase (RDH) and retinal dehydrogenase (RalDH), and the latter alcohol dehydrogenase (ADH) and aldehydedehydrogenase (ALDH).

6.1 Cloning of cDNA and gene of ADH7

Notably, there are several enzymes that have affinity for both retinol and ethanol or retinal and acetaldehyde and contribute to their oxidations such as human ADH 7, corresponding to Class IV ADH in rat. A study on the interaction between the metabolism of retinol and ethanol was opened by the findings of the existence of such enzymes. We cloned the cDNA (Yokoyama et al. 1994) of human ADH7 from a human gastric cDNA library and showed that it had 72% homology to human ADH1, a major ADH, on the cDNA level. We also cloned its gene and demonstrated that it was localized at 4q23-24 of the human genome, i.e. the ADH cluster (Yokoyama et al. 1996). These observations support the view that the enzyme is a member of the ADH family. We also found that the mRNA of ADH7 was exclusively expressed in human gastric mucosa among organs examined at that time (Yokoyama et al. 1995a). At present, ADH7 is known to be generally expressed in human upper digestive organs (Yin et al. 1993). We also reported SNP of ADH7 at exon 7 (Yokoyama et al. 1995b), however, its significance is still unknown. Recently, SNP at codon 92 of ADH7 cDNA (glycine/alanine change rs1573496) has been implicated in a higher incidence of head and neck cancer (Hashibe et al. 2008).

6.2 RA supply from vitamin A in the gastrointestinal tract

To know the significance of ADH7, we examined retinol metabolism in the esophagus and stomach using a high pressure liquid chromatography (HPLC) system by which 3 isoforms, i.e. *all-trans*, 9-*sis* and 13-*cis* of retinol, retinal, and RA were simultaneously quantified (Yokoyama et al. 2000). Subsequently, we established a new HPLC condition to quantify these isoforms more precisely (Miyagi et al. 2001, Figure 7). Using this technique, we demonstrated that RA could be produced when specimens of rat esophageal mucosa (Crabb et al. 2001) and human gastric mucosa (Yokoyama et al. 2001) were incubated with *all-trans* retinol in the presence of NAD. These pathways were designated as NAD-dependent *in situ* RA supply systems. Levels of RA production from retinol were shown to be dependent on ADH7 activities in human gastric mucosa (Matsumoto et al. 2001). We also demonstrated that Helicobacter pylori infection decreased the levels of ADH7 activities as well as the activity levels were inversely associated with the severity of morphological changes in the mucosa (Matsumoto et al. 2005).

6.3 Feature of an NAD dependent *in situ* RA supply system in rat esophageal mucosa

As ADH7, an NAD-dependent enzyme, is expressed in esophageal mucosa and has affinity to retinol, the enzyme is expected to contribute to the first step of an NAD-dependent *in situ* RA supply system in esophageal mucosa. Since ADH7 also has affinity to ethanol, it is postulated that ethanol can hamper the system in a competitive manner. When specimens of esophageal mucosa prepared from normal rats were incubated with retinol in the presence of NAD and various concentrations of ethanol, ethanol of 1 M or more was shown to attenuate RA production in the condition (Shiraishi-Yokoyama et al., 2003). The ethanol concentration which hampered the RA supply was comparable to the established Km value for ethanol of rat Class IV ADH, i.e. at a molar level (Allali-Hassani et al., 1996), RA production was thought to be competitively disturbed in the model (Shiraishi-Yokoyama et al., 2003).

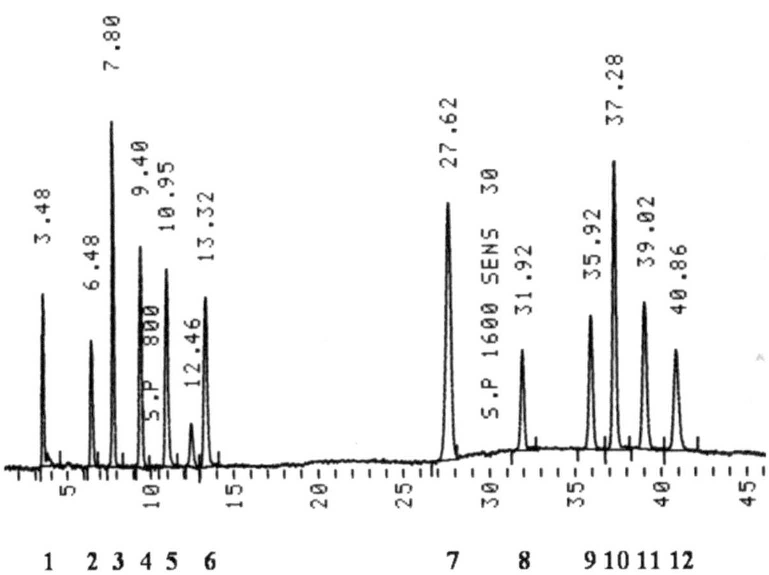

(1) 13-*cis* retinal, (2) 9-*cis* retinal, (3) all-*trans* retinal, (4) 13-*cis* RA, (5) 9-*cis* RA, (6) all-*trans* RA, (7) internal-standard, (8) 13-*cis* retinol, (9) all-*trans* retinol (10) all-*trans* 4-oxo RA, (11) 9-*cis* 4-oxo RA, (12) 13-*cis* 4-oxo RA. Various retinoid isoforms were successfully separated using a HPLC technique established in our laboratory. It allowed us to quantify them up to 2.5 ng/ml. The details are described in the article of Miyagi et al. 2001.

Fig. 7. Simultaneous quantification of various retinoids by a HPLC technique.

Using a similar experimental design, we also found that acetaldehyde of 50 μM and more hampered RA production from retinal in the esophageal mucosa of the rat, suggesting that an enzyme having affinity to both acetaldehyde and retinal participates in the second step of the NAD dependent *in situ* RA supply system in esophageal mucosa (Shiraishi-Yokoyama et al. 2006). One of the candidates having such characteristics was ALDH1A1, and this assumption was supported by our observation that the acetaldehyde concentration that hampered RA supply in the model was comparable to the reported Km value for acetaldehyde of rat ALDH1A1, i.e. 30 μM (Crabb et al., 2004). This also supports the view that RA production was competitively disturbed by acetaldehyde. The finding that catalytic activity for *all-trans* retinal of rat esophageal mucosa was 5.3 μM/min, which was consistent with that of rat ALDH 1A1 for *all-trans* retinal, i.e, 0.6-10 μM (Kathmann et al., 2000; Montplaisir et al., 2002), also suggested that RA production in the model was due to ALDH1A1.

We recently demonstrated that predominant ADHs in rat esophageal mucosa were Class I, III, and IV ADHs in mRNA levels (Yokoyama et al. 2010), which agreed with the expression pattern of ADHs in rat esophageal mucosa as examined in protein levels (Vaglenova et al. 2003). As Class IV ADH exhibits the highest affinity for retinol among these ADHs (Moreno and Pares, 1991), the view that Class IV ADH is involved in the NAD-dependent *in situ* RA supply system in rat esophageal mucosa is plausible. Moreover, we also demonstrated that the predominant ALDHs in rat esophageal mucosa were ALDH 1A1 and 3A1 in mRNA levels (Yokoyama et al. 2010). Since ALDH1A1 has the potential for catalyzing retinal to RA, whereas ALDH3A1 has no affinity for retinal (Yoshida et al., 1992, Bhat et al., 1996, Moore et al., 1998), this finding is compatible with the view that ALDH1A1 constitutes the NAD-dependent *in situ* RA supply system in rat esophageal mucosa.

We also confirmed that the expression levels of mRNA of both Class IV ADHs and ALDH 1A1 in the mucosal-layer of the rat esophagus were significantly higher than those in its muscle-layer (Yokoyama et al. 2010). Similar observations for Class IV ADH in the esophagus (Haselback and Duester, 1997, Vaglenova et al., 2003) and ALDH1A1 in the alveolar wall (Hind M et al., 2002) were reported. It is likely that the NAD-dependent RA supply system predominantly exists in the mucosal-layer, compared to the muscle-layer, in the rat esophagus and is supposed by the fact that a large quantity of RA is required in the epidermis compared to muscle (Randolph and Siegenthaler, 1999).

6.4 An NAD dependent *in situ* RA supply system in human esophageal mucosa

Since the expression pattern of isoforms of ADHs and ALDHs in human esophageal mucosa (Yin et al. 2003) is identical to that of the rat, it is postulated that an NAD-dependent *in situ* RA supply system whose structural feature is similar to that of rat esophageal mucosa exists in human esophageal mucosa, and responsible enzymes for the pathway are expected as ADH7 and ALDH1A, corresponding to rat Class IV ADH and ALDH1A1, respectively. When it is premised on this assumption, various clinical characteristics of esophageal cancers seen in alcoholics can be explained fairly satisfactorily.

The Km value for ethanol of human ADH7 is 25mM (Kedishvili et al., 1995), markedly different from that of rat Class IV ADH. Since this ethanol level habitually appears in alcoholics, the first step of the NAD-dependent *in situ* RA supply system in the human esophagus could be hampered, causing a reduction in RA supply in them. It is of interest to know the effect of above mentioned ADH7 SNP rs1573496, which is implicated in the higher incidence of head and neck cancer (Hashibe et al. 2008), on RA supply. On the other hand, the Km value for acetaldehyde of human ALDH1 is 41 μM (Kathmann et al., 2000), comparable to that of rat ALDH1A1. Importantly, acetaldehyde of such a level actually appears in alcoholics with the *ALDH 2*2* allele. This suggests that the second step of the NAD-dependent *in situ* RA supply system in the human esophagus is further hampered in such subjects (Figure 8).

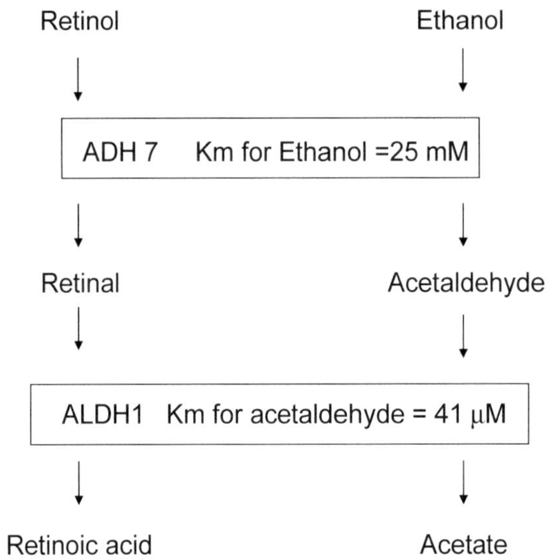

The *in situ* RA supply system in human esophageal mucosa may comprise ADH7 and ALDH1. Since they also have affinity for ethnaol and acetaldehyde, respectively, the system may also participate in ethanol metabolism. Considering their Km values for ethanol and acetaldehyde, when esophagus is exposed to ethanol at a concentration of more than 25 mM, and acetaldehyde at a concentration of more than 41 μM, which can occur in alcoholics and in alcoholics with the ALDH2*2 allele, respectively, RA supply from retinol is hampered, resulting in the development of a RA deficiency. Importantly, multiple lines of evidence suggest that a RA deficiency causes carcinogenesis.

Fig. 8. Metabolism of retinol and ethanol via the *in situ* RA supply system in human esophageal mucosa.

6.5 Features of the *in situ* RA supply system in esophageal mucosa and clinical aspects of esophageal cancers related to ethanol consumption

In this chapter, the relationship between RA and carcinogenesis is summarized and we refer to the possibility that an intracellular RA deficiency leads to carcinogenesis. On the other hand, our observations that an NAD dependent *in situ* RA supply system comprising Class IV ADH and ALDH1A1 exists and ethanol metabolism hampers RA supply in rat esophageal mucosa are introduced. Moreover, we mention the plausibility that human esophageal mucosa also has a similar system comprising ADH7 and ALDH1A. Incorporating these views, our hypothesis is that RA supply in esophageal mucosa is hampered by excessive ethanol consumption and this is a causative factor in the development of esophageal cancer in alcoholics. In this section, whether this hypothesis can fit with the clinical characteristics of esophageal cancer in alcoholics is discussed.

6.5.1 The *in situ* RA supply system and organ specificities in cancers related to ethanol consumption

As mentioned in section 2.1, there are organ specificities in cancers related to ethanol consumption. The present hypothesis suggests that the *in situ* RA supply system in esophageal mucosa comprises ADH7 and ALDH1A, and ethanol metabolism hampers these enzymes, resulting in a compromised intracellular RA level and the development of malignancy. It must be noted that this hypothesis can be applied to organs comprising RA target cells but not to those comprising non RA target cells. Moreover, several enzymes which have affinities for retinol and/or retinal but not for ethanol and/or acetaldehyde, such as families of p450, RDH, and retinal dehydrogenase (Lee et al. ,1991; Drager et al., 1998) has been identified. The present hypothesis can be neither applied to organs of which *in situ* RA supply systems comprise such enzymes since ethanol metabolism does not disturb RA supply in them. Thus, organ specificity of the structural feature of the *in situ* RA supply system may, at least in part, account for the organ specific susceptibilities to malignancy caused by ethanol consumption.

6.5.2 The *in situ* RA supply system and genetic variations in cancers related to ethanol consumption

In section 6.4, we discussed the possibility that ethanol and acetaldehyde of physiological concentrations may hamper the NAD-dependent *in situ* RA supply system in the human esophagus. This indicates that ethanol hampers RA supply via this system and acetaldehyde further affects it. This schema is compatible with the clinical feature that prevalence of esophageal cancer increases in alcoholics and is even higher in alcoholics carrying ALDH2*2 allele (Yokoyama et al. 1996), as described in section 2.2. A recently prevailing explanation as to how acetaldehyde causes esophageal cancer is that acetaldehyde binds to DNA and/or chromatin, forming an acetaldehyde adduct, thereby altering their functions (Yu et al. 2011). However, no distinct difference has been confirmed between esophageal cancers which develop in alcoholics with or without acetaldehyde accumulation, namely in those with or without the ALDH2*2 allele, suggesting that the esophageal cancers which develop in both types of alcoholics have a common pathogenesis. Thus, the hypothesis that both ethanol and acetaldehyde hamper the *in situ* RA supply system, causing carcinogenesis, is easier to accept than that a specific effect of acetaldehyde causes carcinogenesis.

6.5.3 The *in situ* RA supply system and field cancerization in cancer related to ethanol consumption

As emphasized in section 5.4, the reduction in RAR-β2 gene expression has been shown to be related to carcinogenesis in various organs, including the esophagus. Furthermore, as mentioned in section 4 and 5, RA deficiency may cause this reduction in RAR-β2 expression. Interestingly, a significant overlap is observed between cancers related to a lack of RAR-β2 expression and those related to excessive alcohol consumption, as recognized by IARC (Table 1). This overlap is consistent with the present hypothesis that ethanol consumption disturbs the *in situ* RA supply system, resulting in the reduction of RAR-β2 expression and carcinogenesis. As mentioned in section 2.3, some types of cancers in the esophagus develop via field cancerization. One of the distinct features of the field cancerization is the accumulation of mutant p53 not only in cancer cells, but also pre-malignant lesions. Such features were recently demonstrated in the esophageal mucosa of alcoholics (Yokoyama et al. 2011). As mentioned in section 5.4, the lack of RAR-β2 expression has been implicated in the development of field cancerization as well as in p53 accumulation.

Cancers related to RAR–β2 suppresion (from statements of Xu et al. 2007)	Cancers related to alcohol consumption (from statements of Bann et al. 2007)
Oral cavity	Oral cavity
Head and neck	Head and neck
Esophagus	Esophagus
Brest	Brest
Lung	
Pancreas	
Prostate	
	Liver
	Colon and rectum

Table 1. Cancers related to RAR-β2 suppression and alcohol consumption.

6.5.4 The *in situ* RA supply system and strain difference in susceptibility to ethanol with respect to carcinogenesis

As mentioned in section 2.4, thus far, there are limited animal models in which cancers were produced by ethanol administration alone. Although Soffritti et al. could produce multiple cancers in rats by ethanol administration for long periods (Soffritti et al. 2002), there was limited development of esophageal cancer in their model. Since the Km value for ethanol of rat Class IV ADH is a non-physiological level and accumulation of acetaldehyde does not usually occur in rats, it is expected that ethanol consumption does not hamper the *in situ* RA supply system in the esophageal mucosa of the rat and this can explain why ethanol alone does not produce esophageal cancer in their model. The structural feature of the *in situ* RA supply system may also account for the strain difference in susceptibility to ethanol with respect to carcinogenesis.

7. Conclusion

There is much evidence to show that reduction of RAs is associated with the development of malignancy. Most cancers must develop via multiple processes including genetic alterations, dysregulation of cell growth, differentiation, cell function, and cell loss, and change of cell phenotype, and RAs are involved in all these events. Furthermore, the reduction of RAs may down-regulate immune mechanisms against malignant cells. Among the multiple effects of RA, the relationship between the reduction of signals via RAR–β2, one of the RA receptors, and carcinogenesis is of major interest lately. The current observations suggest that RA deficiency may reduce the expression of RAR-β2.

In mammals, RA is synthesized from retinol, a type of alcohol, ingested from food. Recently, it has become clear that RA can be synthesized from retinol, which is delivered by blood vessels, via a two step oxidation pathway in a RA target cell. We recently demonstrated that such a pathway which can produce RA from retinol in an NAD dependent manner exists in rat esophageal mucosa, and designated it as an NAD dependent *in situ* RA supply system. Furthermore, we demonstrated that the pathway comprised Class IV ADH and ALDH1A1 and was hampered by ethanol, a substance of the former as well as by acetaldehyde, that of the latter. Considering the expression patterns of ADH and ALDH in the human and rat esophagus, it is fully plausible that a similar pathway, one comprising ADH7 and ALDH1A exists in human esophageal mucosa. Since their Km values for ethanol and acetaldehyde are at physiological concentrations, we hypothesized that the metabolism of excessive ethanol consumption disturbs the pathway, resulting in a deficiency in RA, and the development of malignancy in esophageal mucosa. This hypothesis can account for clinical characteristics of cancers in alcoholics, including organ specificity, genetic specificity, and strain specificity. Moreover, this hypothesis is also compatible with the fact that esophageal cancer develops in a field cancerization manner in alcoholics. Further studies based on this hypothesis may be beneficial for understanding the pathogenesis of esophageal cancer seen in alcoholics, which must be important for having strategies of its prevention, diagnosis and treatment.

8. References

Allali-Hassani, A.; Martinez, S.E.; Peralba, J.M.; Vaglenova, J.; Vidal, F.; Richart, C.; Farrés, J. & Parés, X. (1997). Alcohol dehydrogenase of human and rat blood vessels. Role in ethanol metabolism. *FEBS Leterts*, Vol. 405, No.2-3 (July) pp.26-30.

Bann, R.; Straif, K.; Grisse, Y.; Bouvard, V.; Altieri, A.& Cogliano, V. (2007) on behalf of the WHO International Agency for Research on Cancer Monograph Working Group Carcinogenicity of alcoholic beverages. *The Lancet Oncology*, Vol.8, No. 4 (April) pp 292-293

Baron, J.M.; Heise, R.; Blaner, W.S.; Neis, M.; Joussen, S.; Dreuw, A.; Marquardt, Y.; Saurat, J.H.; Merk, H.F.; Bickers, D.R. & Jugert, F.K. (2005) Retinoic acid and its 4-oxo metabolites are functionally active in human skin cells in vitro. *The Journal of Investigative Dermatology*, Vol.125, No.1, (July) pp.143-153.

Bean, G.R.; Scott, V.; Yee, L.; Ratliff-Daniel, B.; Troch, M.M.; Seo, P.; Bowie, M.L.; Marcom, P.K.; Slade, J.; Kimler, B.F.; Fabian, C.J.; Zalles, C.M.; Broadwater, G.; Baker, J.C. Jr, ; Wilke , G. & Seewaldt, V.L. (2005). Retinoic acid receptor-beta2 promoter methylation in random periareolar fine needle aspiration. *Cancer, Epidemiology Biomarkers & Prevention,* Vol.142, No.4, (April) pp.790-798.

Berard, J.; Laboune, F.; Mukuna, M.; Masse, S.; Kothary, R.& Bradley, W.E. (1996) Lung tumors in mice expressing an antisense RARbeta2 transgene. *The FASEB Journal,* Vol. 10, N0.9, (July) pp. 1091-1097.

Bhat, P.V.; Poissant, L. & Wang XL (1996) Purification of partial characterization of bovine kidney aldehyde dehydrogenase able to oxidize retinal to retinoic acid. *Biochemistry & Cell Biology,* Vol. 74, No.5, (May) pp. 695-700.

Boffetta, P.; Hashibe, M.; La Vecchia, C.; ,Zatonski, W.& Rehm, J. (2006). The burden of cancer attributable to alcohol drinking. *International Journal of Cancer,* Vol. 119, No.4, (August) pp. 884-887

Bosron, W.F. & Li, T.K. (1987) Catalytic properties of human liver alcohol dehydrogenase isoenzymes. *Enzyme*, Vol 37, No.1-2 (Febuary) pp. 19-28.

Brennan, P.; Lewis, S.; Hashibe, M.; Bell DA.; Boffetta, P.; Bouchardy, C.; Caporaso, N.; Chen, C.; Coutelle, C.; Diehl, S.R.; Hayes, R.B.; Olshan, A.F.; Schwartz, S.M.; Sturgis, E.M.; Wei, Q. & Zavras, A.I. Benhamou S. (2004) Pooled analysis of alcohol dehydrogenase genotypes and head and neck cancer: a HuGE review. *American Journal of Epidemiology,* Vol. 159, No.1, (January) pp. 1-16.

Clifford J.L.; Menter D.G.; Wang, M.; Lotan, R. & Lippman, S.M. (1999) Retinoid Receptor-dependent and -independent Effects of *N*-(4-Hydroxyphenyl)retinamide in F9 Embryonal Carcinoma Cells *Cancer Research* Vol. 59, No.1 (January) pp.14-18,

Cheung, B.; Hocker, J.E.; Smith, S.A.; Norris, M.D.; Haber, M. & Marshall G.M. (1998) Favorable prognostic significance of high-level retinoic acid receptor beta expression in neuroblastoma mediated by effects on cell cycle regulation. *Oncogene* vol. 17, No.6 (August) pp. 751-759,

Crabb, D.W.; Bergheim, I.,; Bosron, W.,; Lieber, C.S.,; Tsukamoto, H. & Yokoyama, H. Alcohol and Retinoids. (2001) *Alcoholism; Clinical and Experimental Research* Vol.25, No.5 Suppl 1 (May) pp 207S-217S,

Drager, U.C.; Wagner, E. & McCaffery, P. (1998) Aldehyde dehydrogenases in the generation of retinoic acid in the developing vertebrate: A central role of the eye. *The Journal of Nutrition* Vol. 128, No.2 Suppl (February) pp. 463S-466S,

Feron, V.J.; Kruysse, A. &Woutersen, R.A. (1982) Respiratory tract tumours in hamsters exposed to acetaldehyde vapour alone or simultaneously to benzo(a)pyrene or diethylnitrosamine. *European Journal of Cnacer & Clinical Oncology* Vol 18, No.1 (January) pp.13-31,

Gao, H.; Wang, L. D.; Zhou, O.; Hong, J. Y.; Huang, T. Y. & Yang, C. S. (1994) *p53* tumor suppressor gene mutation in early esophageal precancerous lesions and carcinoma among high-risk populations in Henan, China. *Cancer Research* Vol. 54, No.16 (August) pp. 4342-4346

Geradts, J.; Chen, J.Y.; Russell, E.K.; Yankaskas, J.R.; Nieves, L. & Minna, J.D. (1993) Human lung cancer cell lines exhibit resistance to retinoic acid treatment. *Cell Growth & Differentiation* Vol. 4, No.10 (October) pp. 799-809

Gillespie, R.F. & Gudas, L.J. (2007) Retinoid regulated association of transcriptional co-regulators and the polycomb group protein SUZ12 with the retinoic acid response elements of Hoxa1, RARbeta(2), and Cyp26A1 in F9 embryonal carcinoma cells. *Journal of Molecular Biology* Vol. 372, No. 2 (September) pp. 298-316

Goedde, H.W.; Agarwal, D.P.; Fritze, G.; Meier-Tackmann, D.; Singh, S.; Beckmann, G.; Bhatia, K.; Chen, L.Z.; Fang, B. & Lisker, R. (1992) Distribution of ADH2 and ALDH2 genotypes in different populations. *Human Genetics* Vol. 88, No.3 (January) pp. 344-366.

Gudas, L. J.; Sporn, M. B. & Roberts, A. B. (1994). Cellular biology and biochemistry of the retinoids. In: The Retinoids, M. D. Sporn, A. B. Roberts, & D. S. Goodman (Ed), 443-520, Raven Press, New York, USA:

Han J (1993). Highlights of the cancer chemoprevention studies in China. *Preventive Medicine* Vol 22, No.5 (September) pp. 712-722,

Haque, N.; Banik l., & and Ray S.K. (2007) Emerging role of combination of all-trans retinoic acid and interferon-gamma as chemoimmunotherapy in the management of human glioblastoma," *Neurochemistryl Research*, Vol. 32, No. 12 (December) pp. 2203–2209,

Harris C.C.; Sporn, M.B.; Kaufman, D.G. & Smith J.M. (1972) Histogenesis of squamous metaplasis in the hamster tracheal epithelium caused by vitamin A deficiency or benzol[α]pyrene-Ferric oxide. *Journal of the Nutrition Cancer Institute* Vol. 48, No.3 (March) pp. 743-761,

Haselback, R.J. & Duester, G. (1997) Regional restriction of alcohol/retinol dehydrogenases along the mouse gastrointestinal epithelium. *Alcoholism; Clincal and Experimental Research* Vol. 21, No.8, (November) pp. 1484-1490

Hashibe, M.; McKay, J.D.; Curado, M.P.; Oliveira, J.C.; Koifman, S.; Koifman, R.; Zaridze, D.; Shangina, O.; Wünsch-Filho, V.; Eluf-Neto, J.; Levi, J.E.; Matos, E.; Lagiou, P.; Lagiou, A.; Benhamou, S.; Bouchardy, C.; Szeszenia-Dabrowska, N.; Menezes, A.; Dall'Agnol, M.M.; Merletti, F.; Richiardi, L.; Fernandez, L.; Lence, J.; Talamini, R.; Barzan, L.; Mates, D.; Mates, I.N.; Kjaerheim, K.; Macfarlane, G.J.; Macfarlane, T.V.; Simonato, L.; Canova, C.; Holcátová, I.; Agudo, A.; Castellsagué, X.; Lowry, R.; Janout, V.; Kollarova, H.; Conway, D.I.; McKinney, P.A.; Znaor, A.; Fabianova, E.; Bencko, V.; Lissowska, J.; Chabrier, A.; Hung, R.J.; Gaborieau, V.; Boffetta, P. & Brennan, P. (2008) Multiple ADH genes are associated with upper aerodigestive cancers. *Nat Genet.* Vol 40 No.6 (Jun) pp. 707-709

Hind M.; Coccoran, J & Maden, M (2002) Alveolar proliferation, retinoic synthesizing enzymes, and endogeous retinoids in the postnatal mouse lung. *American Journal of Respiratory Cell & Molecular Biology* Vol. 26, No.1 (January) pp. 67-73,

Homann, N.; Stickel, F.; König I.R.; Jacobs, A.; Junghanns, K.; Benesova, M,; Schuppan, D.; Himsel, S.; Zuber-Jerger, I, Hellerbrand, C.; Ludwig D,; Caselmann, W.H. & Seitz HK (2006). Alcohol dehydrogenase 1C*1 allele is a genetic marker for alcohol-associated cancer in heavy drinkers. International Journal of Cancer, Vol 118, No.8 (April), pp.1998-2002.

Hong W.K..; Lippman, S.M., Hittelman, W.N. & Lotan R. Retinoid Chemoprevention of Aerodigestive Cancer: From Basic Research to the Clinic. *Clinical Cancer Research*, Vol.1, No.7 (July) pp. 677- 686..

Houle, B.; Rochette-Egly, C. & Bradley, W.E. (1993) Tumor-suppressive effect of the retinoic acid receptor beta in human epidermoid lung cancer cells. *Proceedings of the National Academic Science of USA*, Vol.90, No.3 (Februay) 985-989.

IJpenberg, A.; Tan, N.S.; Gelman, L.; Kersten, S.; Seydoux, J.; Xu, J.; Metzger, D.; Canaple, L.; Chambon, P.; Wahli, W. & Desvergne, B. (2004) In vivo activation of PPAR target genes by RXR homodimers. *The EMBO Journal*, Vol. 23, No.10, (May) ; 2083-2091,

Kathmann, E.C.; Naylor, S. & Lipsky, J.J. (2000) Rat liver and Phenobarbital-inducible cytosolic aldehyde dehydrogenase are highly homologus protein that function as distinct isozymes. *Biochemistry*, vol. 39, No.36 (September) pp. 11170-11176,

Kedishvili, N.Y.; Bosron, W.F.; Stone, C.L.; Hurley, T.D.; Peggs, C.F.; Thomasson, H.R.; Popov, K.M.; Carr, L.G.; Edenberg, H.J.; & Li, T.K. Expression and kinetic characterization of recombinant human stomach alcohol dehydrogenase. Active-site amino acid sequence explain substrate specificity compared with liver isozymes. *Journal of Biological Chemistry*, vol 270, No. 8 (August) pp 3625-3630.

Kim, J.E.; Kim, B.; Kim, H.; Kim, H; Lee., J.D.; Kim H.J. & Cho, K.Y. (2010) Retinyl retinoate induces hyaluronan production and less irritation than other retinoids. *The journal of Dermatology*, Vol. 37, No.5 (May) pp. 448–454,

Lee, M.O.; Manthey, C.L. & Sladek, N.E. (1991) Identification of mouse liver aldehyde dehydrogenases that catalyze the oxidation of retinaldehyde to retinoic acid. *Biochemical Pharmacology*, Vol. 42 No.6 (August) pp. 1279-1285,

Lee P.P.; Lee, M.T.; Darcy, K.M.; Shudo, K & Ip, M.M. (1995) Modulation of normal mammary epithelial cell proliferation morphogenesis, and functional differentiation by retinoids: A comparison of the retinobenzoic acid derivative RE80 with retinoic acid. *Endocrinology*, No.4 (April) Vol. 136, pp. 1701-1717,

Lefebvre, B.; Brand, C.; Flajollet, S. & Lefebvre, P. (2006) Down-regulation of the tumor suppressor gene RAR-β2 through the PI3K/Akt signaling pathway. *Molecular Endocrinology*, Vol. 20, No.9 (September) pp. 2109-2121,

Lewis, C.M.; Clea, L.R.; Bu, D.W L, Zöchbauer-Müller, S.; Milchgrub, S.; Naftalis, E.Z.; Leitch, A.M.; Minna, J.D. & Euhus, D.M. (2005) Promoter hypermethylation in benign breast epithelium in relation to predicted breast cancer risk. *Clinical Cancer Research*, Vol. 11, No.1 (January) pp. 166-172.

Li M.; Song, S.; Lippman, S.M.; Zhang, X.K.; Liu, X.; Lotan R. & Xu, X.C. (2002) Induction of retinoic acid receptorbeta suppresses cyclooxygenase-2 expression in esophageal cancer cells. *Oncogene*, Vol. 21, No.3 (January) pp. 411–418.

Liang Z.D.; Lippman S.M.; Wu T.T.; Lotan R. & Xu X.C. (2006) RRIG1 mediates effects of retinoic acid receptor beta2 on tumor cell growth and gene expression through binding to and inhibition of RhoA. *Cancer Res* Vol.66, No.14 (July) pp.7111-7118.

Lin, B.; Chen, G.Q.; Xiao, D.; Kolluri, S.K.;Cao, X.; Su, H. & Zhang, X.K. (2000).Orphan receptor COUP-TF is required for induction of retinoic acid receptor beta, growth inhibition, and apoptosis by retinoic acid in cancer cells. *Molecular and Cellular Biology* Vol. 20, No.3 (February) pp. 957-970,

Lieber, C.S. (1984) Alcohol and the liver: 1984 update. *Hepatology*. 1984 Vol 4, no.6 (November-December) pp. 1242-1260,

Lippman, S.M. & Davies, P.J. (1997) Retinoids, neoplasia and differentiation therapy. *Cancer Chemotherapy and Biological Resoponse Modifiers* Vol. 17, pp. 349-362.

Lotan, R. (1993) Retinoids and squamous cell differentiation. In: Retinoids in Oncology, W. K. Hong & R. Lotan (Ed.), pp. 43-72, Marcel Dekker, New York, USA

Lotan, R.; Xu, X.C, ; Lippman, S.M., Ro, J.Y., Lee, J.S., Lee, J.J., & Hong, W.K. (1995) Suppression of retinoic acid receptor b in premalignant oral lesions and its upregulation by isotretinoin. *New England Journal of Medicine* Vol. 332, No.21 (May) pp. 1405-1410,

Matsumoto, M.; Yokoyama, H.; Shiraishi, H.; Suzuki, H.; Kato, S. Miura, S. & Ishii H (2001) Alcohol dehydrogenase activities in the human gastric mucosa: Effects of Helicobacter pylori infection, gender, aging, and part of stomach. *Alcoholism Clincal and Expimental Reseach*, Vol.25, No.6 Suppl, (June) pp. 29S-34S,

Matsumoto, M.; Yokoyama, H.; Suzuki, H.; Shiraishi-Yokoyama, H. & Hibi, T. (2005) Retinoic acid formation from retinol in the human gastric mucosa: role of class IV alcohol dehydrogenase and its relevance to morphological changes. *American Journal of Physiology Gastrointestinal & Liver Physiology* Vol. 289, No.3 (September) pp. G429-G433,

McGregor, F.; Wagner, E.; Felix, D.; Soutar, D.; Parkinson, K.& Harrison, P.R. (1997) Inappropriate retinoic acid receptor-beta expression in oral dysplasias: correlation with acquisition of the immortal phenotype. *Cancer Research*, Vol. 57, no.18 (september) pp 3886-3889,

Mellow, M.H.; Layne, E.A.; Lipman, T.O.; Kaushik, M.; Hosteler, C. & Smith, J.C., Jr (1983) Plasma zinc and vitamin A in human squamous carcinoma of the esophagus. *Cancer* Vol.51, No.9 (May) pp. 615-1620,

Miyagi, M.; Yokoyama, H.; Shiraishi, H.; Matsumoto, M. & Ishii, H (2001), Simultaneous quantification of retinol, retinal, and retinoic acid isomers by high-performance liquid chromatography with a simple graduation. *Journal of Chromatography B Biomedical Science Application,* Vol.757, No.2 (June) pp.365-368,

Moon RC, Mehta RG, Rao KVN. Retinoids and cancer in experimental animals. In: Sporn MB, Roberts AB, Goodmann DS, eds. *The Retinoids, Biology, Chemistry, and Medicine,* 2nd edn. New York: Raven Press, 1994; 537–96.

Moore, S.A.; Baker, H.M.; Blythe, T.J.; Kitson, K.E.; Kitson, T.M.& Baker, E.N. (1998) Sheep liver cytosolic aldehyde dehydrogenase: the structure reveals the basis for the retinal specificity of class 1 aldehyde dehydrogenases. *Structure* Vol.6 No.12, (December) pp. 1541-1551

Moreno, A. & Pares, X. (1991) Purification and characterization of a new alcohol dehydrogenase from human stomach. *J Biological Chemistry,* Vol. 266, No.2 (January) pp. 11228-11233.

Moulas, A.N.; Gerogianni, I.C; Papadopoulos, D. & Gourgoilianis, K.I. (2006) Serum retinoic acid, retinol and retinyl palmitate levels in patients with lung cancer. *Respirology* Vol. 11, No.2 (March) pp. 169–174

Muntoni, A.; Fleming, J.; Gordon, K.E.; Hunter, K.; McGregor, F & Parkinson E (2003) Senescing oral dysplasias are not immortalized by ectopic expression of hTERT alone without other molecular changes, such as loss of INK4A and/or retinoic acid receptor-beta: but p53 mutations are not necessarily required. *Oncogene* Vol. 22, No.49 (October) pp. 7804–7808,

Noguchi, K.; Nakajima, M.; Naito, M. & Tsuruo, T. (1995) Inhibition by differentiation-inducing agents of wild-type p53-dependent apoptosis in HL-60 cells. *Japanese Journal of Cancer Research* Vol. 86, No.2 (February) pp. 217-223.

Ou, C.C.; Hsu, S.C.; Hsieh, Y.H.; Tsou, W.L.; Chuang, T.C.; Liu, J.Y.& Kao, M.C. (2008) Downregulation of HER2 by RIG1 involves the PI3K/Akt pathway in ovarian cancer cells. *Carcinogenesis.* Vol 28. No.2 (February) pp. 299-306

Pasquali, D. ; Bellastella, A. ; Colantuoni, V. ; Vassallo, P. ; Bonavolonta, G. ; Rossi, V. ; Notaro, A. & Sinisi, A.A. (2003) All-trans retinoic acid- and N-(4-hydroxyphenil-retinamide-induced growth arrest and apoptosis in orbital fibroblasts in Graves' disease. *Metabolism* Vol. 52, No.11 (November) pp. 1387–1392,

Randolph, R.K. & Siegenthaler, G. (1999). Vitamin A homeostasis in human epidermis; native retinoid composition and metabolism, in Retinoids. In: *The Biochemical and Molecular Basis of Vitamin A and Retinoid Action,* H. Nau & W.D. Blaner (Ed.) 491-520. Springer, New York, USA.

Rogers, M.; Berestecky, J.M.; Hossain, M.Z.; Guo, H.M.; Kadle, R.; Nicholson, B.J. & Bertram, J.S. (1990) Retinoid-enhanced gap junctional communication is achieved by increased levels of connexin 43 mRNA and protein. *Molecular Carcinogensis,* Vol 3, No.6 pp. 335-343

Ross, S.A.; Ahrens, R.A.& De Luca, L.M. (1994) LM. Retinoic acid enhances adhesiveness, laminin and integrin beta 1 synthesis, and retinoic acid receptor expression in F9 teratocarcinoma cells. *Journal of Cellular Physiology,* Vol. 159, No.2 (May) pp. 263-273.

Santin A.D.; Hermonat P.L.; Ravaggi, A.; Chiriva-Internati, M. Pecorelli, S. ; & Parham, G.P (1998) Retinoic acid up-regulates the expression of major histocompatibility complex molecules and adhesion/costimulation molecules (specifically, intercellular adhesion molecule ICAM-1) in human cervical cancer," *American Journal of Obstetrics and Gynecology*, vol. 179, No.4 (October) pp. 1020–1025,

Shao, Z.M.; Dawson, M.I.; Li, X.S.; Rishi, A.K.; Sheikh, M.S.; Han, Q.X.; Ordonez, J.V.; Shroot, B. & Fontana, J.A. (1995) p53 independent G0/G1 arrest and apoptosis induced by a novel retinoid in human breast cancer cells. *Oncogene*, No.3 (August) Vol. 11, pp. 493-504.

Shin, D. M.; Kim, J.; Ro, J. Y.; Hittelman, J.; Roth, J. A.; Hong, W. K., & Hittelman, W. N. (1994) Activation of *p53* gene expression in premalignant lesions during head and neck tumongenesis. *Cancer Research*, Vol. 54, No.2 (January) pp. 321-326,

Shiraishi-Yokoyama, H.; Yokoyama, H.; Matsumoto, M., & Ishii, H. (2003) The existence of an NAD-dependent pathway for retinoic acid formation from vitamin A (retinol) in rat esophagus and its inhibition by ethanol and histamine 2 (H2) receptor antagonists. *Medical Science Monitor*, Vol. 9, No.12 (December) pp. 403-406.

Shiraishi-Yokoyama, H.; Yokoyama, H.; Matsumoto, M.; Imaeda, H. & Hibi, T. (2006) Acetaldehyde inhibits the formation of retinoic acid from retinal in the rat esophagus. *Scandinavian Journal of Gastroenterology,* Vol.41, No.1 (January) pp. 80-86.

Shmarakov, I.; Fleshman, M.K.; D'Ambrosio, D.N.; Piantedosi, R.; Riedl, K.M.; Schwartz, S.J.; Curley, R.W. Jr.; von Lintig, J.; Rubin, L.P.; Harrison, E.H. & Blaner W.S. (2010) Hepatic stellate cells are an important cellular site for β-carotene conversion to retinoid. Archive of Biochemistory and Biophysiology, Vol 504, No.1 (December) pp.697-708,

Soffritti, M.; Belpoggi, F.; Cevolani, D.; Guarino, M.; Padovani, M. & Maltoni, C. (2002) Results of long-term experimental studies on the carcinogenicity of methyl alcohol and ethyl alcohol in rats. Annalus of New York Academy of Science vol 982, (December) pp.46-69,

Song, S.; Lippman, S.M. ; Zou, Y. ; Ye, X. & Xu, X.C. (2005) Induction of cyclooxygenase-2 by benzo[a]pyrene diolepoxide through inhibition of retinoic acid receptor-β2 expression. *Oncogene* Vol. 24, No.56 (December) pp. 8268–8276

Sun, S.Y.; Yue, P.; Wu, G.S.; El Deiry, W.S.; Shroot, B,; Hong, W.K. & Lotan, R. (1999a) Implication of p53 in growth arrest and apoptosis induced by the synthetic retinoid CD437 in human lung cancer cells. *Cancer Research* Vol 59 Vol.12 (June) , pp. 2829-2833.

Sun, S.Y.; Yue, P.; Wu, G.S.; El Deiry, W.S.; Shroot, B.; Hong, W.K. & Lotan R (1999b). Mechanisms of apoptosis induced by the synthetic retinoid CD437 in human non-small cell lung carcinoma cells. *Oncogene* Vol. 18, No.14, (April) pp. 2357-2365,

Sun, S.Y.; Yue, P.; Shroot, B.; Hong, W.K. & Lotan, R. (1999c) Implication of c-Myc in apoptosis induced by the retinoid CD437 in human lung carcinoma cells. *Oncogene* Vol.18, No.26 (July) pp. 3894-3901

Thomasson, H.R.; Crabb, D.W.; Edenberg, H.J. & Li, T.K. (1993) Alcohol and aldehyde dehydrogenase polymorphisms and alcoholism. *Behavior Genetics*. Vol. 23, No.2 (March) pp.131-136. 1993

Thompson, R.H.; Allison, J.P., & Kwon, E.D. (2006) Anti-cytotoxic T lymphocyte antigen-4 (CTLA-4) immunotherapy for the treatment of prostate cancer,*Urologic Oncology*, vol. 24, No.5 (October) pp. 442–447,

Verma A.K.; Shoemaker,A,; Simsiman, R.; Denning, M.& Zachman, R.D. (1992) Expression of retinoic acid nuclear receptors and tissue transglutaminase is altered in various tissues of rats fed a vitamin A-deficient diet. *The Journal of Nutrition* Vol. 122, No.11 (November) pp. 2144–2152,

Vaglenova, J.; Martínez, S.E.; Porté, S.; Duester, G.; Farrés & J.; Parés, X. (2003) Expression, localization and potential physiological significance of alcohol dehydrogenase in the gastrointestinal tract. *Europian Journal of Biochemistry*, Vol. 270, No.12 (June) pp.2652-2662,

Wallden, B.; Emond, M.; , Swift, M.E.; Disis, M.L. & Swisshelm, K. (2005) Antimetastatic gene expression profiles mediated by retinoic acid receptor beta 2 in MDA-MB-435 breast cancer cells. *BMC Cancer* Vol. 5, No.5 (October) pp. 140-153.

Wan, X.; Duncan, M.D.; Nass, P. & Harmon, J.W. (2001). Synthetic retinoid CD437 induces apoptosis of esophageal squamous HET-1A cells through the caspase-3-dependent pathway. *Anticancer Research* Vol. 21, (July-August) pp. 2657-2663,

Widschwendter, M.; Berger, J.; Daxenbichler. G.; Müller-Holzner, E.; , Widschwendter, A.; Mayr, A.; Marth, C. & Zeimet, A.G. (1997) Loss of retinoic acid receptor beta expression in breast cancer and morphologically normal adjacent tissue but not in the normal breast tissue distant from the cancer. *Cancer Research* Vol. 57, No.19, (October) pp. 4158–4161,

Widschwendter, M.; Berger, J.; Hermann, M.; Müller, H.M.; Amberger, A.; Zeschnigk, M.; Widschwendter, A.; Abendstein, B., & Zeimet, A.G. (2000) Daxenbichler G, Marth C.Methylation and silencing of the retinoic acid receptorh2 gene in breast cancer. *Journal of the National Cancer Institute* Vol. 92, No.10 (May) pp. 826-832

Xu, X.C.; Zile, M.H.; Lippman, S.M.; Lee, J.S.; Lee, J.J.; Hong, W.K.; Lotan, R.; Lippman, S.M.; Lee, J.S.; Lee, J.J. & Hong, W.K. (1995) Anti-retinoic acid (RA) antibody binding to human premalignant oral lesions which occurs less frequently than binding to normal tissue increases after 13-cis-RA treatment in vivo and is related to RA receptor beta expression. *Cancer Research* Vol. 55, No.23 (December) pp. 5507–5511

Xu, X.C.; Lee, J.S.; Lee, J.J.; Morice, R.C.; Liu, X.; Lippman, S.M.; Hong W.K. & Lotan,R (1999), Nuclear retinoid acid receptor beta in bronchial epithelium of smokers before and during chemoprevention. *Journal of the National Cancer Institute* Vol 91, No.15, (August), pp.1317-1321,

Xu, X.C. (2007) Tumor-suppressive activity of retinoic acid receptor-β in cancer *Cancer Letter* Vol. 253, No.1 (August) pp. 14-24

Yen, A.; Roberson, M.S.; Varvayanis,S. & Lee, A.T. (1998) Retinoic acid induced mitogen-activated protein (MAP)/extracellular signal- regulated kinase (ERK) kinase-dependent MAP kinase activation needed to elicit HL-60 cell differentiation and growth arrest. *Cancer Research* Vol. 58, Bo.14 (July) pp. 3163-3172

Yin, S.J.; Chou, F.J.; Chao, S.F.; Tsai, S.F., Liao, C.S.. & Wang S.L. (1993) Alcohol and aldehyde dehydrogenases in human esophagus: comparison with the stomach enzyme activities. *Alcoholism; Clin Exp Res* Vol.17, No.2 (April) pp. 376-381

Yin, S.J.; Chou, C.F. & Lai, C.L. (2003), Human class IV alcohol dehydrogenase: kinetic mechanism, functional roles and medical relevance. *Chemistry Biology Interaction,* Vol. 143-144, (February) pp. 219-227

Yokoyama, A.; Muramatsu, T.; Ohmori, T.; Higuchi, S.; Hayashida, M., & Ishii H. (1996). Esophageal cancer and aldehyde dehydrogenase-2 genotype in Japanese males. *Cancer Epidemiology Biomarker Prevention* Vol. 5, No.3 (November) pp. 99-102,

Yokoyama, A.; Tanaka,Y.; Yokoyama, T.; Mizukami, T.; Matsui, T.; Maruyama, K. & Omori, T. (2011) p53 protein accumulation, iodine-unstained lesions, and alcohol dehydrogenase-1B and aldehyde dehydrogenase-2 genotypes in Japanese alcoholic men with esophageal dysplasia.*Cancer Letter,* Vol 308, No.1 (September) pp.112-117.

Yokoyama, H.; Baraona, E. & Lieber, C.S. (1994) Molecular cloning of human class IV alcohol dehydrogenase cDNA. Biochemistry *Biophysiology Research Communication,* Vol. 203, No.1 (August) pp. 219-224,.

Yokoyama, H.; Baraona, E. & Lieber, C.S. (1996) Molecular cloning and chromosomal localization of ADH7 gene encoding human class IV (σ) ADH. *Genomics* No.2 (January) Vol. 31, pp 243-245,

Yokoyama, H.; Baraona, E., & Lieber, C.S. (1995a) Comparison of the ADH7 gene structure in Caucasian and Japanese subjects. *Biochemistry Biophysiology Research Communication,* Vol. 212, No.3, (July), pp. 875-878,

Yokoyama, H.; Baraona, E., & Lieber, C.S. (1995 b) Upstream structure of human ADH7 gene and the organ distribution of its expression. *Biochemistry Biophysiology Research Communication,* Vol. 216, No.1 (November) pp. 216-222,

Yokoyama, H.; Matsumoto, M.; Shiraishi, H., & Ishii, H.(2000) Simultaneous quantification of various retinoids by high performance liquid chromatography: its relevance to alcohol research. *Alcoholism Clinical Experimental Research* Vol 24, No.4 Supple (April) pp. 26S-29S.

Yokoyama, H.; Matsumoto, M.; Shiraishi, H.; Miyagi, M.; Kato, S. & Ishii, H. (2001) NAD dependent retinoic acid formation from retinol in the human gastric mucosa : Its inhibition by ethanol, acetaldehyde, and H2 blockers. *Alcoholism Clinical Experimental Research* Vol. 25, No.6 (June) 24S-28S,.

Yokoyama, H.; Shiraishi-Yokoyamama, H. & Hibi, T. (2010) Structural features of the NAD-dependent *in-situ* retinoic acid supply system in esophageal mucosa. *Alcoholism Clinical Experimental Research.* Vol. 34 Suppl 1, (February) pp. S39-S44.

Yoshida, A.; Hsu, L.C. & Dave, L. (1992) Retinal oxidation activity and biological role of human cytosolic aldehyde dehydrogenase. *Enzyme* Vol 46, No.4-5, pp. 239-244.

Yu, H.S.; Oyama, T.; Isse, T.; Kitagawa, K.; Pham, T.T.; Tanaka, M., & Kawamoto,T. (2010) Formation of acetaldehyde-derived DNA adducts due to alcohol exposure. *Chemico- Biological Interaction.* Vol. 188, No.3 (December) pp. 367-375.

Zou, C.P. ; Clifford. J.L.; Xu, X.C.; Sacks, P.G.; Chambon, P.; Hong, WK, & Lotan, R. (1994) Modulation by retinoic acid (RA) of squamous cell differentiation, cellular RA-binding proteins, and nuclear RA receptors in human head and neck squamous carcinoma cell lines. *Cancer Res* Vol. 54, No.20 (October), pp. 5479-5487

6

Study on the Dietary Factors of Esophageal Cancer

Guiju Sun[1], Tingting Wang[1], Guiling Huang[1], Ming Su[2], Jiasheng Wang[3], Shaokang Wang[1] and Fukang Liu[1]

[1]School of Public Health, Southeast University,
[2]Chuzhou Distract Center for Disease Control and Prevention,
[3]University of Georgia,
[1,2]China
[3]USA

1. Introduction

Esophageal Cancer (EC) is among upper digestive tract cancers and mainly prevalent in developing and underdeveloped countries. There are about 460,000 new cases of EC annually (World Cancer Research Fund & American Institute for Cancer Research [WRCF], 2007). The etiology of EC is complex, including heredity, environment and food factors, etc. The scientific community is convinced that both genetic and environmental factors play important role in EC's carcinogenesis. Although, inherited high susceptibility to EC accounts for part proportion of cases, exogenous exposures are also important for causing this disease. A number of studies have suggested that dietary factors are significant to the development of EC (De Stefani et al., 2006; Engel et al., 2003; Hung et al., 2004). And there is evidence that different varieties of food and nutrients could play a role in protecting against this disease (Chen et al., 2002; Liaw et al., 2003). In this chapter, evidence of food and nutrients on EC has been collected, and provide advices for the prevention of EC.

2. Meta-analysis of nutrients and EC

Meta-analysis has been a useful tool for providing combine quantitatively the evidence from different studies on specific research questions (Tatsionia & Ioannidis, 2008). In order to summarize the relationship between nutrients and risk of EC, we did meta-analysis of the relationship between dietary factors and occurrence of EC.

2.1 Vegetables and fruits

Vegetables and fruits are sources of a wide variety of micronutrients and are rich in antioxidant substances, among them, β-carotene and vitamin C have been shown to play protective role in the occurrence and development of EC (Michels et al., 2005; Terry et al., 2000). As we all known, vegetables and fruits also contain dietary fiber and other bioactive compounds, which are termed as phytochemicals (Soler et al., 2001). They can play important role in the functions of the plant, such as providing flavour, color, or supporting protection (WCRF, 2007). The phytochemicals include many varieties such as flavonoids, isoflavones, glucosinolates and so on, but they are not essential in the human diet (WCRF, 2007). Many researches either in humans or in laboratory experiments have shown that most of the bioactive compounds have potentially beneficial health effects when they are included in diets (Franceschi et al., 2000; Freedman et al., 2007). However, the bioavailability of these compounds is variable and their ultimate heath effects are needed to study further.

The average vegetable consumption (not including vegetable oil) of global population is 2.6 percent of total daily energy intake (Food and Agriculture Organization of the United Nations, [FAOSTAT], 2006). It is generally high in North Africa, the Middle East, parts of Asia, the USA and Cuba, and in southern Europe. The global average for fruit consumption (based on availability) is 2.7 percent of total daily energy intake (FAOSTAT, 2006). Fruit consumption is generally higher than vegetable consumption, but it shows a great variability in different areas.

The case-control or cohort studies from 1995 to 2011 on vegetables, fruits and EC have been collected with searching tools such as Web of Science, PubMed. The keywords were "esophageal cancer", "diet", "nutrients", "vegetables" and "fruit" , and selected odds ratio (OR) as effect index. All the relevant studies have been identified. The heterogeneity test, a fixed effect model or random effect model has been selected to calculate the combined OR and OR 95% confidence interval (95%CI). The software of Stata 11.0 has been used for the meta-analysis.

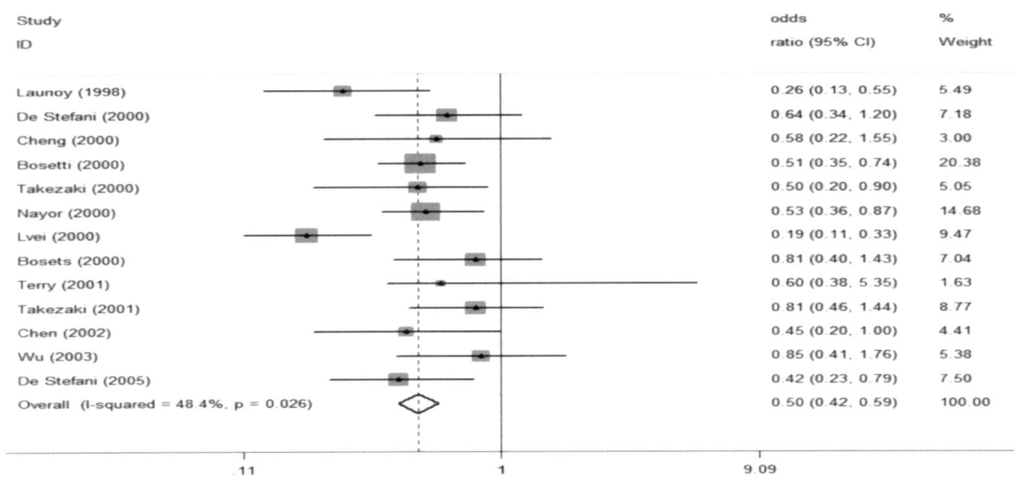

Fig. 1. Forest plot of vegetables and EC, case-control study. The rhombus is stand for the combined OR, and the OR is calculated by highest versus lowest exposure category of vegetables intake.

23 case-control studies and only three cohort studies (Fan et al., 2008; Tran et al., 2005; Zheng et al., 1995) have investigated relation between vegetables and EC, among them, 16 case-control studies have shown decreased risk with increased vegetables intake, which were statistically significant. Only one case-control study has shown an increased risk

(OR=1.54, OR 95%CI: 1.10-2.16) (Takezaki et al., 2001), and six case-control studies were non-significant difference (Bosetti et al., 2000; Chen et al., 2002; Cheng et al., 2000; Zhang et al., 1997; Wu et al., 2003; Yang et al., 2005). The data of studies have suggested an association with reduced risk when increased vegetables intake. According to the different exposures which have been collected from the studies, the OR has been analyzed for two parts, one was the highest versus lowest exposure category, and the other was consumption frequently versus consumption occasionally or less category. The combined OR and OR 95%CI for case-control studies of vegetables and EC were 0.50, 0.42-0.59 (figures 1) and 0.66, 0.61-0.72 (figures 2). The evidence of cohort studies for vegetables and EC has not been enough. Among the three cohort studies, one of which has described association between vegetables and esophageal squamous cell carcinoma (ESCC), esophageal adenocarcinoma (EAC) respectively. The relative risk (RR) and RR 95%CI for ESCC were 0.57, 0.28-1.18 and they were 0.92, 0.57-1.50 for EAC, but both were non-significant statistically (Freedman et al., 2007). The other two cohort studies were also non-significant difference (Fan et al., 2008; Tran et al., 2005). All the studies have been adjusted for confounding factors.

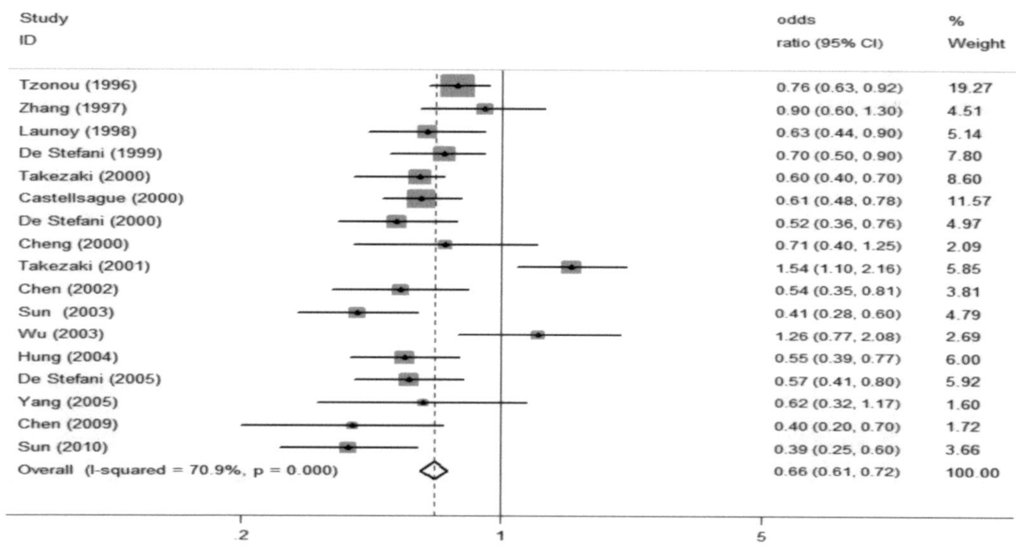

Fig. 2. Forest plot of total vegetables and EC, case-control study. The rhombus is stand for the combined OR, and the OR is calculated by eating frequently versus eating occasionally or less category, the individuals who eat vegetables ≥1 time/d versus those who eat <1 time/ d.

24 case-control studies have investigated association between fruits and EC, 14 of which have shown relationship between fresh fruits consumption and reduced risk of EC (Bosetti et al., 2000; Castellsague et al., 2000; Chen et al., 2009; Cheng et al., 2000; De Stefani et al., 1999; De Stefani et al., 2000; De Stefani et al., 2005; Hung et al., 2004; Sun et al., 2003; Takezaki et al., 2000; Terry et al., 2001; Wang et al., 1999; Wu et al., 2003; Yang et al., 2005), with the other 10 studies reporting results of non-significant difference (Gao et al., 1999; Launoy et al., 1998; Nayar et al., 2000; Phukan et al., 2001; Sharp et al., 2001; Takezaki et al., 2000; Takezaki et al., 2001; Tzonou et al., 1996; Wu et al., 2003; Zhang et al., 1997). Four

cohort studies have shown data on the fresh fruits and EC, RR of the two studies have suggested that fresh fruits intake strongly associated with decreased risk of EC (Fan et al., 2008; Tran et al., 2005). Another one cohort study has shown no relationship between fruits and EC (Zheng et al., 1995). Also one study has found a significant inverse association between total fruits and vegetables intake and ESCC risk (RR: 0.78, 95%CI: 0.67-0.91), but not EAC risk (0.98, 0.90-1.08) (Freeman et al., 2007). The combined OR and OR 95%CI (highest versus lowest exposure category) of case-control studies for fruits and EC were 0.57, 0.49-0.66 (figure 3). And the combined OR and OR 95%CI (eating frequently versus eating occasionally or less category) of case-control studies for fruits and EC were 0.60, 0.55-0.66 (figure 4).

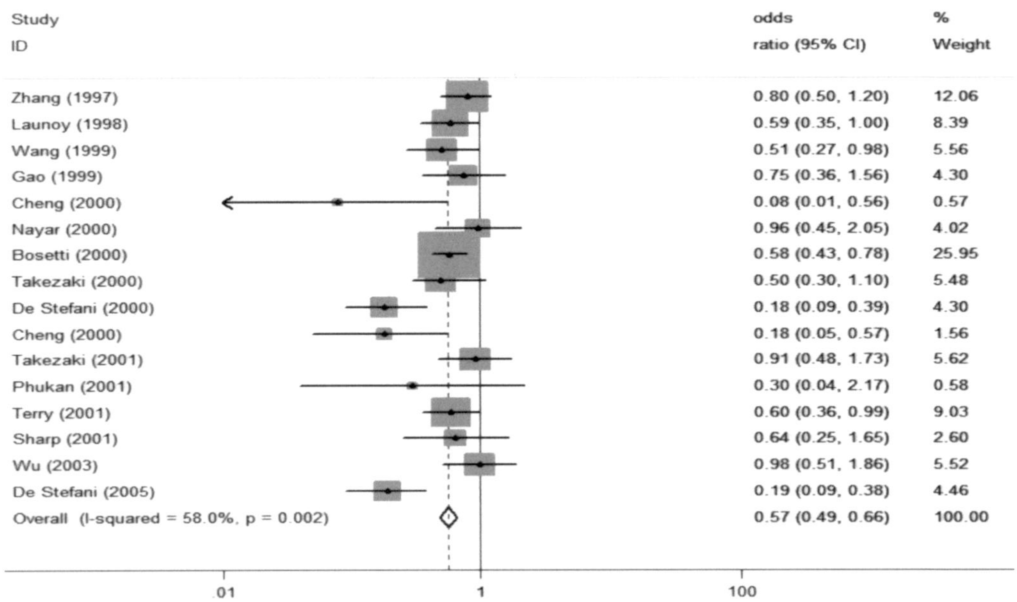

Fig. 3. Forest plot of fruit and EC, case-control study. The rhombus is stand for the combined OR, and the OR is calculated by highest versus against lowest exposure category of fruit intake.

Three case-control studies have investigated vegetables and fruits combined consumption and EC (De Stefani et al., 2000; De Stefani et al., 2005; Zhang et al., 1997). All the data of studies have suggested an association with reduced risk. The results of meta-analysis for the relationship between vegetables, fruits and EC have shown that they could probably protect people from EC.

2.2 Vitamin A

Vitamins are organic molecules, and classified as fat- or water-soluble, which are essential for metabolism but cannot be made in the body. Most vitamins must be supplied from the diet. Vitamin A is a fat-soluble vitamin and can only be digested, absorbed, and transported in conjunction with dietary fats. An important source of vitamin A is from plant foods such as green leafy vegetables and fruits that contain the retinol precursors known as carotenoids,

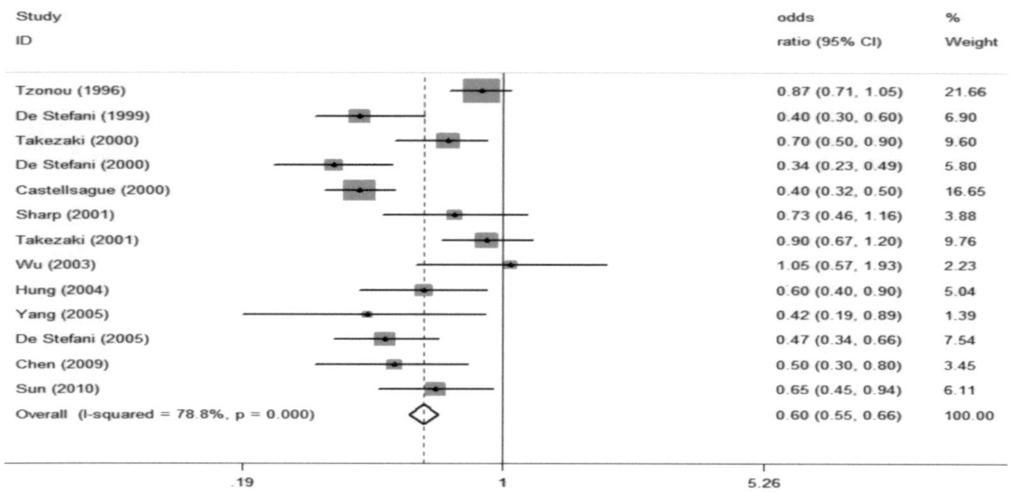

Fig. 4. Forest plot of total fruit and EC, case-control study. The rhombus is stand for the combined OR, and the OR is calculated by eating frequently versus eating occasionally or less category, the individuals who eat fruit ≥1 time/d versus those who eat <1 time/ d.

most importantly β-carotene, which can be converted by the body to retinol, and sometimes are called pro-vitamin A carotenoids. Other sources of vitamin A are from animal foods such as liver, milk and eggs, which can be used by the body directly (WCRF, 2007). Some studies have suggested that vitamin A could play a crucial role in protecting damaged epithelial cells against attack by carcinogens, and esophageal epithelial cells are more sensitive to the deficiency in vitamin A (Poulain et al., 2009).

The meta-analysis has been made respectively for relationship between vitamin A, β-carotene of diet and EC. The case-control or cohort studies from 1995 to 2011 on vitamin A and EC have been collected with searching tools such as Web of Science, PubMed. The keywords were "esophageal cancer", "diet", "nutrients", "vitamin A", "beta- carotene", and selected OR as effect index. Then the method of next step was the same as which has been used for vegetables and EC.

A total of eight case-control studies (Bollschweiler et al., 2002; Chen et al., 2002; De Stefani et al., 1999; Franceschi et al., 2000; Mayne et al., 2001; Terry et al., 2000; Tzonou et al., 1996; Zhang et al., 1997) and one eligible cohort study (Zheng et al., 1995) have investigated vitamin A, retinol and β-carotene of diet, also two cohort studies have investigated retinol and β-carotene in serum (Abnet et al., 2003; Nomura et al., 1997). The evidence for vitamin A and EC was limited; since there have been only three eligible studies before 2001 (De Stefani et al., 1999; Mayne et al., 2001; Tzonou et al., 1996). The combined OR and 95%CI for it were 0.66, 0.49-0.89 (figure 5). Five case-control studies have published data on the β-carotene of diet and EC, and only two eligible studies have shown decreased risk when comparing the highest intake group against the lowest of vitamin A intake. The combined OR and OR 95%CI of meta-analysis were 0.66, 0.54-0.81 (figure 6). A decreased risk associated with high retinol and β-carotene intake were also consistent findings in several studies on EC. The result of meta-analysis has suggested of food containing vitamin A may protect body against EC and need further study.

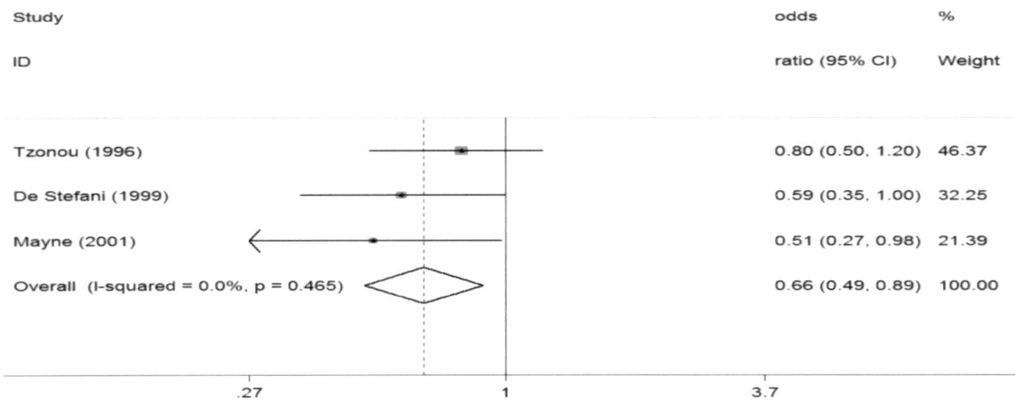

Fig. 5. Forest plot of total vitamin A and EC, case-control study. The rhombus is stand for the combined OR, and the OR is calculated by the 75th percentile versus the 25th percentile of vitamin A intake.

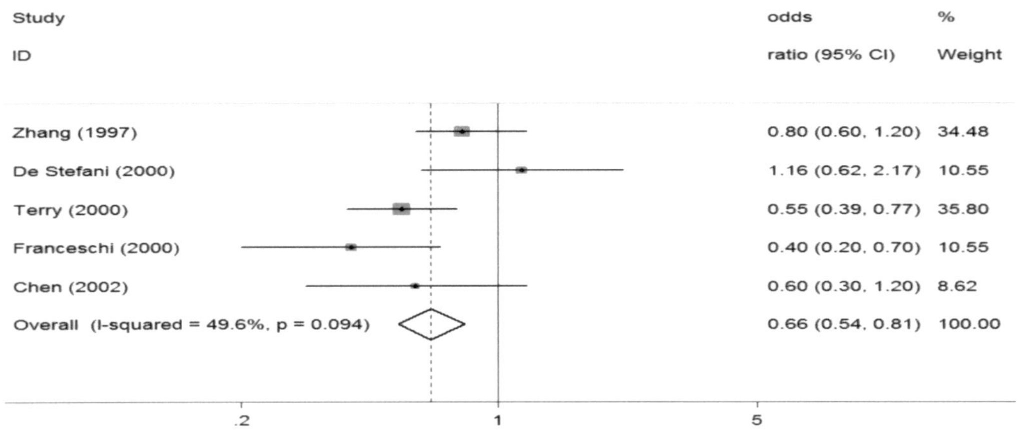

Fig. 6. Forest plot of β-carotene and EC, case-control study. The rhombus is stand for the combined OR, and the OR is calculated by highest versus lowest exposure category of β-carotene intake.

2.3 Folic acid

Folic acid is one of B vitamins which is water-soluble, and is equivalent of pteroylglutamic acid. The main sources of folic acid are lettuce, spinach and tangerine etc vegetables and fruits (WCRF, 2007). Folic acid is involved in a number of metabolic pathways, especially in the synthesis of purines and pyrimidines (Tan et al., 2005). A few studies have suggested that folic acid is important for DNA synthesis and methylation (Axumea et al., 2007; Kima et al., 2009). But limited evidence has supported high folic acid intake may reduce risks of EC overall.

The case-control or cohort studies from 1995 to 2011 on folic acid and EC also have been collected with searching tools such as Web of Science, PubMed. The keywords were "esophageal cancer", "diet", "nutrients", "folic acid", and selected OR as effect index. Then the method of next step was the same as which has been used for vegetables and EC.

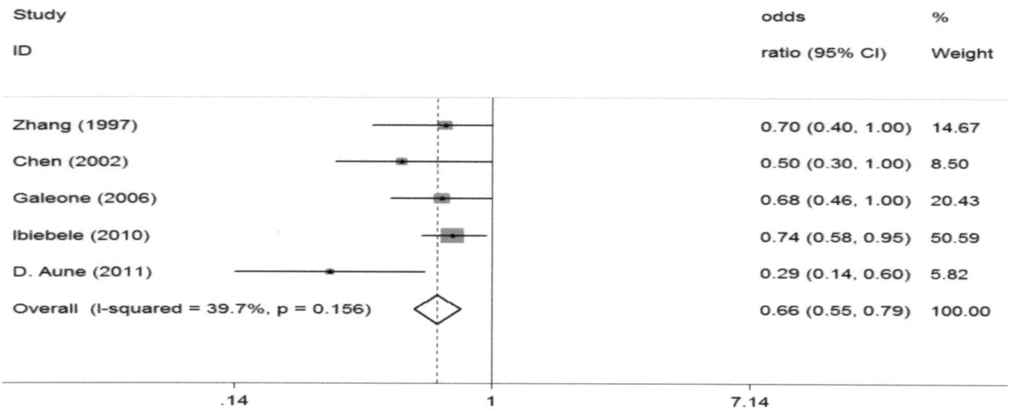

Fig. 7. Forest plot of folic acid and EC, case-control study. The rhombus is stand for the combined OR, and the OR is calculated by highest versus lowest exposure category of folic acid.

A total of eight case-control studies have evaluated the relationship between intake of folic acid from foods and supplements and risk of EC (Aune et al., 2011; Chen et al., 2002; De Stefani et al., 1999; Franceschi et al., 2000; Galeone et al., 2006; Ibiebele et al., 2010; Mayne et al., 2001; Zhang et al., 1997). Of which two case-control studies have reported that dietary folic acid could decrease risk of EC in the highest intake groups when compared to the lowest (Aune et al., 2011; Ibiebele et al., 2010). Only one eligible case-control study has analyzed thymidylate synthase genotype and serum folic acid concentration in patients with ESCC and controls (Tan et al., 2005). The data of meta-analysis have shown that the combined OR was 0.66, and 95%CI was 0.55-0.79 when analyzed the highest versus lowest exposure of folic acid and EC (figure 7). Our result has indicated that folic acid could protect individuals against EC, but still need collect data of further research in population.

2.4 Vitamin C

It is generally that plant foods are important sources of vitamin C. Non-starch vegetables and fruits are rich in vitamin C, which can be directly absorbed by the body. But vitamin C in the foods can be destroyed by heat or exposure to the air, or lost by leaching during cooking (WCRF, 2007). It is biologically demonstrated that vitamin C could protect against EC because it can trap free radicals and reactive oxygen molecules, protecting from lipid peroxidation, reducing nitrates, and stimulating the immune system (Odin, 1997). Moreover, it can recycle other antioxidant vitamins. Many studies have shown that vitamin C could inhibit formation of carcinogens and protect DNA from mutagenic attack (Hercberg et al., 1998). However, evidence supporting a specific mechanism in the esophagus is limited.

The case-control or cohort studies from 1995 to 2011 on vitamin C and EC have been collected with searching tools such as Web of Science, PubMed. The keywords were "esophageal cancer", "diet", "nutrients", "vitamin C", and selected OR as effect index. Then the method of next step was the same as which has been used for vegetables and EC.

Totally, ten case-control (Chen et al., 2002; De Stefani et al., 1999; De Stefani et al., 2000; Franceschi et al., 2000; Kubo et al., 2008; Launoy et al., 1998; Mayne et al., 2001; Terry et al.,

2000; Tzonou et al., 1996; Zhang et al., 1997) and one eligible cohort studies (Zheng et al., 1995) have investigated the relationship between vitamin C of diet and EC. Most of the researches except one (Zhang et al., 1997) have published that a strongly association between high intake of vitamin C and deceased risk of EC. The single eligible cohort study has reported a non-significant reduced risk for the highest intake groups when compared to the lowest after adjustment for smoking, with OR of 0.70 (95%CI: 0.30–1.70). The combined OR and 95%CI of the 75th percentile intake versus the 25th percentile of vitamin C intake were 0.57, 0.52-0.63 (figure 8). Another combined OR and 95%CI (highest versus lowest exposure category) were 0.66, 0.55-0.79 (figure 9). The results of meta-analysis have suggested vitamin C could probably have an effect of prevention of EC.

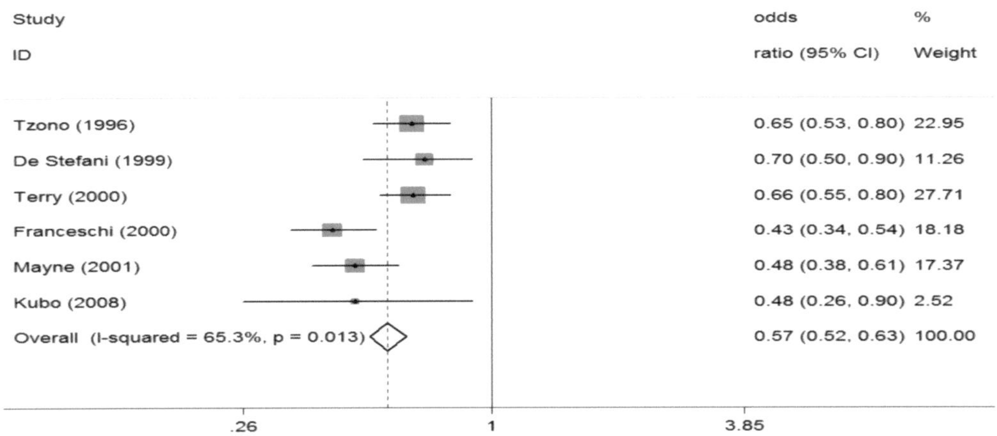

Fig. 8. Forest plot of total vitamin C and EC, case-control study. The rhombus is stand for the combined OR, and the OR is calculated by the 75th percentile versus the 25th percentile of vitamin C intake.

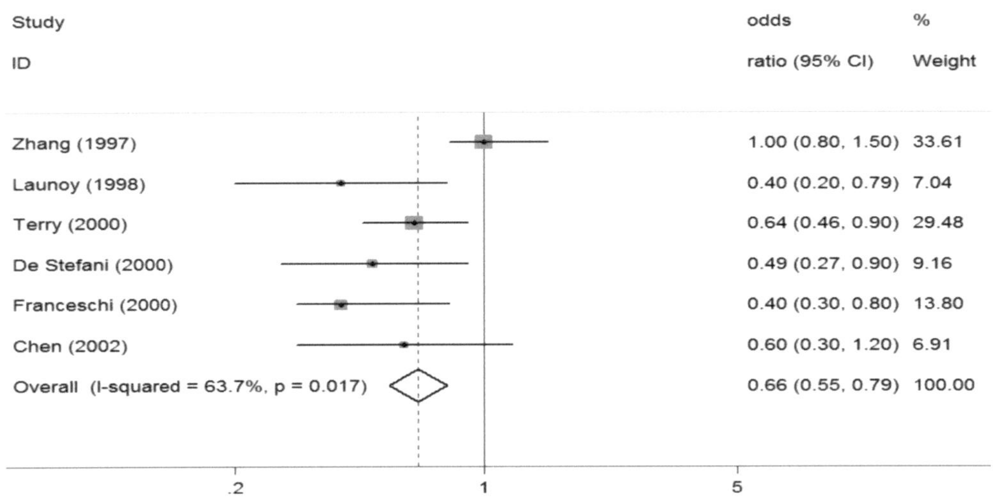

Fig. 9. Forest plot of vitamin C and EC, case-control study. The rhombus is stand for the combined OR, and the OR is calculated by highest versus lowest exposure category of vitamin C intake.

2.5 Vitamin D

Vitamin D is fat-soluble of vitamins, which is a sort of substances showing the biological activity of ergocalciferol (vitamin D_2) and cholecalciferol (vitamin D_3), and 1,25-$(OH)_2D_3$ is the main active form of vitamin D (Reddy et al., 2006). The seafood and liver of animals are rich in vitamin D. Experimental researches have shown that 1,25-$(OH)_2D_3$ could inhibit the proliferation of EC cell EC-9706, and it is important for prevention and treatment of EC (He et al., 2009). The anti-tumor mechanism of 1,25-$(OH)_2D_3$ may be that it could primarily inhibit cycle progression of tumor cells, causing G_1 phase of tumor cells arrest, the cell number of S phase was decreased, and accumulation of G_0/G_1 phase, so that inducing the differentiation and maturity of tumor cells (He et al., 2009) . But there have been not enough evidence to demonstrate the association between vitamin D and EC. Only three eligible case-control studies have investigated the relationship between diet of vitamin D and EC (Franceschi et al., 2000; Launoy et al., 1998; Mayne et al., 2001). Among them, all the results have shown the decreased risk when appropriate intake of vitamin D, but two of which were non-significant difference.

2.6 Vitamin E

Vitamin E is a family of eight compounds collectively referred as tocopherols, of which alpha- and gamma-tocopherol are the most common. Vitamin E is a fat-soluble vitamin. The most important dietary sources of vitamin E are vegetable oils such as soya bean, corn, olive oils, sunflower, and palm. Nuts, sunflower seeds, and wheat germ also contain this vitamin. Vitamin E can act as antioxidants and free radical scavengers (WCRF, 2007). However, few studies have supported it has an anti-cancer effect of esophagus.

The case-control or cohort studies from 1995 to 2011 on vitamin E and EC also have been collected with searching tools such as Web of Science, PubMed. The keywords were "esophageal cancer", "diet", "nutrients", "vitamin E", and selected OR as effect index. Then the method of next step was the same as which has been used for vegetables and EC.

Nine case-control studies (Bollschweiler et al., 2002; Chen et al., 2002; De Stefani et al., 1999; De Stefani et al., 2000; Franceschi et al., 2000; Kubo et al., 2008; Launoy et al., 1998; Mayne et al., 2001; Zhang et al., 1997) and one cohort study (Zheng et al., 1995) have shown the relationship between dietary vitamin E and EC, and two cohort studies have investigated the role of serum vitamin E (Nomura et al., 1997; Taylor et al., 2003). Six case-control studies have reported decreased risk for the highest intake groups when compared to the lowest, which was statistically significant in four, the other studies have reported no effect on EC risk (figure 10). The cohort studies and most case-control studies have shown decreased risk with increased vitamin E intake, but case-control data about serum vitamin E were inconsistent. Both cohort studies have shown decreased risk for the highest level groups of vitamin E intake when compared to the lowest. The combined OR and OR 95%CI of the 75th percentile versus the 25th percentile of vitamin E intake were 0.53, 0.46-0.63 (figure 11).

2.7 Tea

Currently, tea, in the form of green, black or oolong tea, is the most widely consumed beverage in the world. The main active component of tea is polyphenol. In vitro and animal

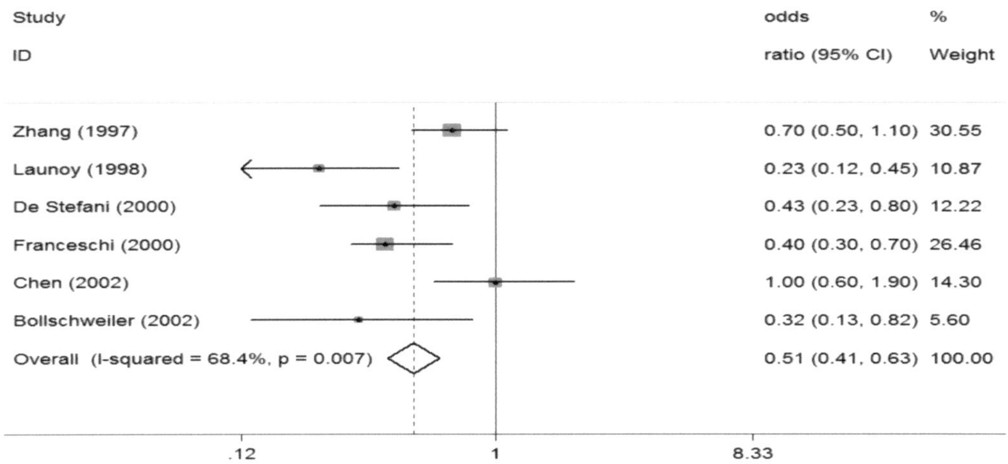

Fig. 10. Forest plot of vitamin E and EC, case-control study. The rhombus is stand for the combined OR, and the OR is calculated by highest versus lowest exposure category of vitamin E intake.

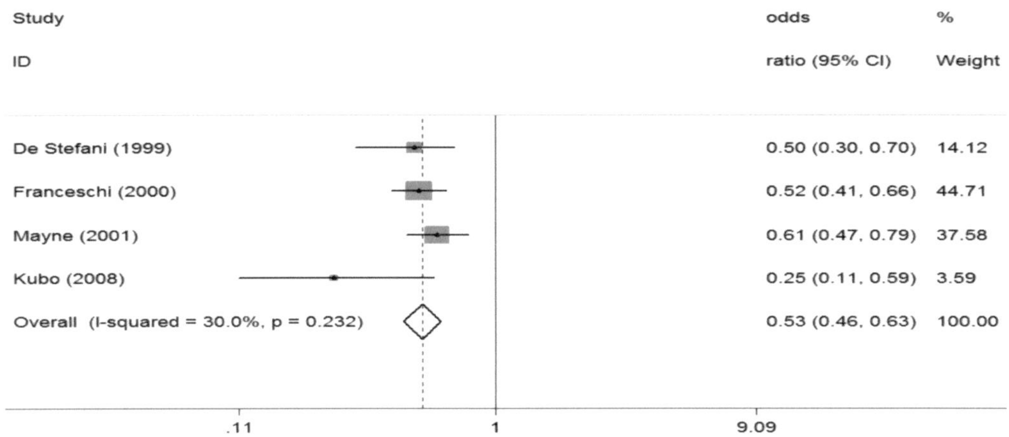

Fig. 11. Forest plot of total vitamin E and EC, case-control study. The rhombus is stand for the combined OR, and the OR is calculated by the 75th percentile versus the 25th percentile of vitamin E intake.

studies have provided strong evidence that polyphenol derived from tea may possess the bioactivity to affect the pathogenesis of different cancers (Khan & Mukhtar, 2007). The association between drinking different tea and risk of EC have been reported in several studies from different parts of the world (Castellsague et al., 2000; Ganesh et al., 2009; Ibiebele et al., 2010; Li et al., 2002). But for different kinds of tea, there has been still little evidence for an association between amount of use and EC risk. Moreover, the majority of studies have shown an increased risk of EC associated with drinking higher temperature tea which was statistically significant in most of them (Wang et al., 2007; Lin et al., 2010).

The case-control or cohort studies from 1995 to 2011 on tea and EC have been collected with searching tools such as Web of Science, PubMed, China National Knowledge Infrastructure.

The keywords were "esophageal cancer", "tea", "green tea", "black tea", "maté" and selected OR as effect index. Then the method of next step was the same as which has been used for vegetables and EC.

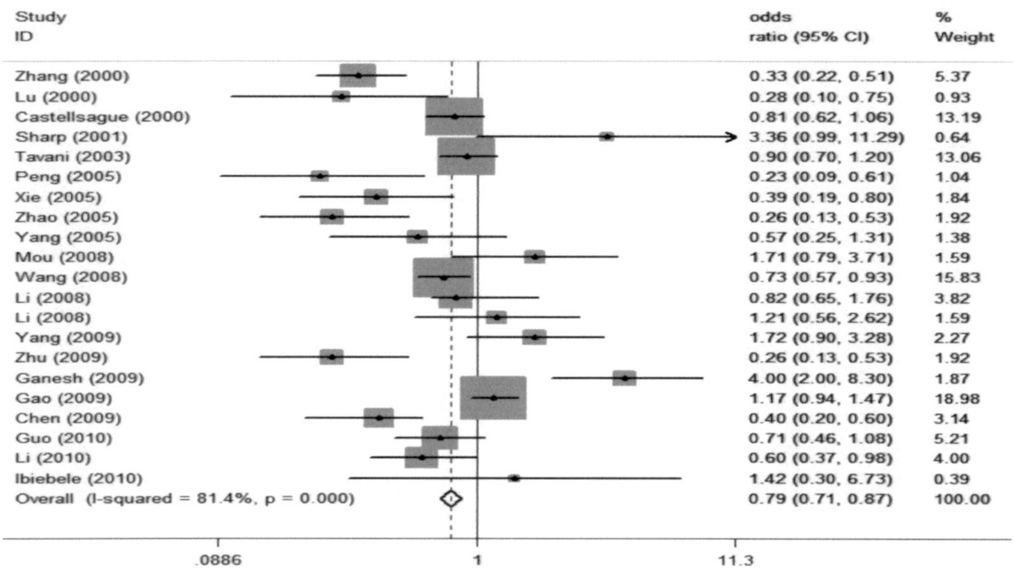

Fig. 12. Forest plot of tea and EC, case-control study. The rhombus is stand for the combined OR, and the OR is calculated by drinking frequently versus drinking occasionally or less category of tea.

A total of 21 case-control studies have published the tea and EC (figure 12). 14 studies have shown decreased EC risk when comparing drinking frequently against drinking occasionally or less category, nine of which the OR were statistically significant (Chen et al., 2009; Li et al., 2010; Lu et al., 20000; Peng et al., 2005; Wang et al., 2008; Xie et al., 2005; Zhang et al., 2000; Zhao et al., 2005; Zhu et al., 2009), but five studies were not statistically significant (Castellsague et al., 2000; Guo et al., 2010; Tavani et al., 2003; Yang et al., 2005; Li, 2008). Another six studies have suggested increased risk of EC with high tea drinking (Gao et al., 2009; Mou et al., 2008; Sharp et al., 2001; Ibiebele et al., 2010; Yang et al., 2009). However, only one eligible study has shown the OR for drinking tea and EC was 4.0, 95%CI was 2.0-8.3 in Indian population (Ganesh et al., 2009). The combined OR and OR 95%CI (drinking frequently versus drinking occasionally or less category) of case-control studies for EC were 0.786, 0.713-0.866. The results have suggested that drinking tea could probably protect body against EC.

2.7.1 Green tea

Green tea is favored in Japan and China, and majority of studies researched on the benefits of green tea were carried out in these countries because of the local customs. The processing of green tea is different from black tea. When producing green tea, freshly harvested leaves are steamed to prevent fermentation, yielding a dry, stable product (WCRF, 2007). Tea polyphenols, which are known as catechins, usually account for 30-42% of the dry weight of green tea (Khan & Mukhtar, 2007).

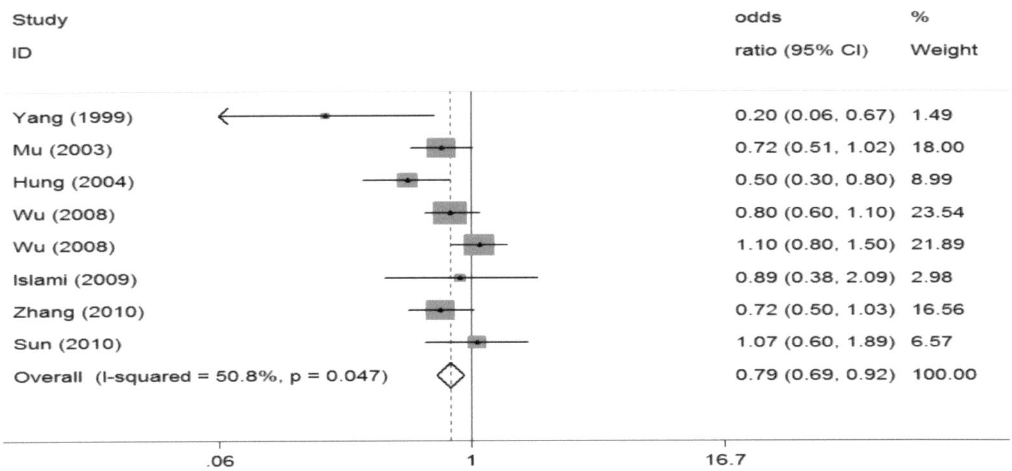

Fig. 13. Forest plot of green tea and EC, case-control study. The rhombus is stand for the combined OR, and the OR is calculated by drinking frequently versus drinking occasionally or less category of green tea.

Seven case-control studies have investigated the association between green tea and EC, and most of them from Chinese population, five studies have shown decreased risk when comparing the drinking great tea group against the non-drinking (Yang et al., 1999; Hung et al., 2004; Islami et al., 2009; Mu et al., 2003; Zhang et al., 2010), of which four were non-significant in statistics. However, two studies have shown that an inverse association between green tea and EC, with no difference in statistics (Sun et al., 2003; Wu et al., 2008). The combined OR and 95%CI of drinking frequently versus drinking occasionally or less category of green tea were 0.79, 0.69-0.92 (figure 13). The results of meta-analysis for green and EC have suggested it has the function for prevention of EC.

2.7.2 Black tea

The black tea composition depends on a technological process known as fermentation, in which about 75% of catechins contained in the tea leaves are crushed to promote enzymatic oxidation and subsequent condensation of tea polyphenols, leading to the formation of oligomeric polyphenols (theaflavins) and polymeric polyphenols (thearubigins) (WCRF, 2007). It is difficult to state a definitive composition for black tea, as it varies with different preparations. Four case-control studies have investigated the relationship between black tea and EC, and the results were not consistent, for two studies have shown increased risk with high drinking of black tea (Chen et al., 2009; Islami et al., 2009), the other two studies have suggested black tea was inversely associated with EC (Gao et al., 2009; Zhang et al., 2010), but all the studies were non-significant statistically (figure 14). The combined OR and 95%CI of drinking frequently versus drinking occasionally or less category of black tea were 1.07, 0.69-1.65. The evidence for black tea is limited and needs further study.

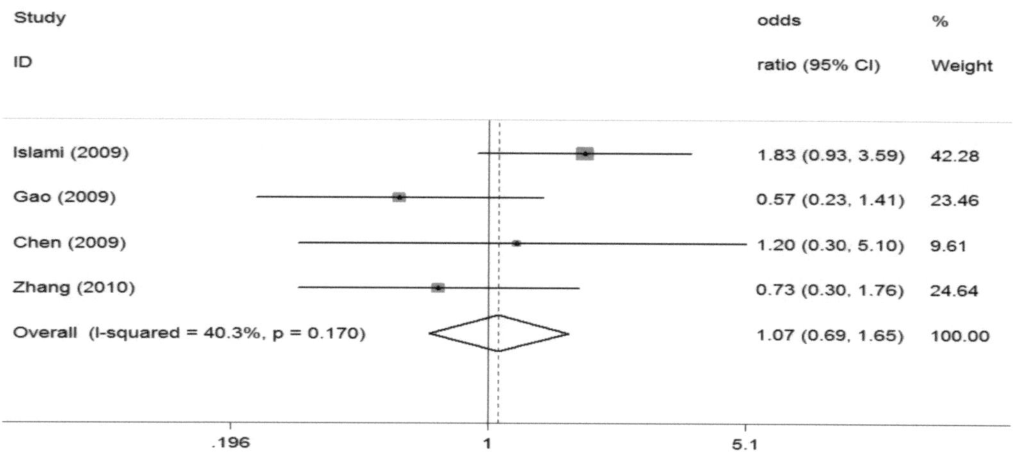

Fig. 14. Forest plot of black tea and EC, case-control study. The rhombus is stand for the combined OR, and the OR is calculated by drinking frequently versus drinking occasionally or less category of black tea.

2.7.3 Maté

Maté, a tea-like infusion of the herb Ilex paraguariensis, is particularly prevalent in southern America, Brazil and in Uruguay. And it is typically drunk scalding hot through a metal straw. This process of heat may damage esophagus (Castellsague et al., 2000). Repeated damage of this nature could lead to cancer of esophagus. Chemical carcinogenesis from constituents of maté has also been postulated.

For maté drinking, the number of studies was limited, but they consistently have shown that EC risk increased with both amount and temperature consumed, and these two were independent risk factors. Three case-control studies have investigated relationship between maté and EC (Castellsague et al., 2000; Sewram et al., 2003; Szymańska et al., 2010). All of them have suggested that an increased incidence of EC with higher maté consumption. Our meta-analysis of case-control data have shown OR was 1.796, 95%CI was 1.363-2.366. The results have shown that maté, an herbal infusion, is probably a cause of EC.

3. A case-control study on the relationship between dietary nutrients intake and EC in China

China is the high EC incidence and mortality country in the world, accounting for more than 50% of new cases in the world, each year about 250,000 cases of newly diagnosed EC, the incidence rate is $19.83/10^5$ and mortality rate is $16.01/10^5$ (Chen et al., 2008; Zhang et al., 2008). The incidence of EC has big regional difference. Chuzhou District, Huaian City, Jiangsu province, China, is a high-incidence area of EC with ESCC incidence over $98/10^5$, which is 7 times higher than the nation's average rate ($13/10^5$) (Hu et al., 2002). Recent years, with the development of the economy, improvement of medical level and enhancement of people's awareness of preventing diseases, incidence of EC has been declining in some of the high-incidence areas in China (Yang et al., 2008), but it is still high in Chuzhou District, Huaian City. The risk factors of EC need to be studied further in this area.

3.1 Subjects and methods

3.1.1 Cases and controls

In the EC high incidence area of Chuzhou District, Huaian City, Jiangsu Province, we have conducted a case-control study of dietary factors and risk of EC. A total of 207 EC cases with newly diagnosed as ESCC by the X-ray, endoscopic or pathological diagnosis in county and above county level hospitals from 2003 to 2008 were considered eligible for the study. The cases were drawn from the local cancer registered system.

Each case was matched within 5 years of age, same sex and nationality by two control subjects who were recruited from the same district. If the people do not want to attend the study, select again randomly, 414 controls were selected in total.

3.1.2 Methods

All the participants were interviewed to fill a structured questionnaire by trained investigators after obtaining written informed consent. The questionnaire included questions about sociodemographic characteristics, occupational history, dietary habits and a detailed food-frequency questionnaire (FFQ) on the intake of 120 food items one year before. Subjects were asked to report how many times they consumed 120 different foods per day, per week, per month or per year and how much per time. This FFQ was considered as representative of this area diet and allowed for the estimation of total energy and nutrients intakes. All data were entered by different persons on two computers using Epidata3.1 software. The total energy and nutrients intake have been calculated using Chinese Food Ingredients Table 2002 (Yang et al., 2002).

3.1.3 Statistical analysis

Single factor logistic analyses for intake of different food groups and interested nutrients were conducted using SPSS 13.0 software to determine differences between controls and cases. Then, unconditional logistic regression was used to calculate OR and corresponding 95%CI for EC compared with controls in relation to daily food group and nutrients intake.

3.2 Results

3.2.1 General status

There were 207 EC cases and matched 414 controls who completed the FFQ after further exclusion of participants with implausible energy intake (<600Kcal/d or >5000Kcal/d). 112 pairs (one pair included one case and two controls) were males and 95 pairs were females. There was no significant difference ($P>0.05$) between cases and controls in age, ethnicity, education level, marital status, etc., and all the cases and controls were farmers (Table 1).

3.2.2 Dietary intakes of foods and nutrients

The daily foods have been divided into 8 categories, 120 species. According to survey data of FFQ, all kinds of food daily intakes were calculated in Table 2 [if the variance of data was heterogeneity, the data were listed with the median (M) and quartile (Q)].

Basic information		Cases	Controls	P value
Age(year)	Male	62.07±7.49	61.83±7.44	0.780
	Female	61.86±8.40	61.80±8.29	0.952
	Total	61.98±7.90	61.82±7.84	0.812
Education level	Illiterate	127	227	0.090
	Primary school	54	103	
	Junior high school	21	60	
	Senior high school and above	5	24	
Marital status	Married	160	342	0.463
	Divorce	1	2	
	Widowed	42	64	
	Spinsterhood	4	6	

Table 1. Comparison of the basic information between cases and controls.

Food kinds	Cases	Controls	P value
Cereals	528.01±276.51	501.73±226.65	0.365
Livestock and poultry meat	38.90±43.08	24.02±32.87	0.008
Fish and shrimp	13.22±22.88	11.38±17.04	0.652
Egg, milk and products	27.95±44.38	27.40±39.56	0.384
Beans and products	79.79±70.30	69.45±77.82	0.341
Vegetables	214.26±227.26	247.70±167.12	0.967
Fruits	39.52±64.17	30.15±42.99	0.201
Allium vegetables	4.11±6.52	8.49±12.16	0.004
Salted and smoked products	34.38±44.86	37.78±46.05	0.718

Table 2. Foods dietary intakes of cases and controls (g/d, M±Q).

As shown in table 2, the large proportion of daily diet was plant-based foods such as cereals, vegetables and so on in both cases and controls. Because the data was not normally distributed, the wilcoxon signed rank test (non-parametric test method for two related samples) was used to compare the differences of various foods intakes between cases and controls. The daily intake of Allium vegetables of controls was significantly higher than that of cases ($P<0.05$), while the daily intake of livestock and poultry meat of controls was significantly lower than that of cases ($P<0.05$). Logistic regression analysis found that not eating garlic (OR=2.006, 95% CI: 1.451-2.774) and liking eating fat meat (OR=1.796, 95%CI: 1.249-2.584) were the risk factors for esophageal cancer.

The nutrients daily intakes for cases and controls were listed in table 3.

Nutrients	Cases	Controls	P value
Energy(KJ)	5460.27±3533.35	6191.34±3150.04	0.006
Protein(g)	50.02±35.08	57.33±30.89	0.045
Fat(g)	29.03±27.89	33.35±26.62	0.222
Carbohydrates(g)	213.70±140.49	253.84±109.67	0.002
Dietary Fibre(g)	11.87±11.21	13.63±10.12	0.088
Vitamin A(μgRE)	579.92±622.39	555.91±388.17	0.266
Thiamine(mg)	0.66±0.58	0.78±0.59	0.006
Riboflavin(mg)	0.74±0.62	0.78±0.44	0.267
Niacin(mg)	16.27±8.07	18.52±8.27	0.000
Vitamin C(mg)	67.09±77.45	75.52±51.83	0.393
Vitamin E(mg)	11.53±12.64	14.30±12.63	0.063
Calcium(mg)	388.35±351.61	444.40±318.82	0.049
Phosphorus(mg)	889.70±595.75	1041.79±522.61	0.016
Potassium(mg)	1499.53±1252.12	1602.00±933.45	0.235
Sodium(mg)	1312.31±1575.14	1442.03±1404.18	0.657
Magnesium(mg)	273.79±207.08	320.38±183.14	0.007
Iron(mg)	21.27±13.85	21.96±9.87	0.623
Zinc(mg)	11.26±6.20	11.71±5.72	0.093
Selenium(mg)	25.37±21.18	27.69±16.81	0.576
Copper(μg)	1.62±1.33	1.78±1.00	0.734

Table 3. The nutrients daily intakes of cases and controls(M±Q).

As shown in table 3, there were no significant difference between the daily intake of fat, dietary fiber, vitamin A, riboflavin, vitamin C, vitamin E, potassium, sodium, iron, zinc, selenium, and copper between cases and controls using wilcoxon signed rank test ($P>0.05$). Meanwhile, the daily intakes of energy, protein, carbohydrate, thiamine, niacin, calcium, phosphorus, magnesium of controls were significantly higher than that of the cases ($P<0.05$).

Nutrients	Intake level	P	OR	95%CI
Energy (KJ)	< 4353.18			
	4353.18-5902.73	0.006	0.456	0.260-0.801
	5902.73-7732.61	0.000	0.321	0.182-0.566
	> 7732.61	0.002	0.414	0.235-0.727
Protein (g)	< 39.06			
	39.06-54.73	0.106	0.633	0.364-1.101
	54.73-73.35	0.005	0.447	0.256-0.780
	> 73.35	0.012	0.492	0.282-0.858

Nutrients	Intake level	P	OR	95%CI
Carbohydrates (g)	< 173.88			
	173.88-230.01	0.009	0.471	0.268-0.829
	230.01-298.76	0.000	0.260	0.146-0.463
	> 298.76	0.002	0.411	0.233-0.725
Thiamine (mg)	< 0.45			
	0.45-0.73	0.859	1.051	0.609-1.814
	0.73-1.07	0.037	0.556	0.320-0.966
	> 1.07	0.043	0.565	0.325-0.983
Niacin (mg)	< 13.13			
	13.13-17.44	0.001	0.369	0.209-0.653
	17.44-21.68	0.001	0.369	0.209-0.653
	> 21.68	0.000	0.262	0.147-0.468
Calcium (mg)	< 288.65			
	288.65-419.98	0.042	0.563	0.323-0.980
	419.98-625.11	0.003	0.429	0.245-0.749
	> 625.11	0.012	0.491	0.281-0.857
Phosphorus (mg)	< 716.61			
	716.61-961.22	0.014	0.498	0.285-0.870
	961.22-1274.97	0.000	0.364	0.207-0.639
	> 1274.97	0.008	0.469	0.268-0.821
Magnesium (mg)	< 210.65			
	210.65-305.14	0.140	0.660	0.380-1.146
	305.14-409.08	0.015	0.504	0.289-0.876
	> 409.08	0.012	0.493	0.283-0.859

Table 4. ORs of nutrients different intake levels for the EC risk.

ORs of significant nutrients for EC were showed in Table 4. The highest intake quartiles of energy, protein, carbohydrate, thiamine, niacin, calcium, phosphorus and magnesium were associated with decrease in risk for EC compared with the lowest quartiles, the ORs were 0.414 (95%CI: 0.235-0.727), 0.492 (95%CI: 0.282-0.858), 0.411 (95%CI: 0.233-0.725), 0.565 (95%CI: 0.325-0.983), 0.262 (95%CI: 0.147-0.468), 0.491 (95%CI: 0.281-0.857), 0.469 (95%CI: 0.268-0.821), and 0.493 (95%CI: 0.283-0.859) respectively.

3.3 Discussion

3.3.1 Allium vegetables

In China, the Allium vegetables include garlic, onions, leeks, green Chinese onions, garlic sprouts, and garlic bolt and so on. These vegetables are rich in vitamins, minerals and phytochemicals. Many studies have indicated that Allium vegetables have anticarcinogenic effect which is attributed to organosulfur compounds [e.g., diallyl sulfide, diallyl disulfide

(DADS), diallyl trisulfide (DATS), S-allyl cysteine (SAC), S-allylmercaptocysteine (SAMC), ajoene, etc.] (Stan et al., 2008). Our results indicated that the daily intake of Allium vegetables of controls was significantly higher than that of cases (P<0.05) and not eating garlic was a risk factor for EC, OR=2.006 (95%CI: 1.451-2.774). Our result was similar to before reports (Chen et al., 2009; Galeone et al., 2006; Takezaki et al., 2001).

3.3.2 Meat

This study found that the daily intake of livestock and poultry meat of cases was significantly higher than that of controls. The logistic regression analysis indicated that who like eating fat meat was a risk factor for EC, OR =1.796 (95%CI: 1.249-2.584). Eating meat and animal fat may promote the mechanism of EC with total fat and saturated fatty acid intake increased. Our result was consistent to other reports (Navarro Silvera et al., 2011; Silvera et al., 2008).

3.3.3 Dietary nutrients intakes

In recent years, researchers pay more attention to the relationship between nutrients and EC. Nutrients deficiency may play an assistant role in the process of carcinogenesis. We have found that the nutritional status of residents in Chuzhou area was poor compared with the low EC incidence area (Wang et al., 2005). In this case-control study we found that the energy, protein, carbohydrates intakes of cases were lower than that of controls (P<0.05). The highest intake quartiles of energy, protein, carbohydrate were associated with decreased risk for EC compared with the lowest quartiles, the ORs were 0.414 (95%CI 0.235-0.727), 0.492 (95%CI 0.282-0.858), and 0.411 (95%CI 0.233-0.725) respectively. Some reports have suggested that high carbohydrate and energy intakes and obesity can account for at least some of the rise in EAC (Thompson et al., 2008). In our study the cases were all ESCC and the energy intake of the participants was low. The percentage of participants whose energy intake reached the Chinese RNI was only 10% which was vulnerable to suffer from energy malnutrition. This may result in that the high energy intake is the protective factor for EC in this area. Protein is the material basis of all life. Inadequate intake of protein leads to physical decline, decreased immunity, prone to various diseases. Chen reported that greater intakes of dietary protein and carbohydrate were inversely associated with risk of EAC (Chen et al., 2002).

Many reports have supported that low vitamin intake may partly explain the high incidence of EC among inhabitants in high incidence areas (Bravi et al., 2011; De Stefani et al., 2006; Ibiebele et al., 2011; Malekshah et al., 2010). This study indicated that the highest intake quartiles of thiamine and niacin were both associated with decreased risk for EC compared with the lowest quartiles, the ORs were 0.565 (95%CI: 0.325-0.983) and 0.262 (95%CI: 0.147-0.468) respectively. The results suggested that inadequate intake of thiamine and niacin may be a risk factor for EC and were consistent with previous reports (Franceschi et al., 2000; Siassi et al., 2000).

Among minerals, the anti-cancer role of selenium and zinc were the research focus and some researchers reported that selenium and zinc were preventive factors for occurrence of EC (Cai et al., 2006; Lu et al., 2006; Wei et al., 2004). However our results did not find the relationship between selenium, zinc and EC. We found calcium, phosphorus, and magnesium had protective action for occurrence of EC. There were reports that high phosphorus intake may decrease the risk of EC (Franceschi et al., 2000; Launoy et al., 1998; Siassi et al., 2000).

4. Conclusions

The role of food and nutrients for EC causation has been a subject of considerable research. The results of our meta-analysis studies suggested that: 1) increased dietary vegetables and fruits decrease the risk of EC; 2) high intake of dietary vitamin A, β-carotene, folic acid and vitamin E were associated with decreased risk of EC; 3) drinking green tea was a protective factor against EC and maté drinking may be a risk factor for EC.

The case-control study suggested that: 1) increased dietary Allium vegetables intake such as garlic was associated with decreased risk of EC, while increased fat meat, livestock and poultry meat intake was associated with increased risk of EC; 2) high dietary intakes of energy, protein, carbohydrate, thiamine, niacin, calcium, phosphorus and magnesium may decrease the risk of EC in this area.

We need more studies especially cohort studies to explore the effects of foods and nutrients on the occurrence of EC. Moreover, the mechanism of the actions needs to be studies further too.

5. Acknowledgement

The authors would like to thank the National Natural Science Fund (30800914), China, and grant CA94683 from NCI for financially supporting this research.

6. References

Abnet, C. C., Qiao Y. L. & Mark, S. D. et al. (2003). Prospective study of serum retinol, β-carotene, β-cryptoxanthin, and lutein/zeaxanthin and esophageal and gastric cancers in China. Cancer Causes and Control, Vol.14, No.7, (April 2003), pp. 645-655

Aune, D., Deneo-Pellegrini, H. & Ronco, A. L. et al. (2011). Dietary folate intake and the risk of 11 types of cancer: a case-control study in Uruguay. *Annals of Oncology*, Vol.22, No.2, (May 2010), pp.444-451

Axumea, J., Smith, S. S. & Pogribny, I. P. et al. (2007).The methylenetetrahydrofolate reductase 677TT genotype and folate intake interact to lower global leukocyte DNA methylation in young Mexican American women. *Nutrition Research*, Vol.27, (December 2006), pp.13-17

Bollschweiler, E., Wolfgarten, E. & Nowroth, T. et al. (2002). Vitamin intake and risk of subtypes of esophageal cancer in Germany. *Journal of Cancer Research and Clinical Oncology*, Vol.128, No.10, (August 2002), pp.575-580

Bosetti, C., Vecchic C. L. & Franceschi, S. et al. (2000). Food groups and risk of squamous cell esophageal cancer in northern Italy. *International Journal of Cancer*, Vol.87, No.2, (December 1999), pp.289-294

Bravi, F., Edefonti, V. & Randi, G. et al. (2011). Dietary patterns and the risk of esophageal cancer. Annals of Oncology, Vol.22, No.7, (Jun 2011), online

Cai, L., You, N. C. & Lu, H. et al. (2006). Dietary selenium intake, aldehyde dehydrogenase-2 and X-ray repair cross-complementing 1 genetic polymorphisms, and the risk of esophageal squamous cell carcinoma. *Cancer*, Vol.106, No.11, (November 2005), pp.2345-2354

Castellsague, X., Munoz, N. &De Stefani, E. et al. (2000). Influence of mate drinking, hot beverages and diet on esophageal cancer risk in south America. *International Journal of Cancer*, Vol.88, No.4, (April 2000), pp.658–664

Chen, H. L., Tucker, K. L. & Graubard, B. I. et al. (2002). Nutrient Intakes and Adenocarcinoma of the Esophagus and Distal Stomach. *Nutrition and Cancer*, Vol.42, No.1, (2002), pp.33-40

Chen, Y. K., Lee, C. H. & Wu, I. C. et al. (2009). Food intake and the occurrence of squamous cell carcinoma in different sections of the esophagus in Taiwanese men. *Nutrition*, Vol.25, No.7-8, (February 2009), pp.753–761

Chen, H. L., Ward, M. H. & Graubard, B. I. et al. (2002). Dietary patterns and adenocarcinoma of the esophagus and distal stomach. *The American Journal of Clinical Nutrition*, Vol.75, No.1, (July 2001), pp.137-144

Chen, W. Q., Zhang, S. W. & Kong, L. Z. et al. (2008). Cancer Mortality Report of 34 Cancer Registries in China, 2004. *Bulletin of Chinese Cancer*, Vol.17, No.11, (2008), pp.913-916

Cheng, K. K., Sharp, L. & Day N. E. et al. (2000). A case–control study of oesophageal adenocarcinoma in women: a preventable disease. *British Journal of Cancer*, (January 2000) Vol.83, No.1, pp.127–132

De Stefani, E., Boffetta, P. & Deneo-Pellegrini H. ,et al. (2005). The role of vegetable and fruit consumption in the aetiology of squamous cell carcinoma of the oesophagus: A case-control study in Uruguay. *International Journal of Cancer*, Vol.116, No.1, (December 2004), pp.130–135

De Stefani, E., Brennan, P. & Deneo-Pellegrini, H. et al. (2000). Vegetables, Fruits, Related Dietary Antioxidants, and Risk of Squamous Cell Carcinoma of the Esophagus: A Case-Control Study in Uruguay. *Nutrition and Cancer*, Vol.38, No.1, (2000), pp.23-29

De Stefani, E., Deneo-Pellegrini, H. & Mendilaharsu, M. et al. (1999). Diet and risk of cancer of the upper aerodigestive tract-I. Foods. *Oral Oncology*, Vol.35, No.1, (May 1998), pp. 17-21

De Stefani, E., Ronco, A. L. & Deneo-Pellegrini, H. et al. (1999). Diet and risk of cancer of the upper aerodigestive tract - II. Nutrients. *Oral Oncology*, Vol.35, No.1, (December 1998), pp.22-26

De Stefani, E., Ronco, A. L. & Boffetta, P. et al. (2006). Nutrient intake and risk of squamous cell carcinoma of the esophagus: a case-control study in Uruguay. *Nutrition and Cancer*, Vol.56, No2, (2006), pp.149-157

Engel, L. S., Chow, W. H. & Vaughan, T. L. et al. (2003). Population Attributable Risks of Esophageal and Gastric Cancers. *Journal of the National Cancer Institute*, Vol.95, No.18, (2003), pp.1404-1413

Fan, Y. H., Yuan, J. M. & Wang, R. W. et al. (2008). Alcohol, Tobacco and Diet in Relation to Esophageal Cancer: The Shanghai Cohort Study. *Nutrition and Cancer*, Vol.60, No.3, (June 2008), pp.354–363

Franceschi, S., Bidoli, E. & Vecchia, C. L. et al. (2000). Role of Macronutrients, Vitamins and Minerals in the Aetiology of Squamous-Cell Carcinoma of the Oesophagus. *International Journal of Cancer*, Vol.86, No.5, (January 2000), pp.626-631

Freedman, N. D., Park Y. & Subar, A. F. et al. (2007). Fruit and vegetable intake and esophageal cancer in a large prospective cohort study. *International Journal of Cancer*, Vol.121, No.12, (July 2007), pp.2753-2760

Galeone, C., Pelucchi, C. & Levi, F. et al. (2006). Folate intake and squamous-cell carcinoma of the oesophagus in Italian and Swiss men. *Annals of Oncology*, Vol.17, No.3, (November 2005), pp.521–525

Galeone, C., Pelucchi, C. & Levi, F. et al. (2006). Onion and garlic use and human cancer. *American Journal of Clinical Nutrition*, Vol.84, No.5, (July 2006), pp.1027-1032

Ganesh, B., Talole, S. D. & Dikshit, R. (2009). Tobacco, alcohol and tea drinking as risk factors for esophageal cancer: A case-control study from Mumbai, India. *Cancer Epidemiology*, Vol.33, No.6, (September 2009), pp.431-434

Gao, C. M., Takezaki, T. & Ding, J. H. et al. (1999). Protective effect of allium vegetables against both esophageal and stomach cancer: a simultaneous case-referent study of a high-epidemic area in Jiangsu Province, China. *Japanese Journal of Cancer Research*, Vol.90, No.6, (June 1999), pp.614-621.

Gao, Y., Hu, N. & Giffen, C. et al. (2009). Jasmine tea consumption and upper gastrointestinal cancer in China. *Cancer Causes Control*, Vol.20, No.10, (June 2009), pp.1997–2007

Guo, H. L., Zuo, S. Q. & Fang, B. et al. (2010). A case-control study on the risk factors for esophageal Neoplasms. *Modern Preventive Medicine*, Vol.37, No.9, (October 2009), pp.1601-1604

He, F. C., Zhang, L. & Gao, D. L. et al. (2009). Effect of Vitamin D3 on EC9706 cells proliferation, xenograft tumor growth and expression of NDRG1 protein. *Journal of ZhengZhou University*, Vol. 44, No.1, (2009), pp.42-45

Hung, H. C., Huang, M. C. & Lee, J. M. et al. (2004). Association between diet and esophageal cancer in Taiwan. *Journal of Gastroenterology and Hepatology*, Vol.19, No.6, (August 2003), pp.632–637

Hu, S. X., Zhou, X. N. & Sun, N. S. et al. (2002). The spatial analysis of GIS for cancer in Jiangsu Province. *Chinese Journal of Epidemiology*, Vol.23, No.1, (2002), pp.73-75

Hercberg, S., Galan, P. & Preziosi, P. et al. (1998). The potential role of antioxidant vitamins in preventing cardiovascular diseases and cancer. *Nutrition*, Vol.14, No.6, (1998), pp.513-520

Ibiebele, T. I., Hughes, M. C. & Pandeya, N. et al. (2011). High Intake of Folate from Food Sources Is Associated with Reduced Risk of Esophageal Cancer in an Australian Population. *The Journal of Nutrition*, Vol.141, No.2, (November 2010), pp.274-283

Ibiebele, T. I., Taylor, A. R, & Whiteman, D. C. et al. (2010). Eating habits and risk of esophageal cancers: a population-based case–control study. *Cancer Causes Control*, Vol.21, No.9, (April 2010), pp.1475-1484

Islami, F., Pourshams, A. & Nasrollahzadeh, D. et al. (2009). Tea drinking habits and oesophageal cancer in a high risk area in northern Iran: population based case-control study. *British Medical Journal*, Vol.338, (December 2008), pp.b929-b936

Khan, N. & Mukhtar, H. (2007). Tea polyphenols for health promotion. *Life Sciences*, Vol.81, (June 2007), pp.519-533

Kima, J. M., Hong, K. & Lee, J. H. et al. (2009). Effect of folate deficiency on placental DNA methylation in hyperhomocysteinemic rats. *Journal of Nutritional Biochemistry*, Vol.20, (January 2008), pp. 172-176

Kubo, A., Levin, T. R. &.Block, G. et al. (2008). Dietary antioxidants, fruits, and vegetables and the risk of Barrett's esophagus. *American Journal of Gastroenterology*, Vol.103, No.7, pp.1614-1623

Launoy, G., Milan, C. & Faivre, J. (1998). Diet and Squamous-Cell Cancer of the Oesophagus: A French Multicentre Case-Control Study. *International Journal of Cancer*, Vol.76, No.1, (November 1997), pp.7-12

Liaw, Y. P., Huang, Y. C. & Yeh, Y.C. (2003). Nutrient intakes in relation to cancer mortality in Taiwan. *Nutrition Research*, Vol.23, No.12, (August 2003), pp.1597-1606

Lin, L., Dong, L. H. & Zhou, J. M. et al. (2010). A case control study on the relationship between Wuyishan cliff tea and esophageal cancer. *Cancer Research and Clinic*, Vol.22, No.5, (August 2009), pp.323-325

Li, K., Yu, P. & Zhu, Y .F. (2002). Relation ship between Congou tea and esophageal cancer in Chaoshan region of Guangdong, China. *Chinese Journal of Disease Control Prevention*, Vol.6, No.1, (April 2001), pp.47-49

Li, D. H. (2008). Comparative Research on Risk Factors of Esophagus Cancer. *Journal of Henan University of Science & Technology (Medical Science)*, Vol.12, No.4, (December 2008), pp.267-268

Li, H., Qu, C. Y. & Bai, L. X. (2008). Case control study on the risk factors in behavior and life style of esophageal carcinoma. *Chinese Journal of Disease Control Prevention*, Vol.12, No.3, (December 2007), pp.211-214

Lu, J. B., Lian, S. Y. & Sun, X. B. et al. (2000). A case-control study on the risk f actors of esophageal cancer in Linzhou. *Chinese Journal of Epidemiology*, Vol.21, No.6, (April 2000), pp.434-436

Lu, H., Cai, L. & Mu, L. N. et al. (2006). Dietary mineral and trace element intake and squamous cell carcinoma of the Esophagus in a Chinese population. *Nutrition and Cancer*, Vol.55, No.1, (2006), pp.63-70

Malekshah, A. F., Kimiagar, M. & Pourshams, A. (2010). Vitamin deficiency in Golestan Province, northern Iran: a high-risk area for esophageal cancer. *Archives of Iranian Medicine*, Vol.13, No.5, (July 2010), pp.391-394

Mayne, S. T., Risch, H.A. & Dubrow, R. et al. (2001). Nutrient Intake and Risk of Subtypes of Esophageal and Gastric Cancer. *Cancer Epidemiology, Biomarkers Prevention*, Vol.10, (August 2001), pp.1055-1062

Michels, K. B., Fuchs, C. S. & Giovannucci, E. (2005). Fiber intake and incidence of colorectal cancer among 76,947 women and 47,279 men. *Cancer Epidemiol Biomarkers Prevention*, Vol.14, (2005), pp.1619-1625

Mou, Z. Y., Zeng, G. & Liu, D. W. et al. (2008). Risk Factors Associated with High Occurence of Esophageal Cancer in Xingtang County, Hebei Province. *Chinese Journal of Natural Medicine*, Vol 10. No.1, (Janurary 2007), pp.19-21

Mu, L. N., Zhou, X. F. & Ding, B. G. et al. (2003). A case-control study on drinking green tea and decreasing risk of cancers in the alimentary canal among cigarette smokers and alcohol drinkers. *Chinese Journal of Epidemiology*, Vol.24, No.3, (October 2002), pp.192-195

Nayar, D., Kapil, U. & Joshi, Y. K. et al. (2000). Nutritional risk factors in esophageal cancer. *Journal of Associated Physicians of India*, Vol.48, pp.781-787

Navarro Silvera, S. A., Mayne, S. T. & Risch, H. A. et al. (2011). Principal component analysis of dietary and lifestyle patterns in relation to risk of subtypes of esophageal and gastric cancer. *Annals of Epidemiology*, Vol.21, No.7, (2011), pp.543-550

Nomura, A. M. Y., Ziegler, R. G. & Craft, N.E. et al. (1997). Serum Micronutrients and Upper Aerodigestive Tract Cancer. *Cancer Epidemiology, Biomarkers Prevention*, Vol.6, (May 1997), pp.407-412

Odin, A. P. (1997). Vitamins as antimutagens: Advantages and some possible mechanisms of antimutagenic action. *Mutation Research*, Vol. 386, No.1, (1997), pp.39-67

Peng, X. E., Zhou, Z. J. & Shi, X. S. et al. (2005). Case- control study on risk factors of esophageal cancer in Anxi county. *Chinese Journal of Public Health*, Vol.21, No.1, (May 2004), pp.10-12

Phukan, R. K., Chetia, C. K. & Ali, M. S. et al. (2001). Role of dietary habits in the development of esophageal cancer in Assam, the northeastern region of India. *Nutrition Cancer*, vol.39, No.2, (2001) pp.204-209

Poulain, S., Evenou, F. & Carré, M. C. et al. (2009). Vitamin A/retinoids signalling in the human lung. *Lung Cancer*, Vol.66, No.1, (March 2009), pp. 1-7

Reddy, C.D., Patti, R. & Guttapalli, A. et a1. (2006). Anticancer effects of the novel 1 α, 25-dihydroxyvitamin D3 hybrid analog QW1624F2-2 in human neuroblastoma. *Journal of cellular biochemistry*, Vol.97, No.1, (September 2005), pp.198-206

Sewram, V., De Stefani, E. & Brennan, P. et al. (2003). Maté Consumption and the Risk of Squamous Cell Esophageal Cancer in Uruguay. *Cancer Epidemiology, Biomarkers & Prevention*, Vol. 12, (March 2003), pp.508-513

Sharp, L., Chilvers, C. E.D. & Cheng, K. K. et al. (2001). Risk factors for squamous cell carcinoma of the oesophagus in women: a case-control study. *British Journal of Cancer*, Vol.85, No.11, (September 2001), pp.1667-1670

Silvera, S. A. N., Mayne, S. T. &, Risch H. et al. (2008). Food group intake and risk of subtypes of esophageal and gastric cancer. *International Journal of Cancer*, Vol.123, NO.4, (December 2007), pp. 852-860

Siassi, F., Pouransari, Z. & Ghadirian, P. (2000). Nutrient intake and esophageal cancer in the Caspian littoral of Iran: a case-control study. *Cancer Detection and Prevention*, Vol.24, No.3, pp.295-303

Soler, M., Bosetti, C. & Franceschi S. et al. (2001). Fiber intake and the risk of oral, pharyngeal and esophageal cancer. *International Journal of Cancer*, Vol.91, No.3, (September 2000), pp.283-287

Stan, S. D., Kar, S. & Stoner, G. D. et al. (2008). Bioactive Food Components and Cancer Risk Reduction. *Journal of Cellular Biochemistry*, Vol.104, No.1, (2008), pp.339-356

Sun, X. B., Meilan, H. & Moler, H. et al. (2003). Risk factors for oesophageal Cancer in Linzhou, China: a case-control study. *Asian Pacific Journal of Cancer Prevention*, Vol.4, No.3, (2003), pp.119-124

Szymańska, K., Matos, E. & Hung, R. J. et al. (2010). Drinking of maté and the risk of cancers of the upper aerodigestive tract in Latin America: a case-control study, *Cancer Causes Control*, (June 2010), Vol.21, pp.1799-1806

Takezaki, T., Shinoda, M. & Hatooka, S. et al. (2000). Subsite-specific risk factors for hypopharyngeal and esophageal cancer (Japan). *Cancer Causes and Control*, Vol.11, No.7, (February 2000), pp.597-608

Takezaki, T., Gao, C. M. & Wu, J. Z. et al. (2001). Dietary Protective and Risk Factors for Esophageal and Stomach Cancers in a Low-epidemic Area for Stomach Cancer in Jiangsu Province, China: Comparison with Those in a High-epidemic Area. *Japanese Journal of Cancer Research*, Vol.92, No.11, (November 2001), pp.1157–1165

Tatsionia, A., & Ioannidis, J.P.A. (2008). Meta-Analysis. *International Encyclopedia of Public Health*, (20 August 2008), pp.442-450

Tan, W., Miao, X. & Wang, L. et al. (2005). Significant increase in risk of gastroesophageal cancer is associated with interaction between promoter polymorphisms in thymidylate synthase and serum folate status. *Carcinogenesis*, Vol.26, No.8, (March 2005), pp.1430-1435

Tavani, A., Bertuzzi, M. & Talamini. R, et al. (2003). Coffee and tea intake and risk of oral, pharyngeal and esophageal cancer. *Oral Oncology*, Vol.39, No.7, (April 2003), pp.695-700

Taylor, P. R., Qiao, Y. L. & Mark, S. D. et al. (2003). Prospective Study of Serum Vitamin E Levels and Esophageal and Gastric Cancers. *Journal of the National Cancer Institute*, Vol.95, No.18, (September2003), pp.1414-1416

Tran, G. D., Sun, X. D. & Abnet, C. C. et al. (2005). Prospective Study of Risk Factors for Esophageal and Gastric Cancers in the Linxian General Population Trial Cohort in China. *International Journal of Cancer*, Vol.113, No.3, (June 2004), pp. 456-463

Terry, P., Lagergren, J. & Ye, W. et al. (2000). Antioxidants and cancers of the esophagus and gastric cardia. *International Journal of Cancer*, Vol.87, No.5, (March 2000), pp.750–754

Thompson, C. L., Khiani, V. & Chak, A. et al. (2008) Carbohydrate consumption and esophageal cancer:an ecological assessment. *The American Journal of Gastroenterology*, Vol.103, (August 2007), pp. 555-561

Tzonou, A., Lipworth, L. & Trichopoulos, D. et al. (1996). Diet and Risk of Esophageal Cancer by Histologic Type in a Low-Risk Population. *International Journal of Cancer*, Vol.68, No.3, (July 1996), pp.300-304

Wang, J. M., Xu, B. & Rao, J. Y. et al. (2007). Diet habits, alcohol drinking, tobacco smoking, green tea drinking, and the risk of esophageal squamous cell carcinoma in the Chinese population. *European Journal of Gastroenterology & Hepatology*, Vol.19, No.2, (2006), pp.171-176

Wang, X. S., Wu, D. L. & Zhang, X. F. et al. (2008). A Population-based 1:1 Matched Case-control Study on Risk Factors for Esophageal Cancer in GanYu. *Chinese Journal of Health Statistics*, Vol.25, No.6, (2008), pp.616-617

Wang, S. K., Sun, G. J. & Xie, Y. et al. (2005). Relationship between nutritional status in populations and different mortality of esophageal cancer and liver cancer. *Chinese Journal of Public Health*, Vol.21 No.11, (November 2005), pp.1337-1339

Wang, M., Guo, C. & Li, M. et al. (1999). A case-control study on the dietary risk factors of upper digestive tract cancer. *Chinese Journal of Epidemiology*, Vol.20, (1999), pp.95-97

Wei, W. Q., Abnet, C. C. & Qiao, Y. L. et al. (2004). Prospective study of serum selenium concentrations and esophageal and gastric cardia cancer, heart disease, stroke, and total death. *The American Journal of Clinical Nutrition*, Vol.79, No.1, (March 2003), pp.80-85

World Cancer Research Fund & American Institute for Cancer Research · (2007) · *Food , Nutrition , Physical Activity , and the Prevention of Cancer : a Global Perspective* · ISBN, 978-0-9722522-2-5, Washington, DC: AICR

Wu, M. T., Wu, D. C., & Hsu, H. K. et al. (2003). Association between p21 codon 31 polymorphism and esophageal cancer risk in a Taiwanese population. *Cancer Letters*, Vol. 201, No.2, (July 2003), pp.175–180

Wu, M., Liu, A. M. & Kampaman, et al. (2009). Green tea drinking, high tea temperature and esophageal cancer in high- and low-risk areas of Jiangsu Province, China: A population-based case–control study. *International Journal of Cancer*, Vol.124, No.8, (October 2008), pp.1907–1913

Xie, Y., Sun, G. J. & Hu, X. et al. (2005). A case - control study of the diet, behavioral factors and esophageal cancer in Chuzhou of Huai'an. *Journal of Hygiene Research*, Vol.34, No.4, (September 2004), pp. 479-480

Yang, C. X., Wang, H. Y. & Wang, Z. M. et al. (2005). Risk Factors for Esophageal Cancer: a Case-control Study in South-western China. *Asian Pacific Journal of Cancer Prevention*, Vol.6, No.1, (2005), pp.48-53

Yang, J., Shan, Y. & Yang, S. J. et al. (2009). Non-conditional Logistic Regression Analysis on the Risk Factors of Esophageal Cancer in LinZhou. *Modern Preventive Medicine*, Vol.36, No.7, (April 2008), pp. 1201-1203

Yang, J. L., Wang, M. R. & Guo, C. H. et al. (1999). Green Tea and Cancer of Esophagus and Stomach : a Case-Control Study. *Chinese Journal of Public Health*, Vol.18, No.6, (March 1999), pp.367-368

Yang, W. X., Lu, S. X. & Liu, G. T. et al. (2008). Etiological Prevention Trial for Esophageal Cancer among High-risk Population in Linzhou City, China. *China Cancer*, Vol.17, No.7, (2008), pp.548-552

Yang, Y. X., Wang, G. Y. & Pan, X. C. (1 December 2002). *The Food Composition of China, 2002*. Beijing University, ISBN 781071180, Beijing.

Zhang, Z. F., Kurtz, R.C. & Harlap, S. et al. (1997). Adenocarcinomas of the Esophagus and Gastric Cardia: The Role of Diet. *Nutrition and Cancer*, Vol.27, No.3, (1997), pp.298-309

Zhang, T. T., Lei, X. & Xu, F. L. (2010). A Case-Control Study on Relationship of Esophageal Cancer with Smoking, Drinking Alcohol Beverage and Drinking Tea. *China Cancer*, Vol.19, No.3, (September 2009), pp.165-167

Zhang, G. S., He, Y. T. & Hou, J. (2000). A case control study on risk factor of esophageal cancer in cixian county. *Sichuan Journal of Cancer Control*, Vol.12, No.2, (Novermber 1999), pp.65-67

Zhang, S. W., Chen, W. Q. & Lei, Z. L. et al. (2008). A Report of Cancer Incidence from 37 Cancer Registries in China, 2004. *Bulletin of Chinese Cancer*, Vol.17, No.11, (2008), pp.909-912

Zhao, J. K., Wu, M. & Liu, A. M. (2005). A Population-based 1:1 Matched Case-control Study on Risk Factors for Esophageal Cancer in a High Cancer Incidence Area of Jiangsu Province. *Chinese Journal of Prevention and control of chronic non-communicable diseases*, Vol.13, No. 1, (November 2004), pp.17-19

Zheng, W., Sellers, T. A. & Folsom, A. R. et al. (1995). Retinol, Antioxidant Vitamins, and Cancers of the Upper Digestive Tract in a Prospective Cohort Study of

Postmenopausal Women. *American Journal of Epidemiology*, Vol.142. No.9, (July 1995), pp.955-960

Zhu, J. Y., Lei, J. & Gao, S. L. (2009). A case-control study on risk factor of esophageal cancer in Urumqi. *Journal of XinJiang Medical University*, Vol.32, No.10, (June 2009), pp.1434-1435

7

Current Therapy for Esophageal Adenocarcinoma

Yoshihiro Komatsu and Michael K. Gibson*
Division of Hematology and Oncology, Department of Internal Medicine,
University of Pittsburgh Medical Center
USA

1. Introduction

Esophageal adenocarcinoma (EAC) affects approximately 17,000 individuals per year in the United States, is increasing in incidence, and is associated with an exceptionally high mortality rate. [1, 2] Overall five-year survival despite aggressive treatment in large, multidisciplinary oncology centers ranges between 15 and 25%. Poor outcome in patients with EAC is reflective of both deficiencies in early detection - the disease is typically diagnosed at an advanced (unresectable) stage - and the inadequacy of available standard therapies across stages. Advanced/recurrent disease is incurable and carries a median survival of 9-12 months. Fully 50% of cases are metastatic at diagnosis, and cure rates with multimodality therapy for locally advanced disease do not exceed 40%--resulting in the majority of these patients eventually requiring palliative chemotherapy. Innumerable regimens have been studied. However, few are validated by phase III trials. Furthermore, trial eligibility ranges between histologies (Squamous cell carcinoma; SCC vs. Adenocarcinoma) as well as location in the upper gastrointestinal tract (distal esophagus, esophagogastric junction [EGJ], stomach). With these limitations in mind, there are a few guiding principles for treatment of advanced/metastatic disease. Chemotherapy is usually given in doublets and is chosen based on projected efficacy, patient performance status/medical co-morbidities, and side effect profile of the agents used. There is significant experience with combinations of cisplatin and 5-fluorouracil (5-FU), particularly with SCC, which are variously validated as better than best supportive care.[3] More recently, with the epidemiologic shift from SCC to EAC, newer regimens focus on GEJ/gastric cancer, use three drugs and sometimes incorporate biologic/targeted therapies.

2. Epidemiology and histology

SCC has become increasingly less common, accounting for fewer than 30% of all esophageal malignancies in North America and many Western European countries.[4] Although EAC is diagnosed predominantly in white men in whom the incidence has risen, EAC also is gradually increasing in men of all ethnic backgrounds and in women also.[5] Several risk

*Corresponding author

factors for EAC have been established such as obesity and high body mass index (BMI).[6-8] Individuals in the highest quartile for BMI had a 7.6-fold increased risk of developing EAC compared with those in the lowest quartile, whereas SCC was not associated with BMI.[9, 10] Gastroesophageal reflux disease (GERD) and Barrett's esophagus are the other two major risk factors for EAC.[11-15] GERD is associated with high BMI and is also a risk factor for Barrett's esophagus. Barrett's esophagus is a condition in which the normal squamous epithelium of the esophagus that damaged by GERD is replaced by a metaplastic, columnar, or glandular epithelium of the esophagus that is predisposed to malignancy.[15] Patients with Barrett's esophagus have 30 to 60 times of greater risk of developing EAC than the general population.[13]

3. Staging

The American Joint Committee on Cancer (AJCC) staging classification has revised in 2010.[16] The tumor (T), node (N), and metastasis (M) classification developed by AJCC 2002 was based on pathologic review of the surgical specimen in patients who had surgery as primary therapy. The revised 2010 AJCC staging classification is based on the risk-adjusted random forest analysis of the data generated by the Worldwide Esophageal Cancer Collaboration (WECC) in 4627 patients who were treated with esophagectomy alone without induction or postoperative therapy. The revised version includes separate stage grouping for SCC and EAC (table 1.). The revised staging system is for the esophageal and EGJ cancers, including cancer within the first 5cm of the stomach that extends into the EGJ or distal thoracic esophagus. T4 disease is sub-classified into T4a (potentially resectable) and T4b (unresectable). Staging and evaluation for respectability requires endoscopic ultrasound (EUS) for T staging (focusing on the possibility of T4 disease), computed tomography (CT), and [18F]-2-deoxy-D-glucose positron emission tomography (FDG-PET), which is often integrated with CT (PET/CT).

3.1 Esophagogastric junction (EGJ)

In the revised AJCC staging system, tumors whose midpoint is in the lower thoracic esophagus, EGJ or within the proximal 5cm of the stomach that extends into the EGJ or esophagus, are classified as adenocarcinoma of the esophagus for the purposes of staging. All other cancers with a midpoint in the stomach lying more than 5cm distal to the EGJ, or those within 5cm of the EGJ but not extending into the EGJ or esophagus are staged using the gastric cancer staging system.

Primary tumor (T)	
TX	primary tumor cannot be assessed
T0	No evidence of primary tumor
Tis	High grade dysplasia
T1	Tumor invades lamina propria, mucularis mucosae, or submucosa

Primary tumor (T)	
T1a	Tumor invades lamina propria, mucularis mucosae
T1b	Tumor invades submucosa
T2	Tumor invades muscularis propria
T3	Tumor invades adventitia
T4	Tumor invades adjacent structures
T4a	Resectable tumor invading plura, pericardium, or diaphragm
T4b	Unresectable tumor invading other adjacent structures, such as aorta, vertebral body, trachea, etc
Regional lymph nodes (N)	
NX	Regional lymph nodes cannot be assessed
N0	No regional lymph node metastasis
N1	Metastasis in 1-2 regional lymph nodes
N2	Metastasis in 3-6 regional lymph nodes
N3	Metastasis in seven or more regional lymph nodes
Distant metastasis (M)	
M0	No distant metastasis
M1	Distant metastasis
Histologic grade (G)	
GX	Grade cannot be assessed - stage grouping as G1
G1	Well differenciated
G2	Moderately differenciated
G3	Poorly differentiated
G4	Undifferentiated - stage grouping as G3 squamous

Adenocarcinoma				
Stage	T	N	M	Grade
0	Tis (HGD)	N0	M0	1, X
IA	T1	N0	M0	1-2, X
IB	T1	N0	M0	3
	T2	N0	M0	1-2, X
IIA	T2	N0	M0	3
IIB	T3	N0	M0	Any
	T1-2	N1	M0	Any
IIIA	T1-2	N2	M0	Any
	T3	N1	M0	Any
	T4a	N0	M0	Any
IIIB	T3	N2	M0	Any
IIIC	T4a	N1-2	M0	Any
	T4b	Any	M0	Any
	Any	N3	M0	Any
IV	Any	Any	M1	Any

Table 1. AJCC 2010 TNM staging of esophagogastric junction (EGJ) adenocarcinoma.

4. Current therapy for resectable esophageal adenocarcinoma

EMR or ablation are good primary treatment options for patients with Tis and T1a tumors where as esophagectomy is still preferred treatment for T1a tumor. For patients with T1b, esophagectomy is the preferred treatment option for those with non-cervical cancer. Chemoradiation therapy is the preferred treatment for patients with cervical cancer.[17]

Primary treatment options for patients with locally advanced resectable esophageal cancer include preoperative chemoradiation therapy, definitive chemoradiation therapy, preoperative chemotherapy, or esphagectomy.

4.1 Chemoradiation therapy

Since the overall poor survival rates of patients who have been treated with resection alone, multiple modalities have been used for the treatment of esophageal cancer. Concomitant chemotherapy and radiation therapy has been studied in the preoperative setting and as definitive nonoperative treatment.

4.1.1 Preoperative concurrent chemoradiation therapy

Preoperative chemoradiation followed by surgery is the most common approach for patients with resectable esophageal cancer. Several trials have directly compared surgery with or without preoperative chemoradiation therapy for patients with potentially resectable esophageal cancer.[18-24] Of the five completed randomized trials compared preoperative concurrent chemoradiation therapy versus surgery alone, only two showed a statically significant survival benefit for chemoradiation therapy.[23, 24] Walsh et al.[23] randomized 113 patients with esophageal or EGJ adenocarcinoma to receive either surgery alone or preoperative chemoradiation therapy. The chemoradiation therapy consisted of two courses of cisplatin (75 mg/m^2 on day 7 of each cycle) and 5-fluorouracil (15mg/kg by bolus days 1 to 5), and radiation therapy was administered in 15 fractions over a three week period to a total of 40 Gy. Only one of the cycles of chemotherapy was actually given concurrently with the radiation. The combined-modality therapy provided a significant improvement in median survival (16 versus 11 months; p =0.01) and in three year survival (32% versus 6 %) compared with surgery alone. These results were criticized because of the lower than expected survival with surgery alone.

In the phase III multicenter CROSS trial from the Netherlands[24], 364 patients with potentially resectable (T2-3, N0-1, M0) esophageal or EGJ cancer were randomized to surgery alone or weekly paclitaxel 50 mg/m2 plus carboplatin [AUC =2] on days 1, 8, 15, 22, and 29, administered with concurrent radiotherapy with 41.4 Gy in 23 fractions over five weeks. Surgery was conducted within 6 weeks of completing chemoradiation therapy. The median survival of patients who received preoperative chemoradiation therapy and surgery was 49 months, compared to 26 months for those who received surgery alone. When adjusted for baseline covariates, the hazard ratio was 0.66 (p = 0.008). After a median follow-up of 32 months, the 1-,2- and 3-year survival rates were 82 percent, 67 percent and 59 percent, respectively, for chemoradiation therapy plus surgery verses 70 percent, 52 percent, and 48 percent for surgery alone with 0.67 of hazard ratio (p = 0.011). In a preliminary report presented at the 2010 ASCO meeting, preoperative chemoradiation therapy was well tolerated, with the only grade 3 or higher toxicity being leucopenia (7%). The complete (R0) resection rate was higher with chemoradiation therapy (92 vs. 65%), and 33 % of those treated with chemoradiation therapy had a pCR.

In contrast, three other trials have not shown a significant survival advantage for this approach. In the trial from University of Michigan[19], 100 patients with locoregional esophageal or EGJ cancer were randomly assigned to surgery with or without preoperative chemoradiation therapy with cisplatin, 5-FU and vinblastine. A pCR was observed in 28 percent of patients after preoperative treatment. At a median follow-up of 8.2 years, the median survival was similar (16.9 vs. 17.6 months for multimodality therapy and surgery respectively). However, three-year survival was nearly twice higher in chemoradiation therapy (30% vs. 16%), although there was no statistically significant.

The CALGB 9781 trial[24] was a prospective randomized Intergroup trial comparing trimodality therapy with surgery alone in 500 patients with stage I through III esophageal or EGJ cancer. Patients were staged with upper endoscopy, barium esophagram, and CT. Staging EUS and thoracoscopy/laparoscopy were encouraged. Due to poor accrual, the study fell short prematurely with only 56 patients enrolled. Those patients were randomized to undergo either surgery alone or concurrent chemoradiation therapy with cisplatin and 5-fluorouracil. A pCR was achieved in 10 of 25 assessable patients in the trimodality therapy (40%), and neither perioperative morbidity nor mortality was increased compared to surgery alone. Patients receiving trimodality therapy also had a better 5-year survival rate (39% vs. 16%), although the difference was not statistically significant.

The benefit of preoperative chemoradiation therapy in smaller resectable tumors was addressed in the French FFCD 9901 trial[25], which randomly assigned 195 patients with stage I or II esophageal or EGJ cancer to preoperative chemoradiation therapy (cisplatin plus 5-FU and concurrent radiation therapy [45Gy]) versus surgery alone. In a preliminary report of an interim analysis, at a median follow-up of 69 months, preoperative chemoradiation therapy did not improve median overall survival (32 vs. 44 months with surgery alone), and it was associated with significantly more serious adverse events (65% vs. 35%) and a significantly higher rate of perioperative mortality (7.3% vs. 1.1%). Full publications of these data are awaited.

A meta-analysis of randomized trials comparing preoperative chemoradiation therapy versus surgery alone included 1116 patients enrolled on nine trials[26]. When compared to surgery alone, there was only a nonsignificant trend towards improved survival with chemoradiation therapy (odds ratio 0.79, 0.77, and 0.66 for one-, two- and three-year mortality, respectively). The improvement in three-year survival was statistically significant when the analysis was restricted to trials of concurrent chemoradiation therapy (odds ratio for mortality 0.45, 95% CI 0.26-0.79). A second meta-analysis of 10 randomized comparing preoperative chemoradiation therapy and surgery alone showed same conlusion[27]. Compared to surgery alone, preoperative chemoradiation therapy was associated with significantly better two-year all cause mortality (hazard ratio 0.81, 95% CI 0.70-0.93). This corresponded to a 13 percent absolute difference in survival at two years.

In brief summary, with several trials and at least two meta-analyses demonstrating better survival with preoperative concurrent chemoradiation, the majority of patient potentially resectable localized cancer of the thoracic esophagus and EGJ now undergo some form of combined modality therapy rather than local therapy alone.

4.1.2 Preoperative sequential chemoradiation therapy

Several trials comparing sequentially administered chemotherapy and radiation therapy followed by surgery to surgery alone have failed to show any survival advantage to combined modality therapy.[18, 20, 21]

4.1.3 Definitive chemoradiation therapy

In randomized studies, the addition of cisplatin-based chemotherapy to radiation therapy significantly improves survival over radiation alone, however, the available data are almost exclusively in SCC, and none of the trials have performed adequate pretreatment staging to reliably correlate outcome with locoregional tumor extent such as locally advanced unresectable versus potentially operable disease.[28-30]

In the RTOG 85-01 trial, patients with locoregional thoracic esophageal SCC or AC received 4 cycles of 5-FU and cisplatin. Radiation therapy (50Gy) was administered concurrently with day 1 of chemotherapy[28]. The control therapy arm was radiation therapy alone which was higher dose (64Gy) than I the combined modality therapy arm. Patients who were randomly assigned to receive combined modality therapy showed a significant improvement in both median survival (14 vs. 9 months) and 5-year overall survival (27% vs. 0%) with projected 8- and 10-year survival rates of 22% and 20%, respectively[29]. As a result of this trial, definitive chemoradiation therapy became the standard care for patients with inoperable disease even though 90 percent of patients had SCC.

The US Intergroup Study 0123 (INT 0123) was designed as the follow-up trial to RTOG 85-01[31]. The trial compared two different radiation doses (50.4 Gy or 64.8 Gy) used with the same chemotherapy regimen as RTOG 85-01 (cisplatin and 5-FU). 236 Patients with nonmetastatic SCC (85%) and AC (15%) of the thoracic esophagus were randomly assigned. No significant difference was observed in median survival (13.0 vs. 18.1 months), two-year survival (31% vs. 40%), and locoregional failure or locoregional persistence of cancer (56% vs. 52%) between the high-dose and standard-dose radiation therapy groups. High-dose radiation therapy was significantly more toxic.

After the results of these studies, definitive chemoradiation therapy with 5-FU and cisplatin using the radiation therapy dose of 50.4 Gy was established as the standard approach for patients with esophageal cancer.

4.1.4 Postoperative chemoradiation therapy

In a phase II nonrandomized trial evaluating postoperative concurrent chemoradiation with cisplatin and 5-FU in patients with poor prognosis esophageal and EGJ cancers, the projected rates of 4-year overall survival, freedom from recurrence, distant metastatic control, and locoregional control were 51%, 50%, 56%, and 86%, respectively[32]. However, the efficacy of postoperative chemoradiation therapy has not been compared with surgery alone in a randomized trial involving patients with esophageal cancer.

The Intergroup trial SWOG 9008/INT-0116 investigated the effect of surgery and postoperative chemoradiation therapy on the survival of patients with resectable adenocarcinoma of the stomach (80%) or EGJ (20%)[33]. 556 patients were randomly assigned to surgery plus postoperative chemoradiation therapy (leucovorin and 5-FU) or surgery alone. Median overall survival in the surgery alone was 27 months compared with 36 months in the postoperative chemoradiation group. The postoperative chemoradiation group had better 3-year survival rates (50% vs. 41%) and significantly improved overall survival for all patients. A major criticism of this study is that surgery was not part of this protocol. Moreover, 54% of patients had a D0 resection, 36% had a D1 resection, and only 10% had a D2 resection. However, the results of this study have established postoperative chemoradiation therapy as a reasonable option of patients with EGJ adenocarcinoma.

4.2 Chemotherapy

4.2.1 Preoperative chemotherapy

Several randomized trials have evaluated the benefit of preoperative chemotherapy in patients with esophageal cancer limited to the primary and regional nodes by clinical assessment[34-39].

In the US Intergroup trial 0113, 467 patients with potentially resectable esophageal or EGJ cancer were randomly assigned to surgery alone or preoperative chemotherapy with cisplatin and 5-FU followed by surgery[34]. The majority of patients had adenocarcinoma (55%) and outcomes were similar for both histologies. The preliminary results did not show any survival benefit between the groups. In a later update of long-term outcomes (median follow-up with 8.8 years), preoperative chemotherapy decreased the incidence of R1 resection (4% vs. 15% in the surgery alone group), however, no improvement was seen in overall survival between the groups.

In contrast to Intergroup 0113, a couple of trials suggest a survival benefit for preoperative chemotherapy compared to surgery alone. The Medical Research Council (MRC) OEO2 trial randomly assigned 802 patients with AC (69%) or SCC (31%) of the esophagus to surgery alone or preoperative chemotherapy with cisplatin and 5-FU[39]. At a median follow-up of 6 years, disease-free and overall survivals were significantly longer for the preoperative chemotherapy group. The 16 percent reduction in the risk of death favoring chemotherapy translated into a significant improvement in five year survival (23 vs. 17%).

The phase III study conducted by the French Study group (FNLCC ACCORD07-FFCD 9703) compared preoperative chemotherapy (5-FU and cisplatin) followed by surgery with surgery alone[40]. 224 patients with potentially resectable stage II or greater adenocarcinoma of EGJ (n=144), distal esophagus (n=25), or stomach (n=55) were randomly assigned.

At a median follow-up of 5.7 years, 3- and 5- year overall survival rates were 48% and 38%, respectively, for patients with preoperative chemotherapy compared with 35% and 21%, respectively, for those with surgery alone.

In a meta-analysis of eight randomized trials of surgery alone or preoperative chemotherapy followed by surgery for esophageal cancer (1724 patients, any histology, excluding cervical esophageal cancers) suggested a small survival benefit for preoperative chemotherapy group[27]. The hazard ratio for all cause survival at two years favored chemotherapy followed by surgery (hazard ratio for all-cause mortality 0.90, 95% CI 0.81-1.0), a difference which translated into a two-year absolute survival benefit of 7 percent. There was no significant benefit for chemotherapy for patients with SCC, however, with patients with EAC, there was a significant benefit, which was based on data from the United Kingdom MRC OEO2 trial.

4.2.2 Perioperative chemotherapy

Investigators with the MRC conducted a second study of preoperative chemotherapy[38]. In contrast to the previous MRC study (MRC OEO2 trial), they included patients with resectable gastric (74%), EGJ (15%), or distal esophageal adenocarcinoma (11%). This UK MAGIC trial evaluated the effect of perioperative chemotherapy with the ECF (epirubicin, cisplatin, and 5-FU) regimen given before and after surgery in resectable gastroesophageal cancer. A total of 503 patients were randomly assigned to surgery with or without perioperative chemotherapy. Most of the patients had gastric cancer (74%), while small group of patients had adenocarcinoma of lower esophagus (14%) and EGJ (11%). At a median follow-up of four years, 5-year overall survival was significantly better in the perioperative chemotherapy group compared with surgery alone (36 vs. 23%).

5. Current therapy for unresectable and metastatic esophageal adenocarcinoma

The goals of therapy for patients with advanced unresectable and metastatic esophageal cancer are to palliate symptoms, including malignant dysphagia, and improve survival. Patients with advanced adenocarcinoma of esophagus and EGJ can be treated using the regimens included in the gastric cancer guide-lined for advanced gastric cancer. Since the mid 1970s, the incidence of SCC in the United States has been declining, while the incidence of adenocarcinoma in white males rose by 350 percent from 1970s to 1990s[41]. Adenocarcinoma became the dominant histology in the early 1990s. In addition, the incidence of distal gastric adenocarcinoma declined, while the incidence of adenocarcinoma of EGJ and proximal stomach has increased. The increasing incidence has paralleled the rise in incidence of EAC. These histories suggest that adenocarcinomas of the distal esophagus, EGJ and proximal stomach share a common pathogenesis.

5.1 Chemotherapy for advanced unresectable or metastatic esophageal adenocarcinoma

In randomized clinical trials, no consistent benefit was seen for any specific chemotherapy regimen, and chemotherapy showed no survival benefit compared with best supportive care for patients with advanced esophageal cancer[3]. However, palliative chemotherapy may improve quality of life in patients with unresectable or metastatic esophageal cancer.

5.1.1 Single agent

Cisplatin is one of the most active agents, with a single-response rate consistently in the range of 20% or greater[42]. Newer agents such as irinotecan[43-45], docetaxel[46, 47], paclitaxel[48-50], and etoposide[51] have also shown activity as single agents in advanced esophageal cancer.

5.1.2 Combination chemotherapy

The combination of cisplatin and fluorouracil has been one of the most commonly used regimens in both metastatic and localized esophageal cancer due to its activity and well-established toxicity profile. Cisplatin also has been combined with taxanes[50, 52-54], irinotecan[55], mitomycin[56], and gemcitabine[57, 58].

Capecitabine is designed oral fluoropyrimidine that is converted to 5-FU in three-step enzymatic process[59]. In the REAL-2 trial[60], multicenter phase III study assessed by a randomized 2x2 design, 1002 patients with histologically confirmed EAC, SCC, or undifferentiated cancer of esophagus, EGJ, or stomach randomly assigned to receive one of four epirubicin-based regimens ([ECF]; epirubicin, cisplatin, 5-FU, [EOF]; epirubicin, oxaliplatin, 5-FU, [ECX]; epirubicin, cisplatin, capecitabine, [EOX]; epirubicin, oxaliplatin, capecitabine). The primary outcome in this study was non-inferiority in overall survival. The primary endpoint was reached and there was a trend toward better overall survival for the capecitabine and oxaliplatin groups.

Regimens containing irinotecan have been studied. Irinotecan has been combined with cisplatin[61], docetaxel[62], and fluoropyrimidines[63]. Irinotecan plus cisplatin is active and well tolerated in several studies. Combinations of irinotecan and docetaxel with or without cisplatin are active but toxic. Combinations of irinotecan and oxaliplatin are highly efficacious and tolerated[63]. There are no phase III trials comparing an irinotecan-based combination with a cisplatin-based regimen.

Tables show brief regimens listed in the guidelines for metastatic or locally advanced esophageal or EGJ cancers (Table 2 and 3).

First-line therapy
DCF or its modifications (category 1 for docetaxel, cisplatin, and fluorouracil; category 2B for docetaxel, carboplatin, and fluorouracil; category 2A for all other combinations
ECF or its modifications (category 1)
Fluoropyrimidine- or taxane-based regimens, single agent or combination therapy, (category 1 for combination of fluoropyrimidine and cisplatin; category 2A for all other regimens)
Trastuzumab with chemotherapy (category 1 for combination with cisplatin and fluoropyrimidine; category 2B for combination with other chemotherapy agents) for patients who are HER2-neu positive, as determined by a standardized method.

Table 2. First-line therapy for Recurrent and Metastatic Esophageal Cancer.

Second-line therapy
Trastuzumab with chemotherapy (category 1 for combination with cisplatin and fluoropyrimidine; category 2B for combination with other chemotherapy agents) for patients who are HER2-neu-positive, if not used as first-line therapy
Docetaxel or paclitaxel (category 2B)
Irinotecan-based single-agent or combination therapy (category 2B)

Table 3. Second-line therapy for Recurrent and Metastatic Esophageal Cancer.

6. Biological/Targeted therapy

With the recent development of small molecules and antibodies designed form biologic first principles, biologic/targeted therapies are now incorporating with chemotherapy. The most commonly used agents include angiogenesis inhibitors (bevacizumab) and epidermal growth factor receptor inhibitors (panitumumab, cetuximab, erlotinib). Shah et al. carried out a phase II trial of 47 patients to study the addition of the anti-vascular endothelial growth factor monoclonal antibody, bevacizumab, to weekly cisplatin and irinotecan in patients with advanced gastroesphageal cancer.[64] The median survival was 12.3 months (95% CI, 11.3 to 17.2 months), and there was no increase in chemotherapy related toxicity. The ongoing REAL-3 trial is testing epirubicin, oxaliplatin and capecitabine (EOX) with or without panitumumab in previously untreated advanced esophagogastric cancer. Pittsburgh group is carrying a phase II study of irinotecan plus panitumumab as second line treatment for advanced EAC. In the setting of locally advanced disease, ECOG 2205 investigated the addition of cetuximab to chemoradiation therapy for resectable EAC, and ACOSOG Z4051 is enrolling patients with adenocarcinoma to chemoradiation therapy plus panitumumab.

The revolution in biological/targeted therapies offers hope for improvement in survival for patients with advanced EAC. However, historically, the empiric addition of targeted agents such as cetuximab and bevacizumab to cytotoxic chemotherapy has yielded a modest improvement in survival for patients with solid tumors.[65-67] This relative failure of the current approach has led to great interest in either selecting patients for therapies or selecting therapies for patients, usually by tumor profiling and selective preclinical models.[68, 69] This project aims to test a novel direct translational model of target selection and inhibition with the goal of furthering the rational selection of targeted therapies for patients with advanced EAC.

6.1 Trastuzumab

HER2 is another member of the EGFR family that is associated with cell proliferation, migration, and differentiation. HER2 over-expression and/or amplification have been reported in EAC, along with some evidence supporting a prognostic utility. Various phase I and II trial have reported a possible benefit for HER2 blockage[70, 71]. Data from these trials served as the basis for a recent prospective phase III trial (ToGA)[72] that evaluated the therapeutic benefit of blocking this target in a randomized fashion.

In the ToGA trial, more than 594 patients with HER2-positive gastric and gastroesophageal cancer were treated with standard chemotherapy (infusional 5-FU or capecitabine plus cisplatin), either with or without trastuzumab. The tumors of the enrolled patients were either fluorescence in situ hybridization (FISH)-positive or positive for HER2 expression by immunohistochemistry (IHC). At a median follow-up of 17.1 to 18.6 months, median overall survival (the primary endpoint) was significantly improved with the addition of trastuzumab (13.8 vs. 11.1 months). Safety profiles were comparable, with no unexpected adverse events in the trastuzumab group and no difference was seen in symptomatic congestive heart failure between the arms. This establishes trastuzumab plus chemotherapy as a new standard of care for the treatment of patients with HER2-expressing advanced gastric and EGJ adenocarcinoma.

6.2 Cetuximab

As monotherapy, cetuximab, a monoclonal antibody targeting the EGFR, has limited activity as second-line therapy[73]. The safety and efficacy adding cetuximab to first-line chemotherapy has been tested in several studies of advanced esophagogastric cancer[74, 75]. All suggest that this approach is safe and in some cases, objective response rates are over 50 percent and median survival is less than 10 months. Conclusions regarding the clinical utility of cetuximab in patients with advanced esophagogastric cancer need data from randomized phase III trial.

6.3 Gefitinib and erlotinib (small molecule tyrosine kinase inhibitors)

Another means of interfering with EGFR signaling is through the use of orally active tyrosine kinase inhibitors (TKIs), small molecules that block the binding site of the EGFR tyrosine kinase. Small molecule TKIs such as Gefitinib and Erlotinib have been tested as single agents in phase II trials in esophagogastric cancer.

In a phase II study of gefitinib in 36 patients who had failed one prior therapy for advanced esophageal cancer, there was only one partial response, but 10 patients had stable disease for at least eight weeks. Treatment was reasonably well tolerated[76].

In another trial, gefitinib was administered to 27 patients with advanced unresectable EAC. There were three partial responses, and seven had stable disease[77].

In SWOG trial, 70 patients with unresectable or metastatic adenocarcinoma originating in the EGJ or stomach received first line treatment with erlotinib[78]. Six patients had an objective response rate (9 percent, one complete), all of them were EGJ tumors. There was no molecular parameter of EGFR expression or mutations were predictive of clinical outcome. The reason for the apparent differential sensitivity of EGJ and gastric cancer s to EGFR blockade using erlotinib is unclear.

6.4 Bevacizumab

Elevated serum and tumor levels of vascular endothelial growth factor (VEGF) are associated with a poor prognosis in patients with resectable gastric cancer[79, 80]. Adding the anti-VEGF monoclonal antibody bevacizumab to chemotherapy in advanced upper GI cancer has been studied.

In the phase III AVAGAST trial, in which 774 patients with previously untreated locally advanced unresectable or metastatic gastric or EGJ cancer were randomly assigned to capecitabine plus cicplatin with either bevacizumab or placebo[81]. In a preliminary report, there was no significant benefit from bevacizumab in median overall survival (the primary endpoint, 12.1 vs. 10.1 months, hazard ratio 0.87, 95% CI 0.73-1.03) although the use of bevacizumab significantly improved both objective response rate and median progression-free survival.

7. Conclusion

The treatment of esophageal and EGJ cancer has undergone a major evolution over the past decades. However, the optimal therapy for these patients is still controversial. Although several advances have made in staging procedures and therapeutic approaches, esophageal cancer is often diagnosed late. Some forms of multimodal management are essential for treating patients with esophageal cancer. Most of the clinical studies have not differentiated between SCC and adenocarcinoma so that most of approaches are similar for both histologies. However, there are an increasing amount of evidence supports the view that they differ in terms of their epidemiology, biology, and prognosis, etc. In recognition of these differences, the AJCC 2010 TNM staging criteria provides separate stage groupings for SCC and adenocarcinomas of the esophagus and EGJ. For patients with locally advanced resectable adenocarcinoma of esophagus and EGJ (T1b or higher, any N), primary treatment options include preoperative chemoradiation therapy, definitive chemoratiation, preoperative chemotherapy, or esophagectomy. Postoperative treatment is based on their staging. Fluoropyrimidine-based chemoradiation therapy is recommended for patients with node-positive adenocarcinoma of esophagus and EGJ. Perioperative chemotherapy is recommended for patients with completely resected adenocarcinoma of EGJ (MAGIC trial). All patients with residual disease at surgical margins may be treated with fluoropyrimidine-based chemoradiation. For patients with unresectable disease or those with resectable disease who choose not to undergo surgery, fluoropyrimidine- or taxane-based concurrent chemoradiation therapy is recommended. For patients with recurrent and metastatic disease, the goals of chemotherapy are to palliate symptoms and improve survival. Biologic/Targeted therapies have produced encouraging results in the treatment of patients with advanced adenocarcinoma of esophagus and EGJ. The efficacy of these new therapies in combination with chemotherapy still need results from randomized phase III trials.

Considerable advanced have been made in the treatment of adenocarcinoma of esophagus and EGJ. Novel therapeutic modalities, such as targeted therapies, antiangiogenic agents, gene therapy, and etc are being studied in clinical trials. More tailor-made treatment for patients with esophageal cancer may be needed and well-designed clinical trials are awaited to enable further advances.

8. References

[1] Landis SH, Murray T, Bolden S, Wingo PA. Cancer statistics, 1998. *CA Cancer J Clin.* Jan-Feb 1998;48(1):6-29.

[2] Landis SH, Murray T, Bolden S, Wingo PA. Cancer statistics, 1999. *CA Cancer J Clin.* Jan-Feb 1999;49(1):8-31, 31.

[3] Homs MY, v d Gaast A, Siersema PD, Steyerberg EW, Kuipers EJ. Chemotherapy for metastatic carcinoma of the esophagus and gastro-esophageal junction. *Cochrane Database Syst Rev.* 2006(4):CD004063.

[4] Jemal A, Siegel R, Xu J, Ward E. Cancer statistics, 2010. *CA Cancer J Clin.* Sep-Oct 2010;60(5):277-300.

[5] Brown LM, Devesa SS, Chow WH. Incidence of adenocarcinoma of the esophagus among white Americans by sex, stage, and age. *J Natl Cancer Inst.* Aug 20 2008;100(16):1184-1187.

[6] Engel LS, Chow WH, Vaughan TL, et al. Population attributable risks of esophageal and gastric cancers. *J Natl Cancer Inst.* Sep 17 2003;95(18):1404-1413.

[7] Chow WH, Blot WJ, Vaughan TL, et al. Body mass index and risk of adenocarcinomas of the esophagus and gastric cardia. *J Natl Cancer Inst.* Jan 21 1998;90(2):150-155.

[8] Vaughan TL, Davis S, Kristal A, Thomas DB. Obesity, alcohol, and tobacco as risk factors for cancers of the esophagus and gastric cardia: adenocarcinoma versus squamous cell carcinoma. *Cancer Epidemiol Biomarkers Prev.* Mar 1995;4(2):85-92.

[9] Lagergren J, Bergstrom R, Nyren O. Association between body mass and adenocarcinoma of the esophagus and gastric cardia. *Ann Intern Med.* Jun 1 1999;130(11):883-890.
[10] Brown LM, Swanson CA, Gridley G, et al. Adenocarcinoma of the esophagus: role of obesity and diet. *J Natl Cancer Inst.* Jan 18 1995;87(2):104-109.
[11] Chow WH, Finkle WD, McLaughlin JK, Frankl H, Ziel HK, Fraumeni JF, Jr. The relation of gastroesophageal reflux disease and its treatment to adenocarcinomas of the esophagus and gastric cardia. *JAMA.* Aug 9 1995;274(6):474-477.
[12] Lagergren J, Bergstrom R, Lindgren A, Nyren O. Symptomatic gastroesophageal reflux as a risk factor for esophageal adenocarcinoma. *N Engl J Med.* Mar 18 1999;340(11):825-831.
[13] Cossentino MJ, Wong RK. Barrett's esophagus and risk of esophageal adenocarcinoma. *Semin Gastrointest Dis.* Jul 2003;14(3):128-135.
[14] Cameron AJ, Romero Y. Symptomatic gastro-oesophageal reflux as a risk factor for oesophageal adenocarcinoma. *Gut.* Jun 2000;46(6):754-755.
[15] Sharma P. Clinical practice. Barrett's esophagus. *N Engl J Med.* Dec 24 2009;361(26):2548-2556.
[16] Edge SB, Compton CC. The American Joint Committee on Cancer: the 7th edition of the AJCC cancer staging manual and the future of TNM. *Ann Surg Oncol.* Jun 2010;17(6):1471-1474.
[17] Tong DK, Law S, Kwong DL, Wei WI, Ng RW, Wong KH. Current management of cervical esophageal cancer. *World J Surg.* Mar 2011;35(3):600-607.
[18] Bosset JF, Gignoux M, Triboulet JP, et al. Chemoradiotherapy followed by surgery compared with surgery alone in squamous-cell cancer of the esophagus. *N Engl J Med.* Jul 17 1997;337(3):161-167.
[19] Urba SG, Orringer MB, Turrisi A, Iannettoni M, Forastiere A, Strawderman M. Randomized trial of preoperative chemoradiation versus surgery alone in patients with locoregional esophageal carcinoma. *J Clin Oncol.* Jan 15 2001;19(2):305-313.
[20] Nygaard K, Hagen S, Hansen HS, et al. Pre-operative radiotherapy prolongs survival in operable esophageal carcinoma: a randomized, multicenter study of pre-operative radiotherapy and chemotherapy. The second Scandinavian trial in esophageal cancer. *World J Surg.* Nov-Dec 1992;16(6):1104-1109; discussion 1110.
[21] Le Prise E, Etienne PL, Meunier B, et al. A randomized study of chemotherapy, radiation therapy, and surgery versus surgery for localized squamous cell carcinoma of the esophagus. *Cancer.* Apr 1 1994;73(7):1779-1784.
[22] Burmeister BH, Smithers BM, Gebski V, et al. Surgery alone versus chemoradiotherapy followed by surgery for resectable cancer of the oesophagus: a randomised controlled phase III trial. *Lancet Oncol.* Sep 2005;6(9):659-668.
[23] Walsh TN, Noonan N, Hollywood D, Kelly A, Keeling N, Hennessy TP. A comparison of multimodal therapy and surgery for esophageal adenocarcinoma. *N Engl J Med.* Aug 15 1996;335(7):462-467.
[24] Tepper J, Krasna MJ, Niedzwiecki D, et al. Phase III trial of trimodality therapy with cisplatin, fluorouracil, radiotherapy, and surgery compared with surgery alone for esophageal cancer: CALGB 9781. *J Clin Oncol.* Mar 1 2008;26(7):1086-1092.

[25] Mariette C SJ, Maillard E. Surgery alone versus chemoradiotherapy followed by surgery for localized esophageal cancer: analysis of a randomized controlled phase III trial FFCD 9901 [abstract]. *Journal of Clinical oncology.* 2010;28(302s).

[26] Urschel JD, Vasan H. A meta-analysis of randomized controlled trials that compared neoadjuvant chemoradiation and surgery to surgery alone for resectable esophageal cancer. *Am J Surg.* Jun 2003;185(6):538-543.

[27] Gebski V, Burmeister B, Smithers BM, Foo K, Zalcberg J, Simes J. Survival benefits from neoadjuvant chemoradiotherapy or chemotherapy in oesophageal carcinoma: a meta-analysis. *Lancet Oncol.* Mar 2007;8(3):226-234.

[28] Herskovic A, Martz K, al-Sarraf M, et al. Combined chemotherapy and radiotherapy compared with radiotherapy alone in patients with cancer of the esophagus. *N Engl J Med.* Jun 11 1992;326(24):1593-1598.

[29] Cooper JS, Guo MD, Herskovic A, et al. Chemoradiotherapy of locally advanced esophageal cancer: long-term follow-up of a prospective randomized trial (RTOG 85-01). Radiation Therapy Oncology Group. *JAMA.* May 5 1999;281(17):1623-1627.

[30] Wong R, Malthaner R. Combined chemotherapy and radiotherapy (without surgery) compared with radiotherapy alone in localized carcinoma of the esophagus. *Cochrane Database Syst Rev.* 2001(2):CD002092.

[31] Minsky BD, Pajak TF, Ginsberg RJ, et al. INT 0123 (Radiation Therapy Oncology Group 94-05) phase III trial of combined-modality therapy for esophageal cancer: high-dose versus standard-dose radiation therapy. *J Clin Oncol.* Mar 1 2002;20(5):1167-1174.

[32] Adelstein DJ, Rice TW, Rybicki LA, et al. Mature results from a phase II trial of postoperative concurrent chemoradiotherapy for poor prognosis cancer of the esophagus and gastroesophageal junction. *J Thorac Oncol.* Oct 2009;4(10):1264-1269.

[33] Macdonald JS, Smalley SR, Benedetti J, et al. Chemoradiotherapy after surgery compared with surgery alone for adenocarcinoma of the stomach or gastroesophageal junction. *N Engl J Med.* Sep 6 2001;345(10):725-730.

[34] Kelsen DP, Ginsberg R, Pajak TF, et al. Chemotherapy followed by surgery compared with surgery alone for localized esophageal cancer. *N Engl J Med.* Dec 31 1998;339(27):1979-1984.

[35] Ancona E, Ruol A, Santi S, et al. Only pathologic complete response to neoadjuvant chemotherapy improves significantly the long term survival of patients with resectable esophageal squamous cell carcinoma: final report of a randomized, controlled trial of preoperative chemotherapy versus surgery alone. *Cancer.* Jun 1 2001;91(11):2165-2174.

[36] Surgical resection with or without preoperative chemotherapy in oesophageal cancer: a randomised controlled trial. *Lancet.* May 18 2002;359(9319):1727-1733.

[37] Roth JA, Pass HI, Flanagan MM, Graeber GM, Rosenberg JC, Steinberg S. Randomized clinical trial of preoperative and postoperative adjuvant chemotherapy with cisplatin, vindesine, and bleomycin for carcinoma of the esophagus. *J Thorac Cardiovasc Surg.* Aug 1988;96(2):242-248.

[38] Cunningham D, Allum WH, Stenning SP, et al. Perioperative chemotherapy versus surgery alone for resectable gastroesophageal cancer. *N Engl J Med.* Jul 6 2006;355(1):11-20.

[39] Allum WH, Stenning SP, Bancewicz J, Clark PI, Langley RE. Long-term results of a randomized trial of surgery with or without preoperative chemotherapy in esophageal cancer. *J Clin Oncol.* Oct 20 2009;27(30):5062-5067.

[40] Boige V PJ, Saint-Aubert B. Final results of a randomized trial compareing preoperative 5-fluorouracil (F)/cisplatin (P) to surgery alone in adenocarcinoma of stomach and lower esophagus (ASLE): FNLCC ACCORD07-FFCD9703 trial [abstract]. *Journal of Clinical oncology.* 2007;25.

[41] Devesa SS, Blot WJ, Fraumeni JF, Jr. Changing patterns in the incidence of esophageal and gastric carcinoma in the United States. *Cancer.* Nov 15 1998;83(10):2049-2053.

[42] Leichman L, Berry BT. Experience with cisplatin in treatment regimens for esophageal cancer. *Semin Oncol.* Feb 1991;18(1 Suppl 3):64-72.

[43] Muhr-Wilkenshoff F, Hinkelbein W, Ohnesorge I, et al. A pilot study of irinotecan (CPT-11) as single-agent therapy in patients with locally advanced or metastatic esophageal carcinoma. *Int J Colorectal Dis.* Jul 2003;18(4):330-334.

[44] Enzinger PC, Kulke MH, Clark JW, et al. A phase II trial of irinotecan in patients with previously untreated advanced esophageal and gastric adenocarcinoma. *Dig Dis Sci.* Dec 2005;50(12):2218-2223.

[45] Burkart C, Bokemeyer C, Klump B, Pereira P, Teichmann R, Hartmann JT. A phase II trial of weekly irinotecan in cisplatin-refractory esophageal cancer. *Anticancer Res.* Jul-Aug 2007;27(4C):2845-2848.

[46] Muro K, Hamaguchi T, Ohtsu A, et al. A phase II study of single-agent docetaxel in patients with metastatic esophageal cancer. *Ann Oncol.* Jun 2004;15(6):955-959.

[47] Albertsson M, Johansson B, Friesland S, et al. Phase II studies on docetaxel alone every third week, or weekly in combination with gemcitabine in patients with primary locally advanced, metastatic, or recurrent esophageal cancer. *Med Oncol.* 2007;24(4):407-412.

[48] Ajani JA, Ilson DH, Daugherty K, Pazdur R, Lynch PM, Kelsen DP. Activity of taxol in patients with squamous cell carcinoma and adenocarcinoma of the esophagus. *J Natl Cancer Inst.* Jul 20 1994;86(14):1086-1091.

[49] Mauer AM, Kraut EH, Krauss SA, et al. Phase II trial of oxaliplatin, leucovorin and fluorouracil in patients with advanced carcinoma of the esophagus. *Ann Oncol.* Aug 2005;16(8):1320-1325.

[50] Ilson DH, Wadleigh RG, Leichman LP, Kelsen DP. Paclitaxel given by a weekly 1-h infusion in advanced esophageal cancer. *Ann Oncol.* May 2007;18(5):898-902.

[51] Harstrick A, Bokemeyer C, Preusser P, et al. Phase II study of single-agent etoposide in patients with metastatic squamous-cell carcinoma of the esophagus. *Cancer Chemother Pharmacol.* 1992;29(4):321-322.

[52] Ilson DH, Ajani J, Bhalla K, et al. Phase II trial of paclitaxel, fluorouracil, and cisplatin in patients with advanced carcinoma of the esophagus. *J Clin Oncol.* May 1998;16(5):1826-1834.

[53] Ajani JA, Fodor MB, Tjulandin SA, et al. Phase II multi-institutional randomized trial of docetaxel plus cisplatin with or without fluorouracil in patients with untreated, advanced gastric, or gastroesophageal adenocarcinoma. *J Clin Oncol.* Aug 20 2005;23(24):5660-5667.

[54] Van Cutsem E, Moiseyenko VM, Tjulandin S, et al. Phase III study of docetaxel and cisplatin plus fluorouracil compared with cisplatin and fluorouracil as first-line therapy for advanced gastric cancer: a report of the V325 Study Group. *J Clin Oncol.* Nov 1 2006;24(31):4991-4997.
[55] Ilson DH. Phase II trial of weekly irinotecan/cisplatin in advanced esophageal cancer. *Oncology (Williston Park).* Dec 2004;18(14 Suppl 14):22-25.
[56] Ross P, Nicolson M, Cunningham D, et al. Prospective randomized trial comparing mitomycin, cisplatin, and protracted venous-infusion fluorouracil (PVI 5-FU) With epirubicin, cisplatin, and PVI 5-FU in advanced esophagogastric cancer. *J Clin Oncol.* Apr 15 2002;20(8):1996-2004.
[57] Millar J, Scullin P, Morrison A, et al. Phase II study of gemcitabine and cisplatin in locally advanced/metastatic oesophageal cancer. *Br J Cancer.* Nov 14 2005;93(10):1112-1116.
[58] Urba SG, Chansky K, VanVeldhuizen PJ, et al. Gemcitabine and cisplatin for patients with metastatic or recurrent esophageal carcinoma: a Southwest Oncology Group Study. *Invest New Drugs.* Jan 2004;22(1):91-97.
[59] Ajani J. Review of capecitabine as oral treatment of gastric, gastroesophageal, and esophageal cancers. *Cancer.* Jul 15 2006;107(2):221-231.
[60] Assersohn L, Brown G, Cunningham D, et al. Phase II study of irinotecan and 5-fluorouracil/leucovorin in patients with primary refractory or relapsed advanced oesophageal and gastric carcinoma. *Ann Oncol.* Jan 2004;15(1):64-69.
[61] Moehler M, Kanzler S, Geissler M, et al. A randomized multicenter phase II study comparing capecitabine with irinotecan or cisplatin in metastatic adenocarcinoma of the stomach or esophagogastric junction. *Ann Oncol.* Jan 2010;21(1):71-77.
[62] Burtness B, Gibson M, Egleston B, et al. Phase II trial of docetaxel-irinotecan combination in advanced esophageal cancer. *Ann Oncol.* Jul 2009;20(7):1242-1248.
[63] Leary A, Assersohn L, Cunningham D, et al. A phase II trial evaluating capecitabine and irinotecan as second line treatment in patients with oesophago-gastric cancer who have progressed on, or within 3 months of platinum-based chemotherapy. *Cancer Chemother Pharmacol.* Aug 2009;64(3):455-462.
[64] Shah MA, Ramanathan RK, Ilson DH, et al. Multicenter phase II study of irinotecan, cisplatin, and bevacizumab in patients with metastatic gastric or gastroesophageal junction adenocarcinoma. *J Clin Oncol.* Nov 20 2006;24(33):5201-5206.
[65] Cunningham D, Humblet Y, Siena S, et al. Cetuximab monotherapy and cetuximab plus irinotecan in irinotecan-refractory metastatic colorectal cancer. *N Engl J Med.* Jul 22 2004;351(4):337-345.
[66] Hurwitz H, Fehrenbacher L, Novotny W, et al. Bevacizumab plus irinotecan, fluorouracil, and leucovorin for metastatic colorectal cancer. *N Engl J Med.* Jun 3 2004;350(23):2335-2342.
[67] Sandler A, Gray R, Perry MC, et al. Paclitaxel-carboplatin alone or with bevacizumab for non-small-cell lung cancer. *N Engl J Med.* Dec 14 2006;355(24):2542-2550.
[68] Jimeno A, Feldmann G, Suarez-Gauthier A, et al. A direct pancreatic cancer xenograft model as a platform for cancer stem cell therapeutic development. *Mol Cancer Ther.* Feb 2009;8(2):310-314.

[69] Altiok S, Mezzadra H, Jagannath S, et al. A novel pharmacodynamic approach to assess and predict tumor response to the epidermal growth factor receptor inhibitor gefitinib in patients with esophageal cancer. *Int J Oncol.* Jan 2010;36(1):19-27.
[70] Leon-Chong J LF, Kang YK. HER2 positivity in advanced gastric cancer is comparable to breast cancer (Abstract). *Journal of Clinical oncology.* 2007;25:638s.
[71] Liang Z, Zeng X, Gao J, et al. Analysis of EGFR, HER2, and TOP2A gene status and chromosomal polysomy in gastric adenocarcinoma from Chinese patients. *BMC Cancer.* 2008;8:363.
[72] Bang YJ, Van Cutsem E, Feyereislova A, et al. Trastuzumab in combination with chemotherapy versus chemotherapy alone for treatment of HER2-positive advanced gastric or gastro-oesophageal junction cancer (ToGA): a phase 3, open-label, randomised controlled trial. *Lancet.* Aug 28 2010;376(9742):687-697.
[73] Gold PJ GB, Iqbal S. Cetuximab as second-line therapy in patients with metastatic esophageal cancer: a phase II Southwest Oncology Group Study (abstract). *Journal of Clinical oncology.* 2008;26:222s.
[74] Pinto C, Di Fabio F, Siena S, et al. Phase II study of cetuximab in combination with FOLFIRI in patients with untreated advanced gastric or gastroesophageal junction adenocarcinoma (FOLCETUX study). *Ann Oncol.* Mar 2007;18(3):510-517.
[75] Pinto C, Di Fabio F, Barone C, et al. Phase II study of cetuximab in combination with cisplatin and docetaxel in patients with untreated advanced gastric or gastro-oesophageal junction adenocarcinoma (DOCETUX study). *Br J Cancer.* Oct 20 2009;101(8):1261-1268.
[76] Janmaat ML, Gallegos-Ruiz MI, Rodriguez JA, et al. Predictive factors for outcome in a phase II study of gefitinib in second-line treatment of advanced esophageal cancer patients. *J Clin Oncol.* Apr 1 2006;24(10):1612-1619.
[77] Ferry DR, Anderson M, Beddard K, et al. A phase II study of gefitinib monotherapy in advanced esophageal adenocarcinoma: evidence of gene expression, cellular, and clinical response. *Clin Cancer Res.* Oct 1 2007;13(19):5869-5875.
[78] Dragovich T, McCoy S, Fenoglio-Preiser CM, et al. Phase II trial of erlotinib in gastroesophageal junction and gastric adenocarcinomas: SWOG 0127. *J Clin Oncol.* Oct 20 2006;24(30):4922-4927.
[79] Fondevila C, Metges JP, Fuster J, et al. p53 and VEGF expression are independent predictors of tumour recurrence and survival following curative resection of gastric cancer. *Br J Cancer.* Jan 12 2004;90(1):206-215.
[80] Yao JC, Wang L, Wei D, et al. Association between expression of transcription factor Sp1 and increased vascular endothelial growth factor expression, advanced stage, and poor survival in patients with resected gastric cancer. *Clin Cancer Res.* Jun 15 2004;10(12 Pt 1):4109-4117.
[81] Kang Y OA, Van Cutsem E. AVAGAST: a randomized, double-blind, placebo-controlled phase III study of first-line capecitabine and cisplatin plus bevacizumab or placebo in patients with advanced gastric cancer (AGC) (abstract LBA4007). *Journal of Clinical oncology.* 2010;28:950s.

8

Nonsurgical Management of Esophageal Cancer

Malek M. Safa and Hassan K. Reda
Dayton Cancer Center, Dayton, Ohio and University of Kentucky, Lexington, Kentucky, USA

1. Introduction

In the recent past, the incidence of esophageal adenocarcinomas has risen dramatically, whereas the incidence of squamous cell carcinomas has remained relatively steady in the United States (Holmes & Vaughan, 2007). Esophageal adenocarcinoma arises from Barrett's esophagus with an estimated incidence rate of 0.4-0.7 per 100-patients/year. (Sharma et al., 2004; Thomas et al., 2007). Barrett's esophagus without dysplasia and those with low-grade dysplasia generally have low rates of disease progression, but some studies showed that over 8 years, 27% of patients with low-grade dysplasia developed high-grade dysplasia or early esophageal adenocarcinoma. In addition, high-grade dysplasia has a definite risk of disease progression with rates exceeding 10% per year (Miros et al., 1991; Reid et al., 2000). The cornerstone of curative treatment for esophageal cancer has been surgery; however, its role has been challenged in very early stage due to morbidity of the procedure. Many studies have reported outcomes for patients undergoing surgical resection for esophageal cancer. However, the outcome of such studies does not inform clinical decision making for the majority of patients who present to surgeons with esophageal cancer. Esophagectomy for high-grade dysplasia or early esophageal carcinoma has mortality rates ranging from 2.5 to 20.3% and 30-50% of patients may develop serious postoperative complications (Spechler, 2005). For a variety of reasons, the majority of patients with esophageal cancer are actually not suitable for esophagectomy. More than 50% have locally advanced, unresectable or metastatic tumors at diagnosis. Other reasons which preclude esophagectomy include old age, comorbidity, or refusal by the patient. Emerging data suggest that endoscopic therapies are viable therapeutic options with significantly lower morbidities. Currently, in many institutions, for a subset of patients with clinically localized early stage esophageal cancer (T0 or T1 lesions), local endoscopic therapy (excisional biopsy, endoscopic resection, photodynamic, local destruction, thermal laser, polypectomy, electrocautery, cryoablation, or radiofrequency ablation) seems to be an acceptable alternative and produces similar results to surgery.

For more advanced stages of esophageal cancers, the mainstay of nonsurgical treatment is chemotherapy (CT) or radiotherapy (RT), either alone or in combination chemoradiotherapy (CRT). A number of factors have been shown to predict survival in advanced esophageal cancer. These include stage, performance status, weight loss, and presence or absence of metastasis. The stage of the cancer, and in particular the presence of metastatic disease, is the single strongest predictor. The influence of other factors, such as histological type, has been less well established. However, there is data suggesting that standard CRT might be equivalent to surgery alone in terms of survival for patients with squamous cell carcinoma of the esophagus.

In this chapter, we sought to determine the outcome of patients who underwent treatment of esophageal cancer with the various local endoscopic therapies, conventional CT or RT or concurrent CRT, but not surgical resection, as published in the literature. In addition, we reviewed the specific outcomes of patients with and without metastatic disease, and with different histological subtypes.

2. Endoscopic mucosal resection

Endoscopic mucosal resection (EMR) serves both diagnostic and therapeutic roles in the management of Barrett's esophagus and early esophageal cancer. It involves local snare excision of the target lesion. EMR resects a lesion in entirety for histopathological assessment, and if the resection margins are clear, it is curative. It has also been used to completely resect the entire at-risk Barrett's epithelium in order to reduce the risk of recurrence.

Ell et al. (Ell et al., 2007) evaluated the efficacy and safety of localized endoscopic mucosal resection in a total of 100 patients with low-risk early esophageal adenocarcinomas (lesion diameter up to 20 mm; mucosal lesion without invasion into lymph vessels and veins; and histopatholological grade G1 and G2). Complete local remission was achieved in 99 of the 100 patients after 1.9 months and a maximum of three resections. During a median follow-up period of 36.7 months, recurrent or metachronous carcinomas were found in 11% of the patients, but successful repeat treatment with endoscopic resection was possible in all cases. There were no major complications.

To address the problem of disease recurrence, the concept of complete circumferential EMR to remove all underlying Barrett's mucosa upon detection of high-grade dysplasia or early esophageal carcinoma was introduced. In an early study (Seewald et al., 2003), 12 patients with high-grade dysplasia or early esophageal carcinoma underwent circumferential EMR using simple snare resection. During a median follow-up of 9 months, no recurrence of Barrett's esophagus or malignancy was observed. Giovannini et al. (Giovannini et al., 2004) subsequently reported their experience in circumferential EMR in 21 patients with Barrett's esophagus who had either high-grade dysplasia or early esophageal carcinoma. Complete circumferential EMR was achieved in two sessions. Resection was complete in 86% of the patients and Barrett's esophagus was completely replaced by squamous cell epithelium in 75%. Later studies reported similar results with rare complication rates including stricture formation, bleeding and perforations. (Peters et al., 2006; Larghi et al., 2007; Lopes et al., 2007).

In summary, although EMR is feasible, safe and effective for the treatment Barrett's esophagus with high-grade dysplasia and early esophageal carcinoma, more long-term data for a larger number of treated patients are still required in order to establish EMR as a standard alternative treatment to surgery.

3. Photodynamic therapy

Photodynamic therapy (PDT) is one of the most widely studied ablative therapies used in the treatment of Barrett's esophagus. PDT is one of the most acceptable ablative therapies for high-grade dysplasia and early invasive adenocarcinoma with some of the longest follow-up data (Prasad et al., 2007).

3.1 Technique

PDT is a photochemical process that requires multiple steps to achieve tissue destruction. First, a photosensitizer drug is required. The only photosensitizer approved in the United States by the Food and Drug Administration for use in Barrett's high-grade dysplasia is porfimer sodium (Ps) (photofrin). Usually, porfimer sodium is administered intravenously over 3 to 5 minutes at a dose of 2 mg/kg body weight. After systemic injection, the photosensitizer is absorbed by most tissues and retained at higher concentrations in neoplastic tissues (Nishioka, 1998). The second step in the process is the application of light of proper power and wavelength to the target tissue. A variety of tunable dye lasers have been approved to activate photosensitizers. These laser units can generate the desired light and about 2 to 2.5 W of energy output. Visible red light at approximately 630 nm is typically used to activate the photosensitizer. The activated drug interacts with molecular oxygen leading to the generation of singlet oxygen. Subsequent radical reactions can form superoxide and hydroxyl radicals leading to cell membrane damage and apoptosis. It is important to note that laser treatment induces a photochemical, and not a thermal effect. For endoscopic applications, illumination with laser light occurs 40 to 50 hours after injection with porfimer sodium (Overholt et al., 2005). The light is transmitted by optical fiber advanced through the accessory channel of an endoscope. The fibers come in different lengths to better match the length of the lesion being targeted. For treatment of BE with high-grade dysplasia, the light dose recommended is 130 to 200 j/cm fiber. A second endoscopy is advised 96 to 120 hours after porfimer sodium injection to assess mucosal damage and degree of necrosis. If needed, a second light application can be administered to skipped or poorly treated areas (Overholt et al., 2005). The depth of injury of porfimer sodium at wavelength of 630 nm is approximately 5 to 6 mm, depending on tissue blood flow and oxygen levels (Gross & Wolfsen, 2010).

There are other drugs, used mostly in Europe, for PDT applications, including 5-aminolevulinic acid (5-ALA) and m-tetrahydroxyphenyl chlorine (mTHPC). ALA is present in all cells and is the first intermediate of the biochemical pathway resulting in heme synthesis. ALA differs from other drugs in that it is not a preformed photosensitizer but rather a precursor of the endogenously formed photosensitizer protoporphyin IX (Dunn & Lovat, 2008). Advantages of ALA over Ps are the ability to administer it orally; the shorter duration of skin photosensitivity (24-48 hours); and the selective destruction of the mucosa that does not induce development of strictures (Pech et al., 2005). In 2007, 5-ALA was granted drug approval by the Food and Drug Administration for the treatment of patients with Barrett's high-grade dysplasia.

3.2 Clinical applications

Porfimer sodium first received approval in the United States in 1995 for palliation of patients with advanced esophageal carcinoma. This led to a number of studies using Ps-PDT for treatment of dysplastic Barrett's mucosa. Overholt and colleagues reported 100 patients treated with PDT including 73 patients with high-grade dysplasia, 14 patients with low-grade dysplasia, and 13 patients with T1 or T2 adenocarcinoma (Overholt et al., 1999). Patients were followed for a mean of 19 months while on omeprazole. Small residual areas of Barrett's mucosa were treated with Nd: YAG laser. Seventy-three patients received one PDT treatment, twenty-two received two treatments, and five patients received three treatments. The results showed that 92% with low-grade dysplasia, 88% with high-grade dysplasia, and 77% of cancers were eradicated by PDT and focal thermal ablation. In 43% of patients, there was complete elimination of all Barrett's mucosa. The most common complication reported was the development of strictures in 34% of patients.

In another study (Wolfsen et al., 2002), 48 patients (14 patients with T1 cancers and 34 patients with high-grade dysplasia) were treated with only one course of PDT, and any residual Barrett's tissue was subsequently treated with argon plasma coagulation (APC). Complete and successful ablation of all high-grade dysplasia and cancer was achieved in 47 of 48 patients. One patient with persistent cancer underwent curative esophagectomy. Most frequent complications included stricture formation in 11 patients (23%); photosensitivity in 7 patients (15%); and esophageal perforation in 1 patient (2%).

Other studies confirmed the benefits of PDT therapy (Overholt et al., 2003; Wolfsen et al., 2004) which led to the first randomized controlled trial in patients with high-grade dysplasia (Overholt et al., 2005). The study included 30 sites and used a centralized pathology laboratory. A total of 208 patients were entered into the study and randomized in a 2:1 ratio to omeprazole plus PDT (138 patients) versus omeprazole alone (70 patients). Patients could receive up to three courses of PDT. Follow-up consisted of endoscopy and four-quadrant biopsies every 2 cm performed every 3 months until four consecutive quarterly biopsies were negative for high-grade dysplasia, then every 6 months thereafter. The mean follow-up was 24 months. Complete ablation of HGD was achieved in 77% of patients in the omeprazole plus PDT group compared to with 39% in the omeprazole alone group ($p< 0.0001$). Complete eradication of all Barrett's esophagus and dysplasia was seen in 52% of patients in the PDT group compared with 7% in the omeprazole group ($p< 0.0001$). There was also a significant difference in progression to cancer, with 13% of patients in the PDT group developing cancer compared with 28% in the omeprazole group. The most common PDT-related events were photosensitivity reactions (69%), esophageal strictures (36%), vomiting (32%), non-cardiac chest pain (20%), pyrexia (20%), and dysphagia (19%). The results of this study led the Food and Drug Administration to approve the use of PDT with porfimer sodium for the treatment of Barrett's with high-grade dysplasia. A 5-year follow-up of the original study demonstrated the persistent superiority of PDT in eliminating high-grade dysplasia long-term (77% in the treatment group vs. 39% in the omeprazole group). However, only 61 patients of the 102 patients eligible were enrolled in the long-term follow-up phase. Progression to cancer remained significantly lower in the PDT group (15%) compared with 29% in the omeprazole group ($p= .027$). There was also a significantly longer time to progression to cancer favoring PDT ($p= .004$).

Based on these encouraging results, multiple studies evaluated PDT for the treatment of patients with early esophageal cancer who are not candidates for surgical resection. Moghissi and colleagues reported their long-term experience in treating patients with early stage esophageal cancer with PDT (Moghissi et al., 2009). Among 144 patients treated with

PDT, 40 had T1 tumors (35 adenocarcinomas and 5 squamous cell carcinomas). At median follow-up of 76.1 months (range 36-150 months), 3 and 5 years or more survival were 72.5% and 53.8% respectively. In another study, 24 patients with early esophageal cancer were treated with PDT (Maunoury et al., 2005). Seventy-five percent of the patients were treated successfully. At a median follow-up of 21 months, 54% of patients were still alive without recurrence. The authors concluded that PDT should be considered as the treatment of choice in patients with early esophageal cancer who are ineligible for surgical resection.

PDT has also been combined with endoscopic mucosal resection (EMR) for treatment of dysplasia and intramucosal cancers in Barrett's esophagus. In one study (Buttar et al., 2001), 17 patients with either T0 or T1 esophageal adenocarcinoma were treated by EMR followed by PDT therapy. At a median follow-up of 13 months, 16 patients (94%) remained in clinical and histologic remission. Three patients with positive mucosal resection margins remained cancer-free after PDT. In a retrospective study (Prasad et al., 2009) from Mayo Clinic, patients with T1 esophageal adenocarcinoma in Barrett's esophagus were treated either endoscopically (either EMR or EMR followed by PDT therapy) or with esophagectomy. There were 132 patients in the endoscopy-treated group (75 with EMR alone and 57 with EMR plus PDT) and 46 in the surgically treated group. Patients treated by endoscopy were older and had more medical comorbidities than those treated surgically. Remission was successful in 91% of patients treated with EMR plus PDT and in 96% of patients treated with EMR alone. Five-year overall survival was comparable in the endoscopy treated group (83%) and the surgical group (95%). In the endoscopy group, 16 patients had recurrent carcinomas detected during follow-up, and all except one were managed by EMR. The presence of residual dysplastic Barrett's esophagus was a significant factor predicting recurrent carcinoma on univariate analysis.

3.3 Response predictors

There have been a few long-term studies evaluating predictors of response to PDT and risk factors for recurrence of dysplasia. In one retrospective study of 116 patients with Barrett's high-grade dysplasia, and intramucosal adenocarcinoma treated with PDT, pretreatment length of BE was inversely correlated with successful ablation of all Barrett's epithelium. The presence of intramucosal adenocarcinoma or T1 cancer was not associated with higher likelihood of treatment failure (Yachimski et al., 2009). In another study (Badreddine et al., 2010) evaluating 261 patients treated with PDT with and without EMR, significant predictors of recurrence of dysplasia or neoplasia on multivariate analysis were older age, presence of residual nondysplastic Barrett's esophagus, and history of smoking. Biomarkers have been examined as potential predictors of response to PDT. Using fluroscence in situ hybridization, one group found that p16 allelic loss predicted decreased response to PDT (Prasad et al., 2008).

3.4 Complications

The most common side effects reported within hours of PDT include chest pain, nausea, dysphagia and odynophagia. These are commonly treated with analgesics, both topical and systemic. These symptoms usually resolve within 1 to 2 weeks after therapy. Photosensitivity has been reported in as many as 69% of patients treated with PDT. Photosensitivity may last anywhere from 4 to 8 weeks. Patients are also sensitive to strong indoor lighting. Symptoms may range from mild erythema to blistering and even bullae formation. However, by far, the most significant long term toxicity of PDT is stricture formation, reported in up to one third of patients (Overholt et al., 1999, 2005). The underlying mechanism of stricture formation after PDT might be due to deep tissue injury which leads to an aggressive fibrotic response that produces structuring. Risk factors for development of strictures include history of previous esophageal stricture, performance of EMR before PDT, and more than one PDT application in one treatment session (Prasad et al., 2007). Another study identified the following independent predictors of stricture development: longer segment Barrett's, multiple PDT treatments, and evidence of intramucosal carcinoma before PDT (Yachimski et al., 2008). Other less common complications include fever, vomiting, cardiac arrhythmias and development of pleural effusions.

3.5 PDT with 5-ALA

In the only double-blind, randomized placebo-controlled study reported of ALA-PDT, 36 patients with Barrett's esophagus and low-grade dysplasia were randomized to receive oral ALA or placebo (Ackroyd et al., 2000). All patients were treated with green light and maintained on omeprazole. Responses were seen in 89% of patients in the ALA-PDT group, with a median decrease in area in the treated region of 30% (range, 0-60%). In the placebo group, a median area decrease of 0% was seen (range, 0-10%). Furthermore, there was complete eradication of low-grade dysplasia in all 18 patients in the ALA-PDT group, compared with only 6 of 18 (33%) in the placebo group ($p < .001$).

The first long-term study of ALA-PDT in Barrett's esophagus with high-grade dysplasia and T1 adenocarcinoma was reported by Pech and colleagues (Pech et al., 2005). A total of 66 patients (35 with high-grade dysplasia and 31 with intramucosal cancer were treated with ALA-PDT. Median follow-up was 37 months. Complete remission was achieved in 34 (7%) of 35 patients with high-grade dysplasia. Six patients developed a recurrence or a metachronous lesion, but five of these underwent successful repeat treatment. In the intramucosal carcinoma group, complete remission was achieved in all patients but nine patients had recurrence of metachronous carcinoma (29%). Seven patients were successfully treated with ALA-PDT, one went for surgery and one was not a surgical candidate and received palliative treatment 2 years later. The 5-year survival was 97% in the high-grade dysplasia group and 80% in the carcinoma group (Pech et al., 2005).

However, other studies of ALA-PDT have shown somewhat disappointing results (Peters et al., 2005) and high-recurrence rate in patients with early cancer (Pech et al., 2005). This variability in results could be caused by multiple factors including 5-ALA dose; light dose; and type of light used (green vs. red).

In general, 5-ALA has an acceptable safety profile. The most common side effects reported include nausea, vomiting, hoptension and transient photosensitivity and rise in liver enzymes.

3.6 Summary

PDT has been a critically important tool for the advancement of endoscopic therapy for esophageal dysplasia and superficial carcinoma. PDT is an effective method to eradicate high-grade dysplasia and to significantly reduce the risk of progression to cancer in Barrett's esophagus. There are advantages of PDT over other treatment modalities including ease of use, the need for fewer endoscopic sessions; and when compared with surgery, reduced morbidity, mortality and even cost. However, in the era of newer endoscopic ablative methods, PDT faces a number of challenges, such as the well-described complications of prolonged photosensitivity, high rate of stricture formation, and the severe pain and discomfort caused by the photochemical reaction. Therefore, to remain a viable clinical option, PDT candidates should be carefully selected to obtain more uniform results, minimize side effects, and maximize treatment outcomes while reducing complications.

4. Argon plasma coagulation

Argon plasma coagulation (APC) is a noncontact thermal technique using ionized argon gas to deliver a monopolar high-frequency current, which effectively coagulates tissue. APC is applied to tissue until a white coagulum appears, and then the catheter and endoscope are manipulated in a vertical or circumferential linear pattern to coagulate additional tissue. The depth of tissue destruction is thought to be limited due to increased resistance and diminished current flow through coagulated tissue, although perforation has occurred with this technique.

Multiple prospective studies have examined the efficacy and safety of APC for Barrett's ablation. The majority of these studies enrolled patients with Barrett's esophagus without dysplasia, while a few included patients with both low-grade dysplasia and high-grade dysplasia (Attwood et al., 2003; Pereira-Lima, et al., 2000; Ragunath et al., 2005). APC was effective in completely eradicating intestinal metaplasia in 58%- 100% of cases, depending on the series. Recurrence was seen in most studies and was reported in 3%-66% of patients followed. In one trial (Attwood et al., 2003), APC was used in patients with Barrett's esophagus and high-grade dysplasia with a response in 25 of 29 patients (86%).

Serious complications and less severe side effects have been reported. Perforation, often requiring thoracotomy, was reported in 0%-3.6% of cases. Other serious adverse events include stricture formation (0%-15.4%) and major bleeding (0%-3.9%). Chest pain was reported frequently (1.8%-54.5%), and one study reported dysphagia and odynophagia in over half the patients (Pereira-Lima et al., 2000).

Another method of ablation is Multipolar electrocoagulation (MPEC) which requires contact with the mucosa across the electrode contacts at the tip of the catheter. MPEC was evaluated in a prospective multicenter trial of patients with non-dysplastic Barrett's esophagus (Sampliner et al., 2001). Among the 72 patients enrolled, 78% of patients achieved a complete response rate for elimination of Barrett's esophagus. A randomized controlled trial compared APC with MPEC in 52 patients (Dulai et al., 2005). Residual Barrett's esophagus was found in both groups and response rates were similar (MPEC 81% vs. APC 65%, P=0.21).

In summary, most experts do not recommend routine ablation of nondysplastic Barrett's esophagus by APC or other modality at this time. The relatively high incidence of complications, low rate of progression to cancer, and lack of long-term data on the effectiveness of eradication in preventing cancer progression confine ablation of nondysplastic Barrett's esophagus to the research setting in most cases. Ablation of high-grade dysplasia or intramucosal carcinoma in Barrett's esophagus has been studied, but the limited data available in this patient group make it difficult to recommend APC for routine care.

5. Cryotherapy

Cryotherapy is the application of extremely cold temperatures to tissues for medical treatment. Several agents were tried until liquid nitrogen was introduced in 1950 by Allington using a cotton swab applicator for the treatment of skin lesions (Allington, 1950). Cryotherapy destroys biological tissue through a variety of methods. These can be divided into immediate and delayed effects. Rapid freezing causes failure of cellular metabolism due to stress on lipids and proteins. Continued freezing produces extracellular ice, creating a hyperosmotic extracellular environment and drawing fluid from cells. This leads to further damage of cell membrane resulting in cell death.

Cryospray ablation (CSA) uses low-pressure liquid nitrogen spray delivered through a 7-Fr catheter passed through the working channel of a standard upper endoscope. The first report of the CSA device as used in humans related 11 patients with Barrett's esophagus (Johnston et al., 2005). Low-grade dysplasia was present in 5 patients and high-grade dysplasia in 1 patient. In this pilot study, 9 of the 11 patients had complete histologic reversal of Barrett's esophagus, with no dysplasia found at 6-months follow-up. No significant complications occurred and the treatment was well tolerated. In a subsequent pilot study (Dumot et al., 2007) of CSA and endoscopic mucosal resection, 30 high-risk patients were treated with serial cryotherapy sessions every 6 weeks until there was resolution of high-grade dysplasia and intramucosal carcinoma. The overall complete response (CR) of eliminating cancer or downgrading high-grade dysplasia was 73% for high-grade dysplasia and 80% for intramucosal carcinoma.

A retrospective study reported the efficacy of endoscopic spray cryotherapy for esophageal cancer (Greenwald et al., 2010). In this study, there were 79 patients with esophageal carcinoma (60 with T1, 16 with T2, and 3 with T3-T4). Previous treatment including endoscopic resection, photodynamic therapy, esophagectomy, chemotherapy, and radiation therapy failed in 53 subjects (67%). Mean length of follow-up after treatment was 10.6 months overall. Complete response was seen in 31 of 49 (61.2%) patients who finished treatment.

A prospective study evaluated the safety and tolerability of cryotherapy in 77 patients at four academic medical centers in the United States (Greenwald et al., 2008). This group included patients with Barrett's esophagus with high-grade dysplasia, low-grade dysplasia, intramucosal carcinoma and invasive carcinoma. The most common side effects in 323 procedures included chest pain (17.6%), dysphagia (13.3%), odynophagia (12.1%), and sore throat (9.6%). Gastric perforation occurred in one patient with Marfan's syndrome. Three patients developed esophageal strictures.

In conclusion, there is a need for improvement to the current CSA technology. Currently, treatment can be limited by patient tolerance and variables outside of the physician's control. These technological advancements will provide longer spray times applied to thicker lesions, and provide therapeutic effect into deeper tissue levels.

The immune reaction induced by CSA may be the most exciting feature of this therapy. Other heat-based ablation methods such as APC and PDT tend to cause an eschar with denaturated proteins compared to apoptosis induced by CSA, which may lead to immune system stimulation as demonstrated by the inflammatory infiltrate visible on full-thickness histologic specimens.

6. Laser and thermal therapy

Lasers have been studied in Barrett's esophagus and esophageal cancer, including potassium-titanyl-phosphate (KTP), neodymium: yttrium-aluminum-garnet (Nd:YAG), and argon lasers.

KTP laser treatment resulted in complete response in 10 patients with Barrett's esophagus with low-grade dysplasia (4 patients), high-grade dysplasia (4 patients), and intramucosal carcinoma (2 patients) (Gossner et al., 1999). The KTP laser emits a light with 532 nm wavelength that is preferentially absorbed by hemoglobin, making it useful for vascular lesions.

Nd: YAG, emitting light at 1064 nm, provides a deeper penetration as it vaporizes tissue. Nd: YAG laser was used in conjunction with MPEC in six patients with intramucosal carcinoma who were deemed to be high-risk candidates for surgery (Sharma et al., 1999). All patients had a complete initial response and one developed a recurrence at 36 months. In a large prospective randomized trial of 236 patients with advanced esophageal cancer, PDT and Nd: YAG were overall similarly effective in palliation of dysphagia, although PDT has an advantage in upper and mid-thoracic tumors and for long tumors (Lightdale et al., 1995). PDT was associated with fewer side effects (3% vs. 19%) excluding photosensitivity and perforations (1% vs. 7%).

Thermal coagulation with a heat probe was used to treat 13 patients with nondysplastic Barrett's esophagus 2-6 cm long (Michopoulos et al., 1999). Three of the 13 had subsquamous intestinal metaplasia and two had a relapse on follow-up thought to be due to noncompliance with acid suppression medications. One patient developed low-grade dysplasia during surveillance.

7. Radiofrequency ablation

Stepwise circumferential and focal radiofrequency ablation (RFA) using the HALO system is a relatively new endoscopic treatment modality for Barrett's esophagus. Recent studies suggest that this ablation technique is highly effective in removing Barrett's mucosa and associated dysplasia without the aforementioned drawbacks of other ablation techniques (Sharma et al., 2006, 2007, 2008; Fleischer et al., 2008; Shaheen et al., 2008; Gondrie et al., 2008).

7.1 Technique and procedure

The HALO system comprises two distinct ablation systems: the $HALO^{360}$ system for primary circumferential RFA and the $HALO^{90}$ system for secondary focal RFA or primarily as treatment for short-segment Barrett's esophagus. Prior to circumferential RFA, a sizing catheter with a 4-cm long noncompliant balloon at its distal end is used to measure the inner esophageal diameter. Upon activation via a foot switch, the sizing balloon is inflated by the $HALO^{360}$ energy generator, and the mean esophageal inner diameter is automatically calculated for the entire length of the 4-cm long ablation. Focal RFA of Barrett's esophagus may be conducted with the $HALO^{90}$ system, which consists of an endoscope-mounted ablation catheter and an energy generator similar to the $HALO^{360}$ generator, but without the pressure: volume system.

Stepwise circumferential and focal ablation of a Barrett's esophagus generally starts with a circumferential ablation procedure using the $HALO^{360}$ system, which comprises the following steps: recording esophageal landmarks, sizing inner esophageal diameter, selecting the appropriate $HALO^{360}$ ablation catheter, first circumferential ablation pass, cleaning procedure between ablation cycles, and second ablation pass. A minimum of 8 weeks after the first circumferential ablation treatment, patients are rescheduled to undergo a second ablation. Patients with residual circumferential Barrett's esophagus greater than 2 cm in size and/or multiple isles or tongues are treated with a second circumferential ablation. Patients with an irregular Z-line, small tongues, circumferential extent below 2 cm, or diffuse isles are treated with focal ablation using the $HALO^{90}$ system.

Post-treatment care includes proper acid suppressant therapy to minimize patient discomfort and to allow the esophagus to heal optimally and regenerate with squamous epithelium. Patients should be prescribed high-dose proton-pump inhibitors as maintenance medication. Additional H2-receptor antagonists and sucralfate can be prescribed. After RFA, patients are advised to adhere to a liquid diet for 24 hours, then they may gradually expand to a soft and then normal diet. Patients may experience symptoms of chest discomfort, sore throat, difficulty or pain with swallowing, and/or nausea. Proposed analgesic measures are viscous lidocaine, liquid acetaminophen with or without codeine, and antiemetic medication.

Two to three months after the last treatment, the absence of residual Barrett's epithelium is verified by endoscopic inspection. A strict biopsy protocol should be applied with four-quadrant biopsies immediately distal (< 5 mm) to the neosquamocolumnar junction and every 1-2 cm of the neosquamous epithelium. Since no long-term follow-up data after RFA are available thus far, it is recommended to schedule patients for follow-up endoscopy 2 and 6 months after the last treatment and then annually.

7.2 Role of RFA in Barrett's esophagus

Patients with visible abnormalities in a Barrett's esophagus containing intramucosal carcinoma or high-grade dysplasia may be treated with RFA, but only after endoscopic resection of the intramucosal carcinoma or visible lesion. First, endoscopic resection permits optimal histopathological staging of a lesion, enabling patients with intramucosal carcinoma and a low risk of lymph node involvement to be selected for endoscopic treatment (Gondrie et al., 2008; Peters et al., 2008). Second, RFA should be performed on a flat mucosa to ensure that the uniform ablation depth, as uniquely effected by the HALO system, truly reaches as deep as the muscularis mucosae.

Patients with Barrett's esophagus with high-grade dysplasia seem to be ideal candidates for RFA, since eradication of their dysplastic Barrett's esophagus may prevent development of intramucosal carcinoma. Proper selection of these patients is, however, of the utmost importance. Patients should have no visible lesions: these require endoscopic resection for optimal staging and treatment.

Studies in the United States on the use of RFA for low-grade dysplasia have shown an excellent efficacy and safety profile (Sharma et al., 2006, 2008; Shaheen et al., 2008), which has led several centers to accept low-grade dysplasia as an indication for RFA treatment. In Europe, low-grade dysplasia is currently treated by RFA only in clinical trials. These differences are mainly driven by cultural approaches; studies comparing the rate of cancer development in patients treated with RFA and patients undergoing surveillance, as well as future studies on molecular and oncogenic markers that may predict malignant progression, may shed more light on which approach is to be preferred in these patients.

Although RFA seems a very promising ablation modality for Barrett's esophagus, there are still some unclear issues that need to be studied further, especially relating to its long-term efficacy. Since the risk of progression to cancer in patients with nondysplastic Barrett's esophagus is small, RFA is still controversial in such patients. Hopes are set on the future development of biological markers for risk stratification to decide which patients with nondysplastic Barrett's esophagus are at risk of malignant progression and would benefit from RFA.

7.3 Clinical trials

A number of prospective clinical studies were initiated to evaluate the safety and efficacy of RFA in the whole spectrum of Barrett's esophagus patients: nondysplastic Barrett's esophagus (Sharma et al., 2007; Fleischer et al., 2008), low-grade dysplasia (Sharma et al., 2006, 2008; Shaheen et al., 2008), and intramucosal carcinoma (Gondrie et al., 2008; Westerterp et al., 2005).

In the AIM trial reported by Sharma et al., 102 patients with nondysplastic Barrett's esophagus were included and treated with RFA. In the second phase of the trial, complete eradication of intestinal metaplasia at 12 months was achieved in 48 of 70 subjects (70%) using only the $HALO^{360}$ system for circumferential ablation (Sharma et al., 2007). Additional ablation of residual's Barrett's esophagus by the $HALO^{90}$ system resulted in complete clearance of intestinal metaplasia in 97% of patients at 30 months follow-up (Fleischer et al., 2008). None of the patients from the AIM trial presented with esophageal stenosis , and no buried Barrett's glands were found in any of the more than 4000 nonsquamous biopsies obtained during follow-up (Sharma et al., 2007; Fleischer et al., 2008).

In a prospective cohort of 63 patients with low-grade dysplasia (n=39) and high-grade dysplasia (n=24) at the Mayo Clinic with a median follow-up of 24 months, Sharma et al. reported an overall complete response for intestinal metaplasia of 79% and a complete response for dysplasia of 89%. For the low-grade dysplasia cohort, complete response was 87% for intestinal metaplasia and 95% for dysplasia. For the high-grade dysplasia cohort, complete response was 67% for intestinal metaplasia and 79% for dysplasia (Sharma et al., 2006).

For ablation of Barrett's esophagus in patients with low-grade dysplasia and high-grade dysplasia, the strongest evidence that RFA reduces the risk of malignant progression comes from the randomized controlled trial by Shaheen et al. (Shaheen et al., 2009) that was conducted in 19 centers in the United States. A total of 127 patients with dysplastic Barrett's esophagus were randomized to RFA or sham (2:1). In the intention-to-treat analyses, among patients with low-grade dysplasia, complete eradication of dysplasia occurred in 90.5% of those in the ablation group, as compared with 22.7% of those in the control group (P<0.001). Among patients with high-grade dysplasia, complete eradication occurred in 81.0% of those in the ablation group, as compared with 19.0% of those in the control group (P<0.001). Overall, 77.4% of patients in the ablation group had complete eradication of intestinal metaplasia as compared with 2.3% of those in the control group (P<0.001). Patients in the ablation group had less disease progression (3.6% vs. 16.3%, P=0.03) and fewer cancers (1.2% vs. 9.3%, P=0.045). Patients reported having more chest pain after the ablation procedure than after the sham procedure. In the ablation group, one patient had upper gastrointestinal hemorrhage, and five patients (6.0%) had esophageal stricture.

Gondrie et al. reported on a total of 23 patients with high-grade dysplasia and/or intramucosal carcinoma, of whom 13 underwent endoscopic resection of visible lesions prior to RFA (Gondrie et al., 2008). After a median of 1.5 circumferential and 2.6 focal ablation sessions, complete eradication of all dysplasia and intestinal metaplasia was achieved in all patients (100%). There were no adverse events. An important observation from the studies by Gondrie et al. is the possibility of resecting areas of Barrett's mucosa that persist after multiple RFA sessions. This may be a significant advantage compared to other endoscopic ablation techniques that typically result in submucosal scarring, which makes escape treatment with endoscopic resection complicated. Compared to the 0%-56% stricture rate associated with other endoscopic ablation techniques (Overholt et al., 2003; Peters et al., 2005; Hage et al., 2004; Schulz et al., 2000; Van Laethem et al., 2001), the minimal rate of esophageal stenosis reported in the trials discussed above is encouraging. In addition, RFA does not impair the functional integrity of the esophagus (Beaumont et al., 2007). It has been shown that stepwise circumferential and focal ablation of Barrett's esophagus with high-grade dysplasia results in restoration of normal-appearing neosquamous mucosa without any of the oncogenetic abnormalities present before treatment (Gondrie et al., 2007). These important findings were confirmed in another study suggesting that the neosquamous tissue holds no residual malignant potential (Finkelstein & Lyday, 2008).

7.4 Summary

Current data suggest that RFA is an encouraging modality for eradication of Barrett's esophagus, with many appealing aspects. RFA has been proven to be highly effective in eradicating intestinal metaplasia and its associated dysplasia; it has a low complication rate, preserves the functional integrity of the esophagus, and is relatively easy to apply; and the regenerating neosquamous epithelium is free of the pre-existing oncogenetic alterations. There are, however, still some unanswered questions concerning the optimal use of the HALO^{90} catheter, the optimal combination of endoscopic resection with RFA, the presence of buried Barrett's glands following RFA, and whether the effect is maintained on the long run. For patients with intramucosal carcinoma and high-grade dysplasia, RFA appears to be a valid and less invasive alternative to PDT, APC or esophagectomy, albeit after endoscopic resection of intamucosal carcinoma and visible lesions. For patients with low-grade dysplasia or nondysplastic Barrett's esophagus, RFA treatment is more debatable but justified in some selected patients. Further clinical studies, data from long-term follow-up after RFA, and development of biological markers to predict malignant progression of intestinal metaplasia will elucidate the question of which patients should be treated with RFA for eradication of Barrett's esophagus.

8. Primary nonsurgical therapy

There is considerable controversy as to the ideal therapeutic approach for esophageal cancer. Definitive therapy for esophageal cancer is either surgical or nonsurgical. Although the overall results of these two approaches are similar, the patient population selected for treatment with each modality is usually different. For multiple reasons, this results in a selection bias against the nonsurgical group. First, patients with unfavorable prognostic features are more likely selected for treatment with nonsurgical therapy. These features include medical contraindications and primary unresectable or metastatic disease. Second, surgical series report results based on pathologically determined stage, whereas nonsurgical series report results based on clinically determined stage. Pathologic staging has the advantage of excluding some patients with metastatic disease not identified during clinical staging. Third, patients treated without surgery are approached in a palliative rather than a curative fashion. Therefore, the intensity of chemotherapy and the doses of radiation therapy might be suboptimal.

In staging esophageal cancer preoperatively not only CT and EUS are used, but the efficacy of FDG-PET must be emphasized. Studies have examined the effectiveness of PET in the staging of esophageal cancer. After standard staging for esophageal cancer (including CT and endoscopy), undetected metastatic disease was identified by PET in 15% of patients in the series by Flamen et al (Flamen et al., 2002) and in 20% of patients in the series by Downey and associates (Downey et al., 2003). Therefore, PET's use is highly encouraged for all patients who are selected for a nonoperative approach.

8.1 Radiation therapy

The 1992–1994 Patterns of Care study examined 400 patients treated at 61 academic and nonacademic radiation oncology practices to determine practice patterns in the United States (Coia et al., 2000). During that period, treatment approaches included primary chemoradiation, 54%; radiation alone, 20%; preoperative chemoradiation, 13%; postoperative combined modality therapy, 8%; postoperative radiation, 4%; and preoperative radiation, 1%. In another study, Patterns of Care analysis from 1996 to 1999, 414 patients who received radiation therapy as part of definitive or adjuvant management at 59 institutions were surveyed (Suntharalingam et al., 2003). Compared with the 1992–1994 survey, more patients underwent EUS staging (18% vs. 2%; $P < .0001$) and more patients received preoperative chemoradiation (27% vs. 10%; $P = .007$); preoperative chemoradiation was used more frequently in the subset of patients with adenocarcinoma (46% vs. 19%; $P = .0002$), and the use of paclitaxel-based chemotherapy increased (22% vs. 0.2%; $P = .001$). Brachytherapy was used in 6% of patients. In a similar patterns of care study of 767 patients treated in Japan from 1998 to 2001, 220 (28%) received preoperative or postoperative radiation or both, with or without chemotherapy (Gomi et al., 2003).

The effect of histologic type (adenocarcinoma vs. squamous cell carcinoma) is unclear. At present, the data is conflicting, with some series reporting different results by histologic type but other series reporting no difference. Fortunately, the current Intergroup randomized trials stratify patients by histologic type. Until these data are available and more mature, the impact of histologic type cannot be adequately assessed, and it is reasonable to treat both types of lesions in a similar fashion.

8.1.1 Radiation therapy alone

Multiple series have reported the results of external-beam radiation therapy alone for patients with esophageal cancer. Most include patients with unfavorable features such as clinical T4 disease and multiple positive lymph nodes. For instance, in the series of De-Ren, 184 of the 678 patients had stage IV disease (De-Ren, 1989). Overall, the 5-year survival rate for patients treated with conventional doses of radiation therapy alone is 0% to 10% (De-Ren, 1989; Newaishy et al., 1982; Okawa et al., 1989). The use of radiation therapy as a potentially curative modality requires doses of at least 50 Gy at 1.8 to 2.0 Gy/fraction. Shi and colleagues reported a 33% 5-year survival rate with the use of late-course accelerated fractionation to a total dose of 68.4 Gy (Shi et al., 1999). However, in the radiation-therapy-alone arm of the RTOG 85-01 trial in which patients received 64 Gy at 2 Gy/d with modern techniques, all patients were dead of their disease by 3 years (Herskovic et al., 1992; Al-Sarraf et al., 1997).

There is limited experience in the use of radiation therapy alone for patients with superficial (Seki et al., 2001) or clinically determined T1 disease (Nemoto et al., 2002). The trial by Sykes et al. was limited to 101 patients (90% with squamous cell carcinoma) with tumors smaller than 5 cm who received 45 to 52.5 Gy in 15 to 16 fractions. The 5-year survival was 20% (Sykes et al., 1998). Overall, these data indicate that radiation therapy alone should be reserved for palliation or for patients who are medically unable to receive concurrent chemoradiotherapy. The results of definitive chemoradiation are more favorable, and it remains the standard of care.

8.1.2 Radiation therapy techniques

Radiation field design for esophageal cancer requires careful techniques in order to achieve optimal results (Phillips et al., 1998). There are a number of sensitive organs that, depending on the location of the primary tumor, may be in the radiation field. These include skin, spinal cord, lung, heart, intestine, stomach, kidney, and liver. Minimizing the dose to these vital structures while delivering an adequate dose to the primary tumor and local-regional lymph nodes requires patient immobilization and CT-based treatment planning for organ identification, lung correction, and development of dose-volume histograms. Although CT can accurately identify adjacent organs and structures, it may be limited in defining the extent of the primary tumor. Among radiation oncologists, there is significant inconsistency in defining the planning target volume, both in the transverse and longitudinal dimensions. Therefore, in addition to a CT scan, it is always helpful to obtain a barium swallow test at the time of radiation therapy simulation. The integration of other imaging modalities such as EUS, PET, and magnetic resonance imaging into radiation treatment planning remains under investigation.

In one study reported by Tai et al., 12 Canadian radiation oncologists drew cervical esophagus target volumes based on the RTOG 94-05 protocol design both before and after a one-on-one training session (Tai et al., 2002). Pretraining and posttraining survey revealed less variability in the longitudinal positions of the target volumes after training, which illustrates the importance of specialized training. In another study, Nutting et al. compared two-phase conformal radiotherapy with intensity-modulated radiotherapy (IMRT) in five patients who received 55 Gy of radiation plus concurrent chemotherapy (Nutting et al., 2001). Treatment plans using both techniques were carried out and were compared using dose-volume histograms and normal tissue complication probabilities. The IMRT using nine equispaced fields did not add any improvement over conformal radiation because the larger number of fields in the IMRT plan distributed a low dose over the entire lung. In contrast, IMRT using four fields equal to the conformal fields offered an improvement in lung sparing.

In the treatment of esophageal cancer, radiation oncologists usually treat tumors at or above the carina as a cervical primary and the supraclavicular nodes are included in the radiation field. Tumors below the carina but not extending to the gastroesophageal junction are considered mid-esophageal, and the radiation field does not include the supraclavicular or celiac nodes. Tumors that involve the gastroesophageal junction are considered distal and the celiac nodes are included. This simple and practical definition is helpful in designing radiation therapy fields.

The standard radiation dose for patients selected for curative nonoperative chemoradiation is 50.4 Gy at 1.8 Gy/fraction. The radiation field should include the primary tumor with 5-cm superior and inferior margins and 2-cm lateral margins. The primary local-regional lymph nodes should receive the same dose.

For cervical esophageal tumors, patients are placed supine. Field designs include a three-field plan (two anterior oblique fields and a posterior field) or, more commonly, anteroposterior-posteroanterior to 39.6 to 41.4 cGy followed by a left or right opposed oblique pair with photons plus an electron boost to the contralateral supraclavicular area, both to a total dose of 50.4 Gy. For mid-esophageal tumors, patients are placed prone to help exclude the spinal cord from the radiation field and a four-field design is used (anteroposterior, posteroanterior, and opposed lateral fields). For distal tumors, patients are treated supine using the same four-field technique. Caution should be taken to exclude as much of the normal stomach as possible, especially if the patient is receiving radiation preoperatively. CT-based three-dimensional treatment planning should be performed, and all fields should be treated each day. Dose-volume histograms help guide the radiation oncologist in choosing a radiation plan that minimizes the loss of normal organ function.

In the palliative setting there are a variety of radiation treatment regimens. Because the goal is rapid palliation of symptoms, the most common approach is to treat anteroposteriorly and posteroanteriorly, including the primary tumor with 2-cm margins, in ten 3-Gy fractions to a total dose of 30 Gy.

The most critical normal structures that lie in proximity to the esophagus are the spinal cord, heart, lungs, and kidneys. When radiation is combined with chemotherapy, the radiation fractionation should be 1.8 Gy/d. The spinal cord dose should not exceed 45 Gy. All fields should be treated each day. Doses to the heart, lungs, and kidneys depend to a large extent on the volume of these organs in the treatment field. Dose-volume histograms are the most effective way to modify treatment techniques to decrease the acute and long-term radiation-related toxicity. In the rare situations when whole heart irradiation is needed, the dose should be limited to 25 to 30 Gy. In the thorax, radiation fields frequently include substantial volumes of lung, especially with oblique or lateral fields. Decreased pulmonary function occurs after irradiation, particularly if large volumes of lung are exposed to doses greater than 20 Gy. There is progressive decreased ventilatory and diffusing capacity as a result of endothelial degeneration and interstitial fibrosis. Fields that include such substantial volumes of lung should be limited to 20 Gy. Except for the spinal cord, it is acceptable for small volumes of normal tissue in immediate proximity to the esophagus to receive doses as high as 60 Gy. However, because the standard total dose of radiation is 50.4 Gy, this degree of inhomogeneity should be uncommon. Fortunately, even with tumors as distal as the gastroesophageal junction, there is a limited amount of liver and kidney in the treatment fields.

8.2 Combined chemoradiation

There are multiple single-arm, nonrandomized trials of chemoradiation alone and they have included patients with disease at different stages (Seitz et al., 1990; Izquiredo et al., 1993; Coia et al., 1991;Valerdi et al., 1994; Poplin et al., 1996). Few series examined patients with T1 or T2 disease (Seki et al., 2001; Coia et al., 1991; Nemoto et al., 2001). In the series reported by Coia and associates, patients received 60 Gy of radiation therapy concurrently with intravenous 5-FU and mitomycin C (Coia et al., 1991). For stage I and II disease, the local failure rate was 25%, the 5-year actuarial local relapse-free survival and overall survival were 70% and 30% respectively.

Thirteen randomized trials compared radiation therapy alone with chemoradiation. Major trials are summarized in Table 1.

In a pooled analysis of these trials (Wong & Malthaner 2006, 2010), concomitant chemoradiotherapy provided significant overall reduction in mortality at 1 and 2 years. The mortality in the control arms was 62% and 83% respectively. Combined chemoradiotherapy provided an absolute reduction of mortality by 7% and 7% respectively. In addition, there was a reduction in the overall local recurrence rate. The local recurrence rate for the control arms was in the order of 68%. Combined chemoradiothrapy provided an absolute reduction of local recurrence rate of 12%. However, chemoradiation was associated with a significant increase in adverse effects, including life-threatening toxicities.

In the ECOG EST-1282 trial (Araujo et al., 1991),patients who received combined modality therapy had a significantly increased median survival compared with those receiving radiation alone (15 months vs. 9 months; $P = .04$) but experienced no improvement in 5-year survival (9% vs. 7%). However, this was not a pure nonsurgical trial because approximately 50% of patients in each arm underwent surgery after receiving 40 Gy of radiation. The operative mortality was 17%.

Series	Patients (n)	Overall Survival (%)	Median Survival (months)	Local Failure (%)
Herskovic et al. (RTOG) (Herskovic et al., 1992; Al-Sarraf et al., 1997; Cooper et al., 1999)				
Radiation alone	62	0 at 5-yr	9	68
Combined therapy	61	27 at 5-yr 22 at 8-yr	14	47
Combined therapy	69	NR	17	52
Araujo et al. (NCI Brazil) (Araujo et al., 1991)				
Radiation alone	31	6 at 5-yr		84
Combined therapy	28	16		61
Roussel et al. (EORTC) (Roussel et al., 1988)				
Radiation alone	69	6 at 3-yr		
Combined therapy	75	12		
Nygaard et al. (Scandinavia) (Nygaard et al., 1992)				
Radiation alone	51	6 at 3-yr		
Combined therapy	46	0		
Smith et al. (ECOG-EST 1282) (Smith et al., 1998)				
Radiation alone	60	7 at 5-yr	9	
Combined therapy	59	9	15	
Slabber et al. (Pretoria) (Slabber et al., 1998)				
Radiation alone	36		5	
Combined therapy	34		6	

Table 1. **Randomized Trials of Radiation Therapy versus Combined Modality Therapy for Esophageal Cancer.**

The trial that was designed to deliver adequate doses of systemic chemotherapy with concurrent radiation therapy was the RTOG 85-01 trial reported by Herskovic et al. (Herskovic et al., 1992; Al-Sarraf et al., 1997; Cooper et al., 1999). This Intergroup trial primarily included patients with squamous cell carcinoma. Patients received four cycles of 5-FU (1000 mg/m^2/24 h x 4 days) and cisplatin (75 mg/m^2 on day 1). Radiation therapy (50 Gy at 2 Gy/d) was given concurrently with day 1 of chemotherapy. After radiation therapy is finished, cycles 3 and 4 of chemotherapy were delivered every 3 weeks (weeks 8 and 11) rather than every 4 weeks (weeks 9 and 13). This intensification may explain, in part, why only 50% of the patients finished all four cycles of the chemotherapy. The control arm was given radiation therapy alone, albeit at a higher dose (64 Gy) than the chemoradiation arm. Patients who received chemoradiation had a significant improvement in median survival (14 months vs. 9 months) and 5-year survival (27% vs. 0%; *P* <.0001) (81). There was a clear plateau in the survival curve. Minimum follow-up was 5 years, and the 8-year survival was 22% (Cooper et al., 1999). Histologic type did not significantly influence the results: 21% of patients with squamous cell carcinomas (n = 107) were alive at 5 years compared with 13% of patients with adenocarcinoma (n = 23) (*P* was not significant). Although African Americans had larger primary tumors and all were squamous cell cancers, there was no difference in their survival compared with whites (Streeter et al., 1999). The incidence of local failure as the first site of failure (defined as local persistence or recurrence) was also decreased in the combined modality arm (47% vs. 65%). The protocol was closed early due to the positive results; however, after this early closure, an additional 69 eligible patients were treated with the same chemoradiation regimen. In this nonrandomized combined modality group, the 5-year survival was 14% and local failure was 52%.

Chemoradiation not only improves the results compared with radiation alone but also is associated with a higher incidence of toxicity. In the 1997 report of the RTOG 85-01 trial, patients who received chemoradiation had a higher incidence of acute grade 3 toxicity (44% vs. 25%) and acute grade 4 toxicity (20% vs. 3%) compared with those who received radiation therapy alone. Including the one treatment-related death (2%), the incidence of total acute grade 3+ toxicity was 66% (81). The 1999 report examined late toxicity. The incidence of late grade 3+ toxicity was similar in the combined modality arm and in the radiation-alone arm (29% vs. 23%) (94). However, grade 4+ toxicity remained higher in the combined modality arm (10% vs. 2%). Interestingly, the nonrandomized chemoradiation group experienced a similar incidence of late grade 3+ toxicity (28%) but a lower incidence of grade 4 toxicity (4%), and there were no treatment-related deaths.

Based on the positive results from the RTOG 85-01 trial, the standard nonsurgical treatment for esophageal carcinoma became chemoradiation. However, the local failure rate in the RTOG 85-01 chemoradiation arm was still high at 45%, and there is room for improvement. Therefore, new approaches such as intensification of chemoradiation and escalation of the radiation dose have been developed in an attempt to help improve these results.

8.3 Comparison of definitive chemoradiation and surgery

There are a number of trials comparing preoperative chemoradiation with surgery alone. However, there is limited data regarding the direct comparison of the two standard treatments for nonmetastatic esophageal cancer: concurrent chemoradiation and surgery alone. The positive results of RTOG 85-01, demonstrating a 27% 5-year survival rate for patients treated with definitive chemoradiation compared with no 5-year survival after treatment with radiotherapy alone, is a major advance. This treatment option has influenced the selection of patients for nonsurgical management because it provides an acceptable alternative for restoring swallowing function in patients with locally advanced disease for whom surgery would be mainly palliative.

For patients with earlier-stage disease that appears resectable, definitive chemoradiation may also be appropriate treatment; however, prospective randomized trials comparing this approach with surgery, stratified by stage, have yet to be performed. Nonetheless, some series suggest that the nonsurgical approach offers a survival rate that is the same or better than that achievable with surgery alone. For example, the median survival time and 5-year survival rate were 14 months and 27%, respectively, in the chemoradiation arm of RTOG 85-01 and 20 months and 20%, respectively, in INT 0122 (Minsky et al., 1999). In comparison, the median survival in the surgical control arm of the Dutch trial reported by Kok et al (Kok et al., 1997) was 11 months, and the median survival time and 5-year survival rate in the surgical control arm of INT 0113 were 16 months and 20%, respectively. Likewise, the local failure rates were similar. The incidence of local failure as the first site of failure was 45% in RTOG 85-01 and 39% in INT 0122. Although local failure as the first site of failure was 31% in INT 0113, this analysis was limited to patients who underwent a complete resection with negative margins (R0 resection). Because an additional 30% of patients had residual local disease, if one were to score these patients also as having locally persistent disease (as was done in the RTOG 85-01 analysis), the comparable local failure rate with surgery alone would be 30% + 31% = 61%. The treatment-related mortality rates were also similar (2% in RTOG 85-01, 9% in INT 0122, and 6% in INT 0113).

Chiu et al. (Chiu et al., 2005) conducted a prospective randomized trial that compared the efficacy and survival outcome of chemoradiation with that of esophagectomy as a curative treatment. In this multicenter trial, 80 patients with potentially resectable squamous cell carcinoma of the mid or lower thoracic esophagus were randomized to esophagectomy or chemoradiotherapy. Patients treated with chemoradiotherapy received continuous 5-fluorouracil infusion (200 mg/m2/day) from day 1 to 42 and cisplatin (60 mg/m2) on days 1 and 22. The tumor and regional lymphatics were concomitantly irradiated to a total of 50–60 Gy. Salvage esophagectomy was performed for incomplete response or recurrence. Forty-four patients received standard esophagectomy, whereas 36 were treated with chemoradiotherapy. Median follow-up was 6.9 months. There was no difference in either survival or disease-free survival between the two groups. Patients treated with surgery had a slightly higher proportion of recurrence in the mediastinum, whereas those treated with chemoradiation sustained a higher proportion of recurrence in the cervical or abdominal regions.

In summary, the local failure, survival, and treatment-related mortality rates for nonsurgical and surgical therapies are similar. Although the results are comparable, it is clear that both the nonsurgical and surgical approaches have limited success.

8.4 Necessity for surgery after chemoradiation

Two trials examined whether surgery is necessary after chemoradiation. The Federation Francaise de Cancerologie Digestive (FFCD) trial addresses the issue of whether patients who respond midway through chemoradiation should continue with the treatment or undergo surgery (Bedenne et al., 2007). The German Oesophageal Cancer Study Group examined the question of whether chemoradiation followed by surgery is equivalent to nonoperative chemoradiation (Stahl et al., 2005).

In the FFCD 9102 trial, all 445 patients with clinically resectable T3 to 4 N0 to 1 M0 squamous cell carcinoma or adenocarcinoma of the esophagus received chemoradiation; however, the randomization was limited to patients who responded to initial chemoradiation. Patients initially received two cycles of 5-FU and cisplatin plus concurrent radiation (either 46 Gy at 2 Gy/d or a split-course regimen of 15 Gy in weeks 1 and 3) (Bedenne et al., 2007). The 259 patients who had at least a partial response were then randomly assigned to receive surgery or additional chemoradiation, which included three cycles of 5-FU and cisplatin, plus concurrent radiation (either 20 Gy at 2 Gy/d or split-course 15 Gy). There was no significant difference in 2-year survival (34% for those undergoing surgery vs. 40% for those receiving chemoradiation; P = .56) or median survival (18 months for the surgery group vs. 19 months for the chemoradiation group). Two-year local control rate was 66.4% in arm A compared with 57.0% in arm B, and stents were less required in the surgery arm (5% in arm A v 32% in arm B; P < .001). The 3-month mortality rate was 9.3% in arm A compared with 0.8% in arm B (P = .002). Cumulative hospital stay was 68 days in arm A compared with 52 days in arm B (P = .02). The data suggest that patients who initially respond to nonoperative chemoradiation should complete chemoradiation rather than stop and undergo surgery. As measured using the Spitzer index, there was no difference in global quality of life; however, a significantly greater decrease in quality of life was observed in the postoperative period in the surgery arm (7.52 vs. 8.45; P <.01) (Bonnetain et al., 2006).

The German Oesophageal Cancer Study Group compared preoperative chemoradiation followed by surgery with chemoradiation alone (Stahl et al., 2005). In this trial, 177 patients with uT3–4N0–1M0 squamous cell cancers of the esophagus were randomly assigned to receive preoperative therapy (three cycles of 5-FU, leucovorin, etoposide, and cisplatin, followed by concurrent etoposide and cisplatin, plus 40 Gy of radiation) followed by surgery or chemoradiation alone (the same chemotherapy regimen, but the radiation dose was increased to 60 Gy). Despite an improvement in 2-year progression free survival for those who were randomly assigned to receive preoperative therapy followed by surgery compared with those receiving chemoradiation alone (64% vs.41%), there was no significant difference in overall survival.. The results of this trial were updated at ASCO in 2008 which showed no significant improvement in 5-year survival between the two arms but persistent benefit of local control with the surgery arm. Although the difference in the radiation dose in the two arms makes the interpretation of the data difficult, there does not appear to be a benefit to surgery after nonoperative chemoradiation.

8.5 Tumor markers and predictors of response to chemoradiation

It would be important to predict which tumors have a higher likelihood of responding to radiation or chemoradiation. In 38 patients with squamous cell carcinoma who received chemoradiation with or without surgery, tumors without p53 expression and tumors with weak Bcl-X $_L$ expression showed a higher response to chemotherapy (56% and 53%, respectively) than tumors positive for p53 or with strong Bcl-X $_L$ expression (30% and 32%, respectively; P not significant) (Sarbia et al., 1998). After preoperative chemoradiation, patients with p53-negative tumors had a significantly better mean survival than those with p53-positive tumors (31 months vs. 11 months; P = .0378). By multivariate analysis, Pomp et al. found that overexpression of p53 resulted in a decrease in survival in 69 patients with squamous cell carcinoma or adenocarcinoma treated with radiation alone (Pomp et al., 1998). In one study, there was a correlation between decreasing levels of four phospholipids and increasing T stage and grade (Merchant et al., 1999).

Kishi and associates reported that, of 77 patients treated with chemoradiation for squamous cell cancer, those with p53- and metallothionein-positive tumors had a poor response to treatment, whereas strong expression of CDC25B was associated with a good response (Kishi et al., 2002). In 73 patients with T2 to 4 M0 esophageal cancer treated with 60 Gy of radiation plus 5-FU and cisplatin, Hironaka et al. examined pretreatment biopsy specimens for a variety of markers, including p53, Ki-67, EGF receptor, cyclin D1, vascular endothelial growth factor, microvessel density (MVD), thymidylate synthase, dihydropyrimidine dehydrogenase, and glutathione S-transferase (Hironaka et al., 2002). By multivariate analysis MVD, T stage, and performance status were independent prognostic variables (P = .002, .02, and .02, respectively). Patients with high-MVD tumors had a better 3-year survival rate than those with low-MVD tumors (61% vs. 33%; P = .02). Morita et al. found that patients with lymphocyte infiltration around the tumor had a 5-year survival rate of 46% to 76% compared with 28% (P <.05) in patients whose tumors did not have lymphocytic infiltration (Morita et al., 2001). With the further discovery and understanding of various tumor suppressor genes, these data may be used to help select patients for chemoradiation.

8.6 Intensification of chemoradiation

The phase II Intergroup trial 0122 [ECOG PE289/RTOG 90-12] was designed to intensify treatment in the RTOG 85-01 combined modality arm (102). Both the chemotherapy and radiation therapy in INT 0122 were intensified as follows: (1) the 5-FU continuous infusion (1000 mg/m^2/24 hours) was increased from 4 days to 5 days, (2) the total number of cycles of chemotherapy was increased from four to five cycles, (3) three cycles of full-dose neoadjuvant 5-FU and cisplatin were delivered before the start of chemoradiation, and (4) the radiation dose was increased from 50 Gy to 64.8 Gy. In this study, 38 patients with squamous cell carcnoma were eligible. The primary tumor response rate was as follows: 47% complete response, 8% partial response, and 3% stable disease (Kelsen et al., 1990). The first site of clinical treatment failure was local in 39% and distant in 24%. In the total patient group, there were six deaths during treatment, four of which were treatment related (9% of 45 patients). The median survival time was 20 months and the 5-year actuarial survival rate was 20%. Unfortunately, this intensive neoadjuvant approach did not appear to offer a benefit compared with conventional doses and techniques of chemoradiation. Similar toxicities were reported by Ishikura et al. for 139 patients with squamous cell cancers treated with 5-FU, cisplatin, and 60 Gy of radiation (Ishikura et al., 2003).

A limited number of phase I and II trials have tested the use of neoadjuvant chemotherapy before radiation therapy or chemoradiation. Valerdi et al. reported the results for 40 patients with clinical stage II and III squamous cell cancers who received two cycles of neoadjuvant cisplatin, vindesine, and bleomycin (days 1 and 29) followed by 60 Gy of radiation (Valerdi et al., 1994). In contrast with the INT 0122 trial, no chemotherapy was delivered with the radiation therapy. The pathologically determined complete response rate was 53%. After a median follow-up of 78 months, the local failure rate was 62%, the median survival time was 11 months, and the 5-year actuarial survival rate was 15%. These results are similar to those obtained for the RTOG 85-01 combined modality arm with the exception of the higher treatment-related death rate of 5%.

Using a five-drug neoadjuvant regimen, Roca and colleagues treated 55 patients (54 with squamous cell cancer) with bolus cisplatin, 5-FU, leucovorin, bleomycin, and mitomycin C for 15 days followed by 60 Gy of radiation plus concurrent chemotherapy with 5-FU, leucovorin, and cisplatin (Roca et al., 1996). No maintenance chemotherapy was delivered. Patients with lesions at all anatomic sites within the esophagus were eligible and 53% had clinical stage III disease. Although the treatment-related mortality was only 4% and the 3-year survival was 35%, local failure as a component of failure was 42%, which was similar to the 45% rate reported in the RTOG 85-01 chemoradiation arm.

Recent trials using newer regimens for neoadjuvant chemotherapy such as paclitaxel and cisplatin (Bains et al., 2002) or CPT-11 and cisplatin (Ilson et al., 2003) before the start of chemoradiation have reported more favorable results. Bains and associates reported that, of 38 patients who presented with dysphagia, 92% had relief after the completion of two cycles (weeks 1 and 4) of neoadjuvant paclitaxel (175 mg/m^2, 3-hour infusion) and cisplatin (75-mg/m^2 bolus) (Bains et al., 2002). Similar results have been reported by Ilson et al. for 19 patients who received two cycles of neoadjuvant CPT-11 (65 mg/m^2) plus cisplatin (30 mg/m^2) weeks 1, 2, 4, and 5 before the start of chemoradiation (Ilson et al., 2003). Treatment was well tolerated with no grade 3+ nonhematologic toxicity, and only 5% of patients required a feeding tube. Of the 16 patients who presented with dysphagia, 81% had dysphagia relief after the completion of neoadjuvant chemotherapy.

Another potential advantage of neoadjuvant chemotherapy is the early identification of those patients who may or may not respond to the chemotherapeutic regimen being delivered. Ott et al. performed FDG-PET in 35 patients with adenocarcinoma of the gastroesophageal junction or stomach 2 weeks after the start of cisplatin, 5-FU, and leucovorin neoadjuvant chemotherapy, which was followed by surgery; results of the FDG-PET scan were able to predict which patients showed a response to the full course of chemotherapy, as judged from the surgical specimens (Ott et al., 2003). Although this study was investigational, if the nonresponders can be identified early, changing the chemotherapeutic regimen may be helpful.

In summary, although the early trials primarily using neoadjuvant regimens based on 5-FU and cisplatin did not suggest a benefit, more recent trials using paclitaxel- and CPT-11–based regimens reveal higher response rates resulting in improvement of dysphagia.

8.7 Intensification of the radiation dose

Another approach to the dose intensification of chemoradiation is increasing the radiation dose above 50.4 Gy. There are two methods by which to increase the radiation dose to the esophagus: brachytherapy and external-beam radiation therapy.

8.7.1 Brachytherapy

Intraluminal brachytherapy allows the escalation of the dose to the primary tumor while protecting the surrounding structures such as the lung, heart, and spinal cord (Armstrong, 1993). A radioactive source is placed intraluminally via bronchoscopy or a nasogastric tube. Brachytherapy has been used both as primary therapy (usually as a palliative modality)(Moni et al., 1996; Sur et al., 1992, 1998; Jager et al., 1995; Maingon et al., 2000) and as boost after external-beam radiation therapy or combined modality therapy (Armstrong, 1993; Calais et al., 1997; Akagi et al., 1999; Schraube et al., 1997; Okawa et al., 1999). It can be delivered either by high dose rate or low dose rate (Caspers et al., 1993). Although there are technical and radiobiologic differences between the two dose rates, there are no clear therapeutic advantages for either.

Studies that combine brachytherapy with external-beam radiation therapy or chemoradiation report results similar to those for conventional chemoradiation. Calais et al. reported a local failure rate of 43% and a 5-year survival of 18% (Calais et al., 1997). Even for a more favorable subset of patients with clinical T1 to T2 disease, Yorozu et al. reported a local failure rate of 44% and a 5-year survival of 26% (Yorozu et al., 1999).

In the RTOG 92-07 trial, 75 patients with squamous cell cancers (92%) or adenocarcinomas (8%) of the esophagus received the RTOG 85-01 combined modality regimen (5-FU, cisplatin, 50 Gy of radiation) followed by a boost during cycle 3 of chemotherapy with either low dose-rate or high dose-rate intraluminal brachytherapy (Gaspar et al., 1997). Due to low accrual rate, the low dose-rate option was discontinued and the analysis was limited to patients who received the high dose-rate treatment. High dose-rate brachytherapy was delivered in weekly fractions of 5 Gy during weeks 8, 9, and 10. Due to the development of several fistulas, the fraction delivered at week 10 was discontinued. Although the complete response rate was 73%, at a median follow-up of only 11 months, rate of local failure as the first site of failure was 27%. Rates of acute toxicity were 58% for grade 3, 26% for grade 4, and 8% for grade 5 (treatment-related death). The cumulative incidence of fistula was 18% per year and the crude incidence was 14%. Of the six treatment-related fistulas, three were fatal. Given the significant toxicity, this treatment approach should be used with caution.

The American Brachytherapy Society has developed guidelines for esophageal brachytherapy (Gaspar et al., 1997). Its recommendations include the following. For patients treated in the curative setting brachytherapy should be limited to tumors 10 cm or less with no evidence of distant metastasis. Contraindications include tracheal or bronchial involvement, cervical esophagus location, or stenosis that cannot be bypassed. The applicator should have an external diameter of 6 to 10 cm. If combined modality therapy is used (defined as 5-FU–based chemotherapy plus 45 to 50 Gy of radiation) the recommended doses of brachytherapy are 10 Gy in two weekly fractions of 5 Gy each for high dose rate and 20 Gy in a single fraction at 4 to 10 Gy/h for low dose rate. The doses should be prescribed to 1 cm from the source. Finally, brachytherapy should be delivered after the completion of external-beam radiation therapy and not concurrently with chemotherapy.

In summary, for patients treated in the curative setting, the addition of brachytherapy does not appear to improve the results compared with those for radiation therapy or combined modality therapy alone. Therefore, although it seems reasonable to assume that adding intraluminal brachytherapy to radiation or combined modality therapy would provide an additional benefit, whether such a benefit exists remains unclear.

8.7.2 External-beam therapy

There are a limited number of phase II trials examining patient tolerance for external-beam radiation doses of 60 Gy or more when delivered concurrently with chemotherapy. In an analysis performed by Coia and associates, the results for 90 patients with clinical stage I to IV squamous cell carcinomas and adenocarcinomas of the esophagus were reported (Coia et al., 1991). The incidence of grade 3 toxicity was 22% and of grade 4 toxicity was 6%. There were no treatment-related deaths.

Calais et al. reported the results for 53 patients with clinically unresectable disease who received 5-FU, cisplatin, and mitomycin C plus 65 Gy of radiation (Calais et al., 1994). The full dose of radiation could be delivered in 96% of patients. The incidence of World Health Organization grade 3+ toxicity was 30% and the overall 2-year survival rate was 42%. It should be noted that the chemotherapy in this trial was not delivered at doses adequate to treat systemic disease. Because almost all patients in both the INT 0122 trial and the Calais trials (96% and 94%, respectively) who started radiation therapy were able to complete the full dose (64.8 to 65.0 Gy), this higher dose of radiation was used in the experimental arm of the Intergroup esophageal trial INT 0123 (RTOG 94-05). The INT 0123 trial (Minsky et al., 2002) was the follow-up to RTOG 85-01. In this trial, patients with either squamous cell carcinoma or adenocarcinoma who were selected for nonsurgical treatment were randomly assigned to receive a slightly modified RTOG 85-01 combined modality regimen with 50.4 Gy of radiation versus the same chemotherapy with 64.8 Gy of radiation). The modifications to the original RTOG 85-01 chemoradiation arm includes (1) using 1.8-Gy fractions to 50.4 Gy rather than 2-Gy fractions to 50 Gy; (2) treating with 5-cm proximal and distal margins for 50.4 Gy rather than treating the whole esophagus for the first 30 Gy followed by a cone down with 5 cm margins to 50 Gy; (3) cycle 3 of 5-FU and cisplatin did not begin until 4 weeks after the completion of radiation therapy rather than 3 weeks after; and (4) cycles 3 and 4 of chemotherapy were delivered every 4 weeks rather than every 3 weeks. INT 0123 was closed to accrual in 1999 after an interim analysis revealed that it was unlikely that the high-dose arm would achieve superior survival compared with the standard-dose arm. For the 218 eligible patients, there was no significant difference in median survival time (13.0 months vs. 18.1 months) or 2-year survival rate (31% vs. 40%) between the high-dose and standard-dose arms (Minsky et al., 2002) Although 11 treatment-related deaths occurred in the high-dose arm compared with 2 in the standard-dose arm, 7 of the 11 deaths occurred in patients who had received 50.4 Gy or less. To help determine if this unexplained increase in treatment-related deaths in the high-dose arm was the factor responsible for the inferior survival rate, a separate survival analysis was performed that included only patients who received the assigned dose of radiation. Despite this biased analysis, there was still no survival advantage for the high-dose arm. Although the crude incidence of local failure or persistence of local disease (or both) was lower in the high-dose arm than in the standard-dose arm (50% vs. 55%), as was the incidence of distant failure (9% vs. 16%), these differences did not reach statistical significance. At 2 years, the cumulative incidence of local failure was 56% for the high-dose arm versus 52% for the standard-dose arm (P = .71). Therefore, based on results of the INT 0123 trial, the standard dose of external-beam radiation remains 50.4 Gy. The modifications to the original RTOG 85-01 chemoradiation arm outlined earlier did not adversely affect the local control or survival rate in the control arm of INT 0123. Therefore, the radiation doses and field design used in the control arm of INT 0123 should be used.

Radiation can be intensified not only by increasing the total dose but also by using accelerated fractionation or hyperfractionation. Selected series using the latter approach for radiotherapy given as primary treatment (without surgery) are listed in Table 2.

Series	No.	Histologic Type	Treatment	Local Control	Survival	Grade 3+ Toxicity
Girinsky et al. (1997)	88	-	65 Gy (2Gy Bid) +/- 5FU/Cisplatin	48 % 3-y	12% 3-y	13%
Jeremic et al. (1998)	28	Squamous	54 Gy (1.5 Gy Bid)	71%	29% 5-y	50%
			5FU + Cisplatin x 4			
Wang et al. (2002(randomized)	101	Squamous	66 Gy (1.5 Gy Bid)vs.	56% 3-y	38% 3-y	61% esophagitis
			68.4 Gy total, 41.4 Gy (1.8 Gy/d), then 27 Gy (1.5 Gy Bid)	57% 3-y	41% 3-y	10% esophagitis

Table 2. **Results of Primary High-Dose Accelerated Fractionation/Hyperfractionation Combined Modality Therapy: Selected Series.**

Wang et al. randomly assigned 101 patients with squamous cell cancer to receive either continuous accelerated hyperfractionated radiation (66 Gy) or late-course accelerated hyperfractionated radiation (68.4 Gy) (Wang et al., 2002). Compared with patients who received late-course accelerated hyperfractionated radiation, those treated with continuous accelerated hyperfractionated radiation had a significantly higher incidence of grade 3+ esophagitis (61% vs. 10%; P <.001); however, no benefit was seen in local control or survival. Although these approaches are reasonable, most series report an increase in acute toxicity without any clear therapeutic benefit. These regimens remain investigational.

8.8 New combined modality regimens

Because 75% to 80% of patients die of metastatic disease, advances in systemic therapies are necessary for further improvement of results. The most widely used chemotherapeutic regimen to be combined with radiation for the treatment of esophageal cancer is 5-FU and cisplatin. There are new chemotherapeutic agents both in current practice and in development for esophageal cancer. Most are being developed for use in preoperative regimens and are combined with radiation doses of 45 to 50.4 Gy. Incorporation of these agents into chemotherapy regimens prior to chemoradiation or as adjuvant therapy may decrease systemic recurrence. Furthermore, new radiation sensitizers may improve locoregional control.

Multiple studies have tested both cytotoxic and targeted small molecules. Chemoradiation regimens using paclitaxel (Goldberg et al., 2003; Bains et al., 2002; Orditura et al., 2010; Ruppert et al., 2010), docetaxel (Pasini et al., 2005; Spigel et al., 2010), irinotecan (Ruppert et al., 2010; Ilson et al., 2002; Watkins et al., 2011; Sun et al., 2011), oxaliplatin (Spigel et al., 2010; De Vita et al., 2011; Chiarion-Sileni et al., 2009), epirubicin (Sun et al., 2011) and pemetrexed (Jatoi et al., 2010) have shown encouraging results. Biologic agents, such as cetuximab, trastuzumab, erlotinib, celecoxib and bevacizumab (De Vita et al., 2011; Safran et al., 2002; Enzinger et al., 2003; Suntharalingam et al., 2006) are being used as the foundations for new regimens which may enhance chemoradiation and target systemic micrometastases. Whether these investigational approaches offer improved results compared to conventional chemoradiation regimens based on 5-FU and cisplatin is not known.

9. Conclusion

For early esophageal cancer, endoscopic therapies are viable therapeutic options with significantly lower morbidities as compared to surgery. Currently, for a subset of patients with clinically localized early stage esophageal cancer (T0 or T1 lesions), local endoscopic therapy seems to be an acceptable alternative and produces similar results to surgery.

However, it is still unknown which of the endoscopic therapies represents the best alternative to surgical resection.

For more advanced stages of esophageal cancers, concurrent chemoradiation remains the standard nonsurgical treatment. New chemotherapeutic or biologic agents and radiation techniques are still needed to improve the survival of patients undergoing definitive chemoradiation.

10. References

Ackroyd R, Brown NJ, Davis MF, et al. Photodynamic therapy for dysplastic Barrett's oesophagus: a prospective, double blind, randomized, placebo controlled trial. Gut 2000; 47: 612-617.

Akagi Y, Hirokawa Y, Kagemoto M, et al. Optimum fractionation for high-dose-rate endoesophageal brachytherapy following external irradiation of early stage esophageal cancer. Int J Radiat Oncol Biol Phys 1999; 43:525-530.

Allington HV. Liquid nitrogen in the treatment of skin diseases. Calif Med 1950; 72: 153-155.

Al-Sarraf M, Martz K, Herskovic A, et al. Progress report of combined chemoradiotherapy versus radiotherapy alone in patients with esophageal cancer: an intergroup study. J Clin Oncol 1997; 15: 277-284. Erratum in: J Clin Oncol 1997; 15: 866.

Araujo CM, Souhami L, Gil RA, et al. A randomized trial comparing radiation therapy versus concomitant radiation therapy and chemotherapy in carcinoma of the thoracic esophagus. Cancer 1991;67:2258-2261.

Armstrong JG, High dose rate remote afterloading brachytherapy for lung and esophageal cancer. Semin Radiat Oncol 1993; 4:270-277.

Attwood SE, Lewis CJ, Caplin S, et al. Argon beam plasma coagulation as therapy for high-grade dysplasia in Barrett's esophagus. Clin Gastroenterol Hepatol 2003; 1: 258-263.

Badreddine RJ, Prasad GA, Wang KK, et al. Prevalence and predictors of recurrence neoplasia after ablation of Barrett's esophagus. Gastrointest Endosc 2010; 71: 697-703.

Bains MS, Stojadinovic A, Minsky B, et al. A phase II trial of preoperative combined-modality therapy for localized esophageal carcinoma: initial results. J Thorac Cardiovasc Surg 2002; 124:270-277.

Beaumont H, Bergman JJ, Pouw RE et l. Preservation of the functional integrity of the distal esophagus after circumferential ablation of Barrett's esophagus. Gastroenterol 2007; 132: A-A255.

Bedenne L, Michel P, and Binquet C et al. Chemoradiation followed by surgery compared with chemoradiation alone in squamous cancer of the esophagus: FFCD 9102. J Clin Oncol 2007; 25: 1160-1168.

Bonnetain F, Bouche O, and Bedenne L et al. A comparative longitudinal quality of life study using the Spitzer quality of life index in a randomized multicenter phase III trial (FFCD 9102): chemoradiation followed by surgery compared with chemoradiation alone in locally advanced squamous resectable thoracic esophageal cancer. Ann Oncol 2006; 17: 827-834.

Buttar NS, Wang KK, Lutzke LS, et al. Combined endoscopic mucosal resection and photodynamic therapy for esophageal neoplasia within Barrett's esophagus. Gastrointest Endosc 2001; 54: 682-688.

Calais G, Jadaud E, Chapet S, et al. High dose radiotherapy (RT) and concomitant chemotherapy for nonresectable esophageal cancer. Results of a phase II study. *Proc ASCO* 1994; 13:197.

Calais G, Dorval E, Louisot P, et al. Radiotherapy with high dose rate brachytherapy boost and concomitant chemotherapy for stages IIB and III esophageal carcinoma: results of a pilot study. Int J Radiat Oncol Biol Phys 1997; 38: 769-775.

Caspers RJL, Zwinderman AH, Griffioen G, et al. Combined external beam and low dose rate intraluminal radiotherapy in oesophageal cancer. Radiother Oncol 1993; 27:7-12.

Chiarion-Sileni V, Innocente R, Ancona E et al. Multicenter- phase II trial of chemo-radiotherapy with 5-fluorouracil, leucovorin and oxaliplatin in locally advanced esophageal cancer. Cancer Chemother Pharmacol 2009; 63: 1111-1119.

Chiu PW, Chan AC, Ng EK et al. Multicenter prospective randomized trial comparing standard esophagectomy with chemoradiotherapy for treatment of squamous esophageal cancer: results from the Chinese University Research Group for Esophageal Cancer (CURE). J Gastrointest Surg 2005; 9: 794-802.

Coia LR, Engstrom PF, Paul AR, et al. Long-term results of infusional 5-FU, mitomycin-C, and radiation as primary management of esophageal cancer. Int J Radiat Oncol Biol Phys 1991; 20:29-36.

Coia LR, Minsky BD, Berkey BA, et al. Outcome of patients receiving radiation for cancer of the esophagus: results of the 1992–1994 patterns of care study. J Clin Oncol 2000; 18: 455-462.

Cooper JS, Guo MD, Herskovic A, et al. Chemoradiotherapy of locally advanced esophageal cancer. Long-term follow-up of a prospective randomized trial (RTOG 85-01). JAMA 1999; 281:1623-1627.

De Vita F, Orditura M, Ciardiello F et al. A multicenter phase II study of induction chemotherapy with FOLFOX-4 and cetuximab followed by radiation and cetuximab in locally advanced oesophageal cancer. Br J Cancer 2011; 104: 427-432.

De-Ren S. Ten-year follow-up of esophageal cancer treated by radical radiation therapy: analysis of 869 patients. Int J Radiat Oncol Biol Phys 1989; 16: 329-334.

Downey RJ, Akhurst T, Ilson D, et al. Whole body 18FDG-PET and the response of esophageal cancer to induction therapy: results of a prospective trial. J Clin Oncol 2003; 21: 428-432.

Dulai GS, Jensen DM, Fontana L, et al. Randomized trial of argon plasma coagulation vs. multipolar electrocoagulation for ablation of Barrett's esophagus. Gastrontest Endosc 2005; 61: 232-240.

Dumot JA, Vargo JJ, Rice TW, et al. Preliminary results of cryotherapy ablation for esophageal high grade dysplasia (HGD) or intra-mucosal cancer (IMC) in high-risk non-surgical patients. Gastrointest Endosc 2007; 65: AB110.

Dunn J, Lovat L. Photodynamic therapy using 5-aminolaevulinic acid for the treatment of dysplasia in Barrett's oesophagus. Expert Opin Pharmacother 2008; 9: 851-858.

Ell C, May A, Pech O, et al. Curative endoscopic resection of early esophageal adenocarcinoma (Barrett's cancer). Gastrointest Endosc 2007; 65: 3-10.

Enzinger PC, Mamon H, Bueno R, et al. Phase II cisplatin, irinotecan, celecoxib and concurrent radiation therapy followed by surgery for locally advanced esophageal cancer. Proc ASCO 2003; 22:361.

Finkelstein SD, Lyday WD. The molecular pathology of radiofrequency mucosal ablation of Barrett's esophagus. Gastroenterol 2008; 134: A436.

Flamen P, Van Cutsem E, Lerut A, et al. Positron emission tomography for assessment of the response to induction radiochemotherapy in locally advanced oesophageal cancer. Ann Oncol 2002; 13:361-368.

Fleischer DE, Overholt BF, Sharma VK et al. Endoscopic ablation of Barrett's esophagus: a multicenter study with 2.5-year follow-up. Gastrointest Endosc 2008; 68: 867-876.

Gaspar LE, Nag S, Herskovic A, et al. American Brachytherapy Society (ABS) consensus guidelines for brachytherapy of esophageal cancer. Int J Radiat Oncol Biol Phys 1997; 38:127-132.

Gaspar LE, Qian C, Kocha WI, et al. A phase I/II study of external beam radiation, brachytherapy and concurrent chemotherapy in localized cancer of the esophagus (RTOG 92-07): preliminary toxicity report. Int J Radiat Oncol Biol Phys 1997; 37:593-599.

Giovannini M, Bories E, Pesenti C, et al. Circumferential endoscopic mucosal resection in Barrett's esophagus with high grade intraepithelial neoplasia or mucosal cancer: preliminary results in 21 patients. Endoscopy 2004; 36: 782-787.

Girinsky T, Auperin A, Marsiglia H, et al. Accelerated fractionation in esophageal cancers: a multivariate analysis on 88 patients. Int J Radiat Oncol Biol Phys 1997; 38:1013-1018.

Goldberg M, Farma J, Weiner LM et al. Survival following intensive preoperative combined modality therapy with paclitaxel, cisplatin, 5-fluorouracil, and radiation in resectable esophageal carcinoma: A phase I report. J Thorac Cardiovasc Surg 2003; 126: 1168-1173.

Gomi K, Oguchi M, Hirokawa Y, et al. Process and preliminary outcome of a patterns of care study of esophageal cancer in Japan: patients treated with surgery and radiotherapy. Int J Radiat Oncol Biol Phys 2003; 56: 813-822.

Gondrie JJ, Rygiel AM, Sondermeijer CM et al. Balloon-based circumferential ablation followed by focal ablation of Barrett's esophagus containing high-grade dysplasia effectively removes all genetic alterations. Gastroenterol 2007; 132: A-A64.

Gondrie JJ, Pouw RE,Sondermeijer CM et al. Effective treatment of early Barrett's neoplasia with stepwise circumferential and focal ablation using the HALO system. Endoscopy 2008; 40: 370-379.

Gondrie JJ, Pouw RE, Sondermeijer CM et al. Stepwise circumferential and focal ablation of Barrett's esophagus with high-grade dysplasia: results of the first prospective series of 11 patients. Endoscopy 2008; 40: 359-369.

Gossner L, May A, Stolte M, et al. KTP laser destruction of dysplasia and early cancer in columnar-lined Barrett's esophagus. Gastrointest Endosc 1999; 49: 8-12.

Greenwald BD, Horwhat JD, Abrams JA, et al. Endoscopic cryotherapy ablation is safe and well-tolerated in Barrett's esophagus, esophageal dysplasia, and esophageal cancer. Gastrointest Endosc 2008; 67: AB76.

Greenwald BD, Dumot JA, Wolfsen HC, et al. Endoscopic spray cryotherapy for esophageal cancer: safety and efficacy. Gastrointest Endosc 2010; 71: 686-693.

Gross SA, Wolfsen HC. The role of photodynamic therapy in the esophagus. Gastrointestinal Endosc Clin N Am. 2010; 20: 35-53.

Hage M, Siersma PD, van Dekken H et al. 5-aminolevulinic acid photodynamic therapy versus argon plasma coagulation for ablation of Barrett's oesophagus: a randomized trial. Gut 2004; 53: 785-790.

Herskovic A, Martz K, Al-Sarraf M, et al. Combined chemotherapy and radiotherapy compared with radiotherapy alone in patients with cancer of the esophagus. N Engl J Med 1992; 326:1593-1598.

Hironaka S, Hasebe T, Kamijo T, et al. Biopsy specimen microvessel density is a useful prognostic marker in patients with T2-4M0 esophageal cancer treated with chemoradiotherapy. Clin Cancer Res 2002; 8:124-130.

Holmes SR and Vaughan LT. Epidemiology and pathogenesis of esophageal cancer. Seminars in Radiation Oncology 2007; 17: 2-9.

Ilson DH, Minsky B, Kelsen D. Irinotecan, cisplatin and radiation in esophageal cancer. Oncology 2002; 16s:11-15.

Ilson DH, Bains M, Kelsen DP, et al. Phase I trial of escalating-dose irinotecan given weekly with cisplatin and concurrent radiotherapy in locally advanced esophageal cancer. J Clin Oncol 2003; 21:2926-2932.

Ishikura S, Nihei K, Ohtsu A, et al. Long-term toxicity after definitive chemoradiotherapy for squamous cell carcinoma of the thoracic esophagus. J Clin Oncol 2003; 21:2697-2702.

Izquierdo MA, Marcuello E, Gomez de Segura G, et al. Unresectable nonmetastatic squamous cell carcinoma of the esophagus managed by sequential chemotherapy (cisplatin and bleomycin) and radiation therapy. Cancer 1993; 71:287-292.

Jager J, Langendijk H, Pannebakker M, et al. A single session of intraluminal brachytherapy in palliation of esophageal cancer. Radiother Oncol 1995; 37:237-240.

Jatoi A, Soori G, Alberts SR et al. Phase II study of preoperative pemetrexed, carboplatin, and radiation followed by surgery for locally advanced esophageal cancer and gastroesophageal junction tumors. J Thorac Oncol 2010; 5: 1994-1998.

Jeremic B, Shibamoto Y, Acimovic L, et al. Accelerated hyperfractionated radiation therapy and concurrent 5-fluorouracil/cisplatin chemotherapy for locoregional squamous cell carcinoma of the thoracic esophagus: a phase II study. Int J Radiat Oncol Biol Phys 1998; 40:1061-1066.

Johnston M, Eastone JA, Horwhat JD, et al. Cryoablation of Barrett's esophagus: a pilot study. Gastrointest Endosc 2005; 62: 842-848.

Kelsen DP, Minsky B, Smith M, et al. Preoperative therapy for esophageal cancer: a randomized comparison of chemotherapy versus radiation therapy. J Clin Oncol 1990:1352-1361.

Kishi K, Doki Y, Miyata H, et al. Prediction of the response to chemoradiation and prognosis in oesophageal squamous cancer. Br J Surg 2002; 89:597-603.

Kok TC, Lanschot JV, Siersema PD, et al. Neoadjuvant chemotherapy in operable esophageal squamous cell cancer: final report of a phase III multicenter randomized trial. Proc ASCO 1997;16:277.

Larghi A, Lightdale CJ, Ross AS, et al. Long-term follow-up of complete Barrett's eradication endoscopic mucosal resection (CBE-EMR) for the treatment of high grade dysplasia and intramucosal carcinoma. Endoscopy 2007; 39: 1086-1091.

Lightdale CJ, Heier SK, Marcon NE, et al. Photodynamic therapy with porfimer sodium versus thermal ablation therapy with Nd: YAG laser for palliation of esophageal cancer: a multicenter randomized trial. Gastrointest Endosc 1995; 42:507-512.

Lopes CV, Hela M, Pesenti C, et al. Circumferential endoscopic resection of Barrett's esophagus with high grade dysplasia or early adenocarcinoma. Surg Endosc 2007; 21: 820-824.

Maingon P, d'Hombres A, Truc G, et al. High dose rate brachytherapy for superficial cancer of the esophagus. Int J Radiat Oncol Biol Phys 2000; 46:71-76.

Maunoury V. Mordon S., Mariette C., et al. Photodynamic therapy for early oesophageal cancer. Digestive and Liver Disease. 2005; 37: 491-495.

Merchant TE, Minsky BD, Lauwers GY, et al. Esophageal cancer phospholipids correlated with histopathologic findings: a 31P NMR study. NMR Biomed 1999; 12:184-188.

Michopoulos S, Tsibouris P, Bouzakis H et al. Complete regression of Barrett's esophagus with heat probe thermocoagulation: mid-term results. Gastrointest Endosc 1999; 50: 165-172.

Minsky BD, Neuberg D, Kelsen DP, et al. Final report of intergroup trial 0122 (ECOG PE-289, RTOG 90-12): phase II trial of neoadjuvant chemotherapy plus concurrent chemotherapy and high-dose radiation for squamous cell carcinoma of the esophagus. Int J Radiat Oncol Biol Phys 1999; 43:517-523.

Minsky BD, Pajak T, Ginsberg RJ, et al. INT 0123 (RTOG 94-05) phase III trial of combined modality therapy for esophageal cancer: high dose (64.8 Gy) vs. standard dose (50.4 Gy) radiation therapy. J Clin Oncol 2002; 20:1167-1174.

Miros M, Kerlin P, Walker N. Only patients with dysplasia progress to adenocarcinoma in Barrett's esophagus. Gut 1991; 32: 1441-1446.

Moghissi K, Dixon Hons KBA, Thorpe JAC, et al. Photofrin PDT for early stage oesophageal cancer: long term results in 40 patients and literature review. Photodiag and Photodyn 2009; 6: 159-166.

Moni J, Armstrong JG, Minsky BD, et al. High dose rate intraluminal brachytherapy for carcinoma of the esophagus. Dis Esophagus 1996; 9:123-127.

Morita M, Kuwano H, Araki K, et al. Prognostic significance of lymphocytic infiltration following preoperative chemoradiotherapy and hyperthermia for esophageal cancer. Int J Radiat Oncol Biol Phys 2001; 49:1259-1266.

Nemoto K, Yamada S, Hareyama M, et al. Radiation therapy for superficial esophageal cancer: a comparison of radiotherapy methods. Int J Radiat Oncol Biol Phys 2001; 50:639-644.

Nemoto K, Zhao HJ, Goto T, et al. Radiation therapy for limited-stage small-cell esophageal cancer. Am J Clin Oncol 2002; 25: 404-407.

Newaishy GA, Read GA, Duncan W, et al. Results of radical radiotherapy of squamous cell carcinoma of the esophagus. Clin Radiol 1982; 33: 347-352.

Nishioka NS. Drug, light and oxygen: a dynamic combination in the clinic. Gastroenterol 1998; 114: 604-606.

Nutting CM, Bedford JL, Cosgrove VP, et al. A comparison of conformal and intensity-modulated techniques for oesophageal radiotherapy. Radiother Oncol 2001; 61:157-163.

Nygaard K, Hagen S, Hansen HS, et al. Pre-operative radiotherapy prolongs survival in operable esophageal carcinoma: a randomized, multicenter study of pre-operative radiotherapy and chemotherapy. The second Scandinavian trial in esophageal cancer. World J Surg 1992; 16:1104-1109.

Okawa T, Kita M, Tanaka M, et al. Results of radiotherapy for inoperable locally advanced esophageal cancer. Int J Radiat Oncol Biol Phys 1989; 17:49-54.

Okawa T, Dokiya T, Nishio M, et al. Multi-institutional randomized trial of external radiotherapy with and without intraluminal brachytherapy for esophageal cancer in Japan. Int J Radiat Oncol Biol Phys 1999; 45:623-628.

Orditura M, Galizia G, Devita F et al. Weekly chemotherapy with cisplatin and paclitaxel and concurrent radiation therapy as preoperative treatment in locally advanced esophageal cancer: a phase II study. Cancer Invest 2010; 28: 820-827.

Ott K, Fink U, Becker K, et al. Prediction of response to preoperative chemotherapy in gastric carcinoma by metabolic imaging: results of a prospective trial. J Clin Oncol 2003; 21:4604-4610.

Overholt BF, Panjehpour M, Haydek JM. Photodynamic therapy for Barrett's esophagus: follow-up in 100 patients. Gastrointest Endosc 1999; 49: 1-7.

Overholt BF, Panjehpour M, Halberg DL. Photodynamic therapy for Barrett's esophagus with dysplasia and/or early stage carcinoma: long term results. Gastrointest Endosc 2003; 58: 183-188.

Overholt BF, Lightdale CJ, Wang KK, et al. Photodynamic therapy with porfimer sodium for ablation of high-grade dysplasia in Barrett's esophagus: international, partially blinded, randomized phase III trial. Gastrointestinal Endosc 2005; 62: 488-98.

Overholt BF, Wang KK, Burdick S, et al. Five-year efficacy and safety of photodynamic therapy with Photofrin in Barrett's high-grade dysplasia. Gastrointest Endosc 2007; 66: 460-468.

Pasini F, de Manzoni G, Cordiano C, et al. High pathologic response rate in locally advanced esophageal cancer after neoadjuvant combined modality therapy: dose finding of a weekly chemotherapy schedule with protracted venous infusion of 5-fluorouracil and dose escalation of cisplatin, docetaxel and concurrent radiotherapy. Ann Oncol 2005; 16: 1133-1139.

Pech O, Gossner L, May A, et al. Long-term results of photodynamic therapy with 5-aminolevulinic acid for superficial Barrett's cancer and high-grade intraepithelial neoplasia. Gastrointest Endosc 2005; 62: 24-30.

Pereira-Lima JC, Busnello JV, Saul C, et al. High power setting argon plasma coagulation for the eradication of Barrett's esophagus. Am J Gastroenterol 2000; 95: 1661-1668.

Peters F, Kara M, Rosmolen W, et al. Poor results of 5-aminolevulinic acid-photodynamic therapy for residual high-grade dysplasia and early cancer in Barrett esophagus after endoscopic resection. Endoscopy 2005; 37: 418-424.

Peters FP, Kara MA, Rosmolen WD, et al. Stepwise radical endoscopic resection is effective for complete removal of Barrett's esophagus with early neoplasia: a prospective study. Am J Gastroenterol 2006; 101: 1449-1457.

Peters FP, Brakenhoff KP, Curvers WL et al. Histologic evaluation of resection specimens obtained at 293 endoscopic resections in Barrett's esophagus. Gastrointest Endosc 2008; 67: 604-609.

Phillips TL, Minsky BD, Dicker A. Cancer of the esophagus. In: Leibel S, Phillips TL, eds. Textbook of radiation oncology. Philadelphia: WB Saunders, 1998: 601-612.

Pomp J, Davelaar J, Blom J, et al. Radiotherapy for oesophagus carcinoma: the impact of p53 on treatment outcome. Radiother Oncol 1998; 46:179-184.

Poplin EA, Jacobson J, Herskovic A, et al. Evaluation of multimodality treatment of locoregional esophageal carcinoma by Southwest Oncology Group 9060. Cancer 1996; 78:1851-1856.

Prasad GA, Wang KK, Buttar NS, et al. Long-term survival following endoscopic and surgical treatment of high-grade dysplasia in Barrett's esophagus. Gastroenterol 2007; 132: 1226-1233.

Prasad GA, Wang KK, Buttar NS, et al. Predictors of stricture formation after photodynamic therapy for high-grade dysplasia in Barrett's esophagus. Gastrointest Endosc 2007; 65: 60-66.

Prasad GA, Wang KK, Halling KC, et al. Utility of biomarkers in prediction of response to ablative therapy in Barrett's esophagus. Gastroenterol 2008; 135: 370-379.

Prasad GA, Wu TT, Wigle DA, et al. Endoscopic and surgical treatment of mucosal (T1a) esophageal adenocarcinoma in Barrett's esophagus. Gastroenterol 2009; 137: 815-823.

Ragunath K, Krasner N, Raman VS, et al. Endoscopic ablation of dysplastic Barrett's oesophagus comparing argon plasma coagulation and photodynamic therapy: a randomized prospective trial assessing efficacy and cost-effectiveness. Scand J Gastroenterol 2005; 40: 750-758.

Reid BJ, Levine DS, Longton G, et al. Predictors of progression to cancer in Barrett's esophagus : baseline histology and flow cytometry identify low-and high-risk patient subsets. Am J Gastroenterology 2000; 95: 1669-1676.

Roca E, Pennella E, Sardi M, et al. Combined intensive chemoradiotherapy for organ preservation in patients with resectable and non-resectable oesophageal cancer. Eur J Cancer 1996; 32A:429-432.

Roussel A, Jacob JH, Jung GM, et al. Controlled clinical trial for the treatment of patients with inoperable esophageal carcinoma: a study of the EORTC Gastrointestinal Tract Cancer Cooperative Group, in recent results in cancer research. In: Schlag P, Hohenberger P, Metzger U, eds. Berlin: Springer-Verlag, 1988:21-28.

Ruppert BN, Watkins JM, Sharma AK et al. Cisplatin/irinotecan versus carboplatin/paclitaxel as definitive chemoradiotherapy for locoregionally advanced esophageal cancer. Am J Clin Oncol 2010; 33:346-352.

Safran H, DiPetrillo T, Nadeem A, et al. Neoadjuvant Herceptin, paclitaxel, cisplatin, and radiation for adenocarcinoma of esophagus: a phase I study. Proc ASCO 2002; 21:141a.

Sampliner RE, Faigel D, Fennerty B, et al. Effective and safe endoscopic reversal of nondysplastic Barrett's esophagus with thermal electrocoagulation combined with high-dose acid inhibition: a multicenter study. Gastrointest Endosc 2001; 53: 554-558.

Sarbia M, Stahl M, Fink U, et al. Expression of apoptosis-regulating proteins and outcome of esophageal cancer patients treated by combined therapy modalities. Clin Cancer Res 1998; 4:2991-2997.

Schraube P, Fritz P, Wannenmacher MF. Combined endoluminal and external irradiation of inoperable oesophageal carcinoma. Radiother Oncol 1997; 44:45-51.

Schulz H, Miehlke S, Antos D et al. Ablation of Barrett's epithelium by endoscopic argon plasma coagulation in combination with high-dose omeprazole. Gastrointest Endosc 2000; 51: 659-663.

Seewald S, Akaraviputh T, Seitz U, et al. Circumferential EMR and complete removal of Barrett's epithelium: a new approach to management of Barrett's esophagus containing high grade intraepithelial neoplasia and intramucosal carcinoma. Gastrointest Endosc 2003; 57: 854-859.

Seitz JF, Giovannini M, Padaut-Cesana J, et al. Inoperable nonmetastatic squamous cell carcinoma of the esophagus managed by concomitant chemotherapy (5-fluorouracil and cisplatin) and radiation therapy. Cancer 1990; 66:214-219.

Seki K, Karasawa K, Kohno M, et al. The treatment result of definitive radiotherapy for superficial esophageal cancer. Int J Radiat Oncol Biol Phys 2001; 51:264-268.

Shaheen NJ, Sharma P, Overholt BF e tal. A randomized, multicenter, sham-controlled trial of radiofrequency ablation (RFA) for subjects with Barrett's esophagus containing dysplasia: interim results of the AIM dysplasia trial. Gastroenterol 2008; 134: A-A37.

Shaheen NJ, Sharma P, Lightdale CJ et al. Radiofrequency ablation in Barrett's esophagus with dysplasia. N Eng J Med 2009; 360: 2277-2288.

Sharma P. Jaffe PE, Sampliner RE, et al. Laser and multipolar electrocoagulation ablation of early Barrett's adenocarcinoma: long-term follow. Gastrointest Endosc 1999; 49: 442-446.

Sharma P, McQuaid, DentJ, et al. A critical review of the diagnosis and management of Barrett's esophagus: the AGA Chicago workshop. Gastroenterology 2004; 127:310-330.

Sharma VK, Kim HJ, Das A et al. Successful ablation of Barrett's esophagus with dysplasia using the HALO360 ablation system: a single-center experience (abstract). Am J Gastrointest 2006; 101: 535.

Sharma VK, Wang KK, Overholt BF et al. Balloon-based, circumferential, endoscopic radiofrequency ablation of Barrett's esophagus: 1-year follow-up of 100 patients. Gastrointest Endosc 2007; 65: 185-195.

Shi X, Yao W, Liu T. Late course accelerated fractionation in radiotherapy of esophageal carcinoma. Radiother Oncol 1999; 51:21-26.

Slabber CF, Nel JS, Schoeman L, et al. A randomized study of radiotherapy alone versus radiotherapy plus 5-fluorouracil and platinum in patients with inoperable, locally advanced squamous cell cancer of the esophagus. Am J Clin Oncol 1998:21:462-465.

Smith TJ, Ryan LM, Douglass HO, et al. Combined chemoradiotherapy vs. radiotherapy alone for early stage squamous cell carcinoma of the esophagus: a study of the Eastern Cooperative Oncology Group. Int J Radiat Oncol Biol Phys 1998; 42:269-276.

Spechler SJ. Dysplasia in Barrett's esophagus: limitations of current management strategies. Am J Gastroenterology 2005; 100: 927-935.

Spigel DR, Greco FA, Hainsworth JD et al. Phase I/II trial of preoperative oxaliplatin, docetaxel, capecitabine with concurrent radiation therapy in localized carcinoma of the esophagus or gastroesophageal junction. J Clin Oncol 2010; 28: 2213-2219.

Stahl M, Stuschke M, and Wilke H et al.Chemoradiation with and without surgery in patients with locally advanced squamous cell carcinoma of esophagus. J Clin Oncol 2005; 23: 2310-2317.

Streeter OE, Martz KL, Gaspar LE, et al. Does race influence survival for esophageal cancer patients treated on the radiation and chemotherapy arm of RTOG # 85-01? Int J Radiat Oncol Biol Phys 1999;44:1047-1052.

Sun W, Metz JM, Haller DG et al. Two phase I studies of concurrent radiation therapy with continuous-infusion-5fluorouracil plus epirubicin, and either cisplatin or irinotecan for locally advanced upper gastrointestinal adenocarcinomas. Cancer Chemother Pharmacol 2011; 67: 621-627.

Suntharalingam M, Moughhan J, Coia LR, et al. The national practice for patients receiving radiation therapy for carcinoma of the esophagus: results of the 1996–1999 Patterns of Care Study. Int J Radiat Oncol Biol Phys 2003; 56: 981-987.

Suntharalingam M, Dipetrillo T, Safran H et al. Cetuximab, carboplatin and paclitaxel and radiation for esophageal and gastric cancer. Proc J Clin Oncol 2006: 4029.

Sur RK, Singh DP, Sharma SC. Radiation therapy of esophageal cancer: role of high dose rate brachytherapy. Int J Radiat Oncol Biol Phys 1992; 22:1043-1046.

Sur RK, Donde B, Levin VC, et al. Fractionated high dose rate intraluminal brachytherapy in palliation of advanced esophageal cancer. Int J Radiat Oncol Biol Phys 1998; 40:447-453.

Sykes AJ, Burt PA, Slevin NJ, et al. Radical radiotherapy for carcinoma of the oesophagus: an effective alternative to surgery. Radiother Oncol 1998; 48:15-21.

Tai P, van Dyk J, Battista J, et al. Improving the consistency in cervical esophageal target volume definition by special training. Int J Radiat Oncol Biol *Phys* 2002; 53:766-774.

Thomas T, Abrams KR, de Caestecker JS, Robinson RJ. Meta analysis: cancer risk in Barrett's esophagus. Aliment Pharmacol Ther 2007; 26:1465-1477.

Valerdi JJ, Tejedor M, Illarramendi JJ, et al. Neoadjuvant chemotherapy and radiotherapy in locally advanced esophagus carcinoma: long term results. Int J Radiat Oncol Biol Phys 1994; 27:843-847.

Van Laethem JL, Jagodzinski R, Peny MO et al. Argon plasma coagulation in the treatment of Barrett's high-grade dysplasia and in-situ adenocarcinoma. Endosc 2001; 33: 257-261.

Wang Y, Shi XH, He SQ, et al. Comparison between continuous accelerated hyperfractionated and late-course accelerated hyperfractionated radiotherapy for esophageal carcinoma. Int J Radiat Oncol Biol Phys 2002; 54:131-136.

Watkins JM, Zauls AJ, Sharma AK et al. Toxicity, response rates and survival outcomes of induction cisplatin and irinotecan followed by concurrent cisplatin, irinotecan and radiotherapy for locally advanced esophageal cancer. Jpn J Clin Oncol 2011; 41: 334-342.

Westerterp M, Koppert LB, Buskens CJ e tal. Outocme of surgical treatment for early adenocarcinoma of the esophagus or gastro-esophageal junction. Virchows Arch 2005; 446: 497-504.

Wolfsen HC, Woodward TA, Raimondo M. Photodynamic therapy for dysplastic Barrett's esophagus and early esophageal adenocarcinoma. Mayo Clin Proc 2002; 77: 1176-1181.

Wolfsen HC, Hemminger LL, Wallace MB, et al. Clinical experience of patients undergoing photodynamic therapy for Barrett's dysplasia or cancer. Aliment Pharmacol Ther 2004; 20: 1125-1131.

Wong R, Malthaner R. Combined chemotherapy and radiotherapy (without surgery) compared with radiotherapy alone in localized carcinoma of the esophagus. Cochrane Database Syst Rev. 2006. Review. Update in: Cochrane Database Syst Rev. 2010.

Yachimski P, Puricelli WP, Nishioka NS. Patient predictors of esophageal stricture development after photodynamic therapy. Clin Gastroenterol Hepatol 2008; 6: 302-308.

Yachimski P, Puricelli WP, Nishioka NS. Patient predictors of histopathologic response after photodynamic therapy of Barrett's esophagus with high-grade dysplasia or intramucosal carcinoma. Gastrointest Endosc 2009; 69: 205-212.

Yorozu A, Dokiya T, Oki Y, et al. Curative radiotherapy with high-dose-rate brachytherapy boost for localized esophageal carcinoma: dose-effect relationship of brachytherapy with the balloon type applicator system. Radiother Oncol 1999; 51:133-139.

9

Emerging Therapies for Esophageal Cancer

Hajime Orita[1], Malcolm Brock[2] and Koichi Sato[1]
[1]Juntendo University school of Medicine, Shizuoka Hospital, Department of Surgery
[2]Johns Hopkins University school of Medicine, Department of Surgery and Oncology
[1]Japan
[2]USA

1. Introduction

This chapter will review the status of clinical and laboratory research exploring targeted therapies for treatment of esophageal cancer. Therapies that target specific pathways activated in cancers offer the potential for potent anti-cancer effects with minimal host toxicity. This review will not only summarize the status of targeted therapies currently being evaluated in clinical trials for treating esophageal cancer, but also discuss therapies that show promise in pre-clinical studies, including those that target metabolic pathways in cancer.

Esophageal cancer is the sixth most common cause of cancer mortality worldwide, and its incidence is increasing [1, 2]. Although there are different histologic variants of esophageal cancer **(Squamous cell and Adenoma carcinoma)** that have distinctive epidemiologic patters, the major risk factors (smoking, dietary factors) and many clinical features are similar among these histologic variants [3]. More than 90% of esophageal cancers - of all histologic variants - are diagnosed in late stage. In spite of new diagnostic and therapeutic approaches, esophageal cancer has poor prognosis, with 5-year survival rates between 10–13%.

Conventional treatment for esophageal cancer depends largely on stage of the tumor, typically including chemotherapy as well as surgery and radiotherapy. Standard agents include cisplatin, 5-fluoruracil, taxanes, irinotecan, and mitomycin C, but the inability of these agents to effectively treat most cases of esophageal cancer has provided an impetus for the recent attention that has been directed to therapeutics selectively targeting molecular pathways in cancer cells. Gene therapy, such as restoring p53 gene function, has also been explored [4], but because of the discouraging level of progress in this area, gene therapy will not be discussed in this chapter.

2. Targeting the EGFR signaling pathway

Epidermal growth factor receptor (EGFR) is one of the most commonly altered genes in human cancer, with alterations including overexpression, amplification, and mutation. Targeted inhibition of EGFR activity suppresses signal transduction pathways, affecting tumor cell proliferation and resistance to apoptosis. Small molecule tyrosine kinase inhibitors and monoclonal antibodies are among the most common EGFR-targeting agents and have been used clinically for treating various malignancies with EGFR mutations or abnormal expression of the receptor. The outcomes of clinical trials using EGFR inhibitors will be summarized after a general discussion of the molecular biology of this target.

EGFR is a 170 KDa transmembrane glycoprotein situated on the cell surface, which is activated by binding of its specific ligands, including epidermal growth factor and transforming growth factor α (TGFα)[5]. . An EGF-specific receptor was first found on surface of fibroblasts in 1975 [6], but only relatively recently have mutations affecting EGFR been discovered to be involved in the development of cancers [7]. EGFR (also known as ERBB1/HER1) is a member of a family of receptor proteins that contains 3 other members: HER2/ERBB2, HER3/ERBB3, and HER4/ERBB4. All the receptor members of this family have an extracellular ligand-binding region or ectodomain, a single membrane-spanning region, and a cytoplasmic region that contains a tyrosine kinase domain. Binding of the ligand to the ectodomain initiates receptor homo- and hetero-dimerization, resulting in activation of the cytoplasmic tyrosine kinase and stimulation of intracellular signaling pathways. Gene amplification, mutation or structural changes of the receptor kinase can cause carcinogenesis, due to disregulation of cellular proliferation as well as characteristics that support cancer cell invasion and metastasis.

EGFR protein expression can be detected in about 30% to 70% of esophageal carcinomas [8, 9]. Similar to head and neck cancer squamous cell cancers (HNSCC), squamous cell carcinomas of the esophagus have very high frequency of elevated expression of EGFR (70-90%) [10, 11]. High levels of EGFR protein expression have been correlated with worse patient survival in both esophageal carcinoma and HNSCC, although the association has not been robust and results not consistent among various studies[12] [13] [14]. Moreover, a high EGFR gene copy number, which variably correlates with increased EGFR protein expression, also has been reported as a poor prognostic marker [15, 16]. Therefore, EGFR represents a rational target for therapeutics.

2.1 Monoclonal antibodies to target EGFR

There are several potential strategies to target the EGFR, most notably monoclonal antibodies (mAbs) and low molecular weight tyrosine kinase inhibitors (TKIs), which have both demonstrated clinical utility. mAbs bind to the extracellular domain of the receptor and compete with the natural ligands (TGF-αand EGF) binding to the receptor, therefore blocking activation of the receptor. By contrast, TKIs compete with ATP binding to the tyrosine kinase portion of the endodomain of the receptor and thereby abrogate the receptor's catalytic activity. Both strategies appear to be effective at blocking the downstream receptor-dependent signaling pathways, which include activation of MAPK, PI3K/Akt, and Jak/Stat.

In 1983, John Mendelsohn created the chimeric IgG1 Cetuximab('Erbitux', C225), the first epidermal growth factor receptor inhibitors (EGFR-I) [17]. In fact, cetuximab has been approved for the treatment of advanced colorectal cancer (CRC) over the last decade. Both single agent cetuximab as well as the combination with irinotecan have shown activity in patients with CRC [18, 19]. A second-generation EGFR-I, Panitumumab (ABX-EGF) is a fully human IgG2 mAb with high affinity for the EGFR[20].

Cetuximab has also shown efficacy in the treatment of non-small-cell lung cancer (NSCLC)[21-25]and locally advanced head and neck squamous cell carcinoma (HNSCC)[26, 27].

2.2 Clinical trial for targeting EGFR-I

Currently, several trials of EGFR-I with FOLFOX, FOLFIRI are demonstrating efficacy against CRC in various sites around the world [28, 29]. The side effects of IGFR-I therapy include skin rash, diarrhea, and hypomagnesaemia. Skin rash can be especially troubling, and this appears to be associated with depressive psychosis [30-32]. Biomarker analysis from several recent studies demonstrated that patients with KRAS mutated tumors are resistant to monotherapy with cetuximab or Panitumumab [33, 34]. Thus, benefits of adding EGFR-I to chemotherapy is limited to patients with wild-type (WT) KRAS in colorectal carcinoma [35, 36].

Several phase II trials for advanced esophageal cancer are ongoing throughout the world. One trial is the LLEDO G group (Paris) studying the effects of oxaliplatin, leucovorin and fluorouracil-when given together with Cetuximab and radiation therapy (NCT00578201). A second is being conducted at the National Cancer Institute (NCI), studying cetuximab in combination with cisplatin and irinotecan for treatment of patients with metastatic esophageal cancer, gastroesophageal junction cancer, or gastric cancer that did not respond to previous irinotecan and cisplatin (NCT00397904). Finally, a trial centered at Brown University is evaluating the rate of complete pathologic response as determined by surgical resection or post treatment endoscopy (for patients not undergoing resection) for the treatment regimen being tested (NCT00439608). While cetuximab administered as a single agent had minimal clinical activity in patients with advanced esophageal cancers, these ongoing phase 2 clinical trials of EGFR inhibitors in combination with other agents may define a role for these agents in the treatment [37, 38].

Interestingly, no KRAS mutations have been detected in esophageal cancers [39, 40], so mutations of this gene will apparently not cause resistance of esophageal cancers to EGFR-inhibitory therapy.

Shandong Cancer Hospital and Institute (NCT00815308) also studied to determine whether the treatment of locally advanced esophageal squamous cell carcinoma (ESCC) with cetuximab in combination with paclitaxel, cisplatin and radiation could improve clinical outcome. Unfortunately, the results were not encouraging. By contrast, the Hoosier Oncology Group (NCT00319735) investigating cetuximab combined with radiation found promising results. In this study, EGFR inhibitory agents enhanced radiation-induced apoptosis and inhibited radiation-induced damage repair. These interactions may represent the principle effects that contribute to the synergy between EGFR and radiation.

2.3 Tyrosine kinase inhibitors to target EGFR

Tyrosine kinase inhibitors (TKIs) are a class of small molecules that inhibit ATP binding within the tyrosine kinase domain, leading to inhibition of EGFR autophosphorylation and signal transduction. TKIs are now widely used in the treatment of lung cancers and are also being explored for treatment of esophageal cancers. Glivec was the first widely used TKI, used to treat myelogenous leukemia and gastrointestinal stromal tumors (GIST). A protein kinase inhibitor is a type of enzyme inhibitor that specifically blocks the action of one or more protein kinases. Hence, they can be subdivided or characterized by the amino acids whose phosphorylation is inhibited: most kinases act on both serine and threonine, the tyrosine kinases act on tyrosine, and a number (dual-specificity kinases) act on all three. There are also protein kinases that phosphorylate other amino acids, including histidine kinases that phosphorylate histidine residues. They can interfere with the repair of DNA double-strand breaks [41]. TKIs are a class of oral, small molecules that inhibit ATP binding within the TK domain, which completely inhibits EGFR autophosphorylation and signal transduction [63].

There are a large number of TKIs directed to the EGFR family in clinical development for treatment of esophageal cancer. EGFR monoclonal antibodies (mAbs) bind to the extracellular domain of the receptor and compete with their ligands, therefore, blocking activation of the receptor. On the contrary, TKIs compete with ATP binding to the tyrosine kinase portion of the endodomain of the receptor and, thereby, abrogate the receptor's catalytic activity.

Gefitinib (Iressa®) and Erlotinib (Tarceva®) have been approved for treatment in non-small cell lung cancer (NSCLC). Several clinical trials have demonstrated an increase in progression-free survival in EGFR mutant lung cancer patients treated with these agents [42]. More recently, Gefitinib (Iressa®) has been evaluated in esophageal cancer in several phase 2 studies. Rodriguez, C. P.[43] demonstrated 80 advanced esophageal cancer patients for chemoradiotherapy (CRT) plus gefitinib (250 mg/d). Although gefitinib did not worsen CRT toxicity, maintenance therapy proved difficult.

Other study, Altiok S, Gibson MK [44] describe a short-term ex vivo assay to predict response to epidermal growth factor receptor (EGFR) targeted therapy (gefitinib) in adenocarcinoma patients. According to their pharmacokinetics research, after treated with gefitinib (250 mg/day) for 14 days, advanced esophageal adenocarcinoma were correlated with the gefitinib-mediated alteration in proliferating cell nuclear antigen (PCNA) expression, a marker of cell proliferation. PK studies demonstrated constant gefitinib concentrations during the treatment, confirming persistent exposure of target tissue to the drug at sufficient levels to achieve EGFR blockade.

Erlotinib (Tarceva®) is the second generation drug. Ilson, D. H.[45] evaluated 30 patients with measurable, metastatic cancer of the esophageal and gastroesophageal junction received 150 mg erlotinib daily. Erlotinib had limited activity in esophageal cancer (2 of 24(8%) partial responses were observed in the EGFR-positive and no responses were observed in the EGFR-negative cohort. Reponses were limited to patients who had squamous cell carcinoma (2 of 13 patients; 15%; response duration, 5.5-7 months). The time to tumor progression was longer in patients who had squamous cell carcinoma (3.3 months; range, 1-24 months) compared with patients who had adenocarcinoma (1.6 months; range, 1-6 months; P = .026). Therapy was tolerable with the expected toxicity of skin rash (grade 1-2, 67%; grade 3, 10%). and some protracted stable disease were observed in those with squamous cell carcinoma. Efficacy according to EGFR status could not be assessed given the rarity of EGFR-negative tumors.

Recently, Lapatinib (Tykerb), used in the form of lapatinib ditosylate, an orally active drug, starts for breast cancer and other solid tumors treatment [46]. It is a dual tyrosine kinase inhibitor which interrupts the HER2 growth receptor pathway[47]. It is used in combination therapy for HER2-positive breast cancer. It has been approved as front-line therapy in triple positive breast cancer and as an adjuvant therapy when patients have progressed on Herceptin [48, 49]. Phase 1 trials are now ongoing for esophageal cancer. Alvarez H and Maitra A in Hopkins [50] analyzed small molecule inhibitors of Axl function. Axl is a receptor tyrosine kinase (RTK) with oncogenic potential and transforming activity. Blockade of Axl function abrogated phosphorylation of ERBB2 (Her-2/neu) at the Lapatinib residue, indicative of receptor crosstalk. Axl RTK is an adverse prognostic factor in esophageal cancer. The availability of small molecule inhibitors of Axl function provides a tractable strategy for molecular therapy.

3. Targeting the HER2 signaling pathway

Amplification and over-expression of HER-2/neu (c-erbB-2) in esophageal cancer has also been to predict a poor prognosis. Although recognition of gene amplification could be considered as a therapeutic target in esophageal cancer, there is actually a paucity of data regarding HER-2/neu amplification in esophgeal cancer and its implications for clinical management.

HER2/neu (also known as ErbB-2) exists on the cell surface and is a 185 KDa transmembrane glycoprotein with tyrosine kinase activity[51]. It is a member of the ErbB protein family, more commonly known as the epidermal growth factor receptor family. In 1985, this cell surface receptor of the tyrosine kinase gene family was identified and characterized by molecular cloning [52] .HER2 is a cell membrane surface-bound receptor tyrosine kinase and is normally involved in the signal transduction pathways leading to cell growth and differentiation. HER2 gene is relating the development and maintenance of heart and nerve system, and also cell proliferation and differentiation [53, 54]. However, ErbB receptors dimerise on ligand binding, and HER2 is the preferential dimerisation partner of other members of the ErbB family[55]. The HER2 gene is a proto-oncogene located at the long arm of human chromosome 17(17q21-q22)[52].

HER2/neu is a protein associated with aggressiveness in breast cancers. Approximately 30% of breast cancers have an amplification of the HER2/neu gene or overexpression of its protein product. Overexpression of this receptor in breast cancer is associated with increased disease recurrence and worse prognosis [56, 57]. Because of its prognostic role as well as its ability to predict response to trastuzumab (Herceptin), breast tumors are routinely checked for overexpression of HER2/neu same as hormone receptors. HER2 is also overexpressed in other types of cancers, including 25–30% of ovarian cancers [58], 35–45% of pancreatic carcinomas[59, 60], and in 30–80% of esophageal adenocarcinoma [61, 62], and squamous cell carcinoma [63-65].

A drug targeting HER2/neu is the monoclonal antibody trastuzumab (Herceptin). Trastuzumab is effective only in cancers where the HER2/neu receptor is overexpressed. In fact, trastuzumab was clinically shown to have survival benefit in patients with HER-2–overexpressing breast cancer with metastasis [66, 67]. One of the mechanisms of how trastuzumab works after it binds to HER2 is by increasing p27, a protein that halts cell proliferation [68].

The results of a study combining trastuzumab with cisplatin in HER2 positive untreated patients with gastric or gastro-esophageal junction cancer have recently been presented [69].

In this study, capecitabine plus cisplatin or fluorouracil plus cisplatin was given every 3 weeks for six cycles or chemotherapy in combination with intravenous trastuzumab (NCT01041404). 594 patients were randomly assigned to study treatment (trastuzumab plus chemotherapy, n=298; chemotherapy alone, n=296), of whom 584 were included in the primary analysis (n=294; n=290). Median overall survival was 13.8 months (95% CI 12-16) in those assigned to trastuzumab plus chemotherapy compared with 11.1 months (10-13) in those assigned to chemotherapy alone (hazard ratio 0.74; 95% CI 0.60-0.91; p=0.0046). The most common adverse events in both groups were nausea, vomiting, and neutropenia. Rates of overall grade 3 or 4 adverse events (201 [68%] vs. 198 [68%]) and cardiac adverse events (17 [6%] vs. 18 [6%]) did not differ between groups. The authors concluded that Trastuzumab in combination with chemotherapy can be considered as a new standard option for patients with HER2-positive advanced gastric or gastro-esophageal junction cancer.

4. Angiogenesis inhibitors

Agents that inhibit vascular endothelial cell growth factor (VEGF) and the angiogenesis process have also attracted considerable interest for treatment of a variety of cancer types. VEGF is overexpressed in 30%–60% of patients with esophageal cancers. Bevacizumab, a recombinant humanized mAb to VEGF, is the most widely studied anti-angiogenesis agent. Bevacizumab is still undergoing clinical evaluation for esophageal cancer treatment, and this approach could represent an important addition to the treatment of this disease.

Vascular endothelial growth factor (VEGF) is a glycoprotein important for regulating vasculogenesis and angiogenesis. VEGF was first isolated in 1983 from mouse ascites[70] and functions to create new blood vessels for restoring the oxygen supply to tissues when blood circulation is inadequate. VEGF is activated by binding of its ligands VEGFR, leading to stimulation of cell division and differentiation. There are five members of the human VEGF family: VEGF-A (referred to in this chapter as VEGF), VEGF-B, VEGF-C,VEGF-D and placental growth factor (PlGF). In addition, multiple isoforms of VEGF, VEGF-B and PlGF are generated through alternative splicing of pre-mRNA.1 The VEGF family ligands interact with the receptor tyrosine kinases VEGF receptor-1 (VEGFR1), VEGFR2 and VEGFR3. VEGF family interaction with VEGFRs is also regulated by the non-enzymatic co-receptors neuropilin (Nrp)-1 and Nrp2.1. Bevacizumab binds VEGF-A, and inhibit function of VEGFR1, VEGFR2 and Nrp-1.

VEGF is overexpressed in 30%–60% of esophageal cancer tumors, and several studies have demonstrated a correlation among high levels of VEGF expression, advanced stage, and poor overall survival in patients undergoing a potentially curative esophagectomy [96–99]. One recent study suggests that the activation of the EGFR-pathway contributes to angiogenesis in esophageal adenocarcinoma by different mechanisms, including upregulation of VEGF and Neuropilin-1 expression [38]. In another study, Kulke and others found no significant association between VEGF expression and treatment response or overall survival [71]. This discrepancy may be in part explained by the potential induction of VEGF and increased angiogenic activity that may occur with the delivery of preoperative chemoradiotherapy. The treatment-induced development of more aggressive and resistant tumor phenotypes might weaken potential associations among pretreatment VEGF levels, treatment response, and overall survival.

Bevacizumab is a monoclonal antibody that binds to all isoforms of human VEGF and thus functions as a direct angiogenesis inhibitor. This drug has found use in combination therapy for colorectal cancer, with reported survival benefit when used in combination with irinotecan-, oxaliplatin- and 5-fluorouracil-based chemotherapy [38–41]. Bevacizumab has several severe side-effects when used for treatment of colorectal cancer, most notable intestinal perforation, which occurs at a frequency of somewhat less than 5 %. While emergency surgery can rescue patients with colon perforations, esophageal perforations would most likely be lethal to patients, suggesting that this drug will need to be used carefully in patients with esophageal cancers.

5. Metabolic pathways as targets for cancer therapy

Over the past decade, there has been increasing interest in cancer metabolism pathways as targets for cancer therapy. Two potential therapeutic strategies will be discussed with respect to esophageal cancer therapy: first, the potential role of metformin, a drug used for treatment of diabetes, and second the potential role of inhibitors of fatty acid synthase. Metformin is likely to be investigated at a clinical level soon, since this drug is widely available and has an established safety profile. While inhibitors of fatty acid synthase still require pre-clinical development, studies to date provide encouragement that this metabolic pathway could offer a new target for esophageal cancer therapy.

5.1 Metformin for cancer treatment

As a background for testing metformin in treatment of esophageal cancer, it should be noted that type 2 diabetes, is associated with significantly higher risks of developing certain types of cancers and with increased mortality from those cancers [72-74]. Insulin resistance, hyperinsulinemia, oxidative stress, advanced glycation end products, and chronic low-grade inflammations have all been considered to explain the association between diabetes and high cancer incidence. While gastroesophageal reflux and high body mass index (BMI) are well established risk factors [75-77] for esophageal cancers, it has also reported that diabetes is associated with substantial and significant increase in risk of esophageal adenocarcinoma [78-82].

Effective treatment of diabetes might favorably affect cancer incidence and mortality [83-85]. Since the 1960s, metformin (a biguanide) has become the first line anti-hyperglycemic agent in type 2 diabetes (T2DM) treatment worldwide[86], and a large number of observational studies have reported a reduced incidence of neoplastic disease in diabetic patients treated with metformin [87, 88]. It is generally thought that metformin suppresses gluconeogenesis in the liver, leading to decreased production of insulin, a potential cancer cell growth factor. In addition, by activating the enzyme AMPK (AMP activated protein kinase), skeletal muscles are induced to take up glucose from the blood. Moreover, by activating AMPK, metformin inhibits the mammalian target of rapamycin complex 1 (mTORC1) resulting in decreased cancer cell proliferation. Concomitantly, metformin induces activation of LKB1 (serine/threonine kinase 11), a tumor suppressor gene, which is required for the phosphorylation and activation of AMPK [89, 90].

The new encouraging experimental data supporting the anti-cancer effects of metformin urgently require further clinical studies in order to establish its use as a synergistic therapy targeting the AMPK/mTOR signaling pathway. Although few studies have been performed to date, a retrospective study performed in Taiwan evaluating 800, 000 people found that diabetic patients without any drug treatment had twice the level of gastrointestinal cancer incidence (gastric, colorectal, hepatic, pancreatic and esophageal cancer) as metformin-treated diabetics. The authors of this study [78] proposed a metformin dose of 500 mg/ day for a significant decrease in cancer incidence.

Encouraging findings have also been reported in retrospective studies of breast cancer neoadjuvant chemotherapy for locally advanced (inoperable) breast cancer. This treatment has become an accepted alternative to adjuvant chemotherapy in operable early-stage breast cancer, because it allows breast conservation. Importantly, diabetic patients with breast cancer receiving metformin and neoadjuvant chemotherapy were found to have a higher pCR(Pathologic Complete Response) rate than diabetics not receiving metformin [91].

The breast cancer data is particularly relevant to the esophageal cancer situation, because neoadjuvant therapy (combinations of chemotherapy and radiotherapy) is also performed to reduce tumor size before surgery for advanced esophageal cancer. While no data is available for metformin effects in esophageal cancer neoadjuvant therapy, it certainly would be important to evaluate responses retrospectively as well as consider metformin use in non-diabetic patients for esophageal cancer treatment.

Interestingly, Hirsch H et al [92] reported that metformin selectively kills cancer stem cells in four genetically different types of breast cancer. The combination of metformin and a well-defined chemotherapeutic agent, doxorubicin, kills both cancer stem cells and non-stem cancer cells in culture. Furthermore, this combinatorial therapy reduces tumor mass and prevents relapse much more effectively than either drug alone in a xenograft mouse model. These results provide further evidence supporting the combination of metformin and chemotherapeutic drugs to improve treatment of patients with cancers, including esophageal cancer.

5.2 Fatty acid synthase as a target for cancer treatment

It is well-known that anaerobic metabolism predominates in many tumors, and this type of metabolism causes lipid combustion and beta oxidization. Lipids are made from triglyceride and fatty acids by the enzyme, fatty acid synthase. Fatty acid synthase (FAS) is highly expressed in many human cancers. [93]. Because fatty acid synthesis expends energy, it seems reasonable to expect that high FAS activity confers some survival or growth advantage to human cancer.

In esophageal cancer (both squamous cancers and adenocarcinomas), FAS is expressed at very high levels similar to other cancers [94, 95], and high expression is also seen in Barrett's esophagus with dysplasia [96, 97]. (Figure1) It appears that increased expression of FAS is associated with neoplastic transformation and is not typical of esophageal glandular epithelium in general [98]. Our recent study found that esophageal cancers (and likely high-grade precursors) that express high levels of FAS could potentially be treated by therapy directed to inhibit this enzyme.

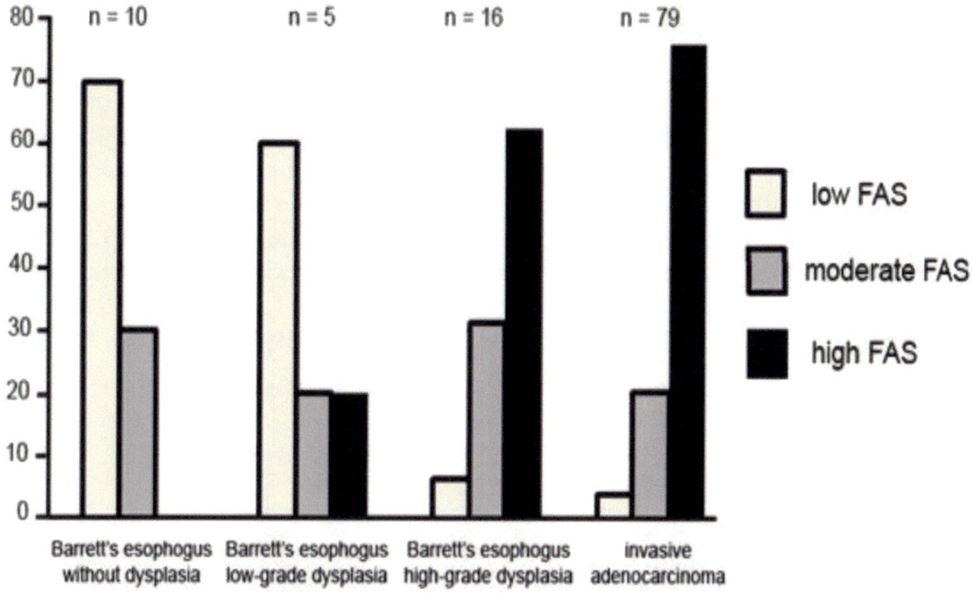

Fig. 1. **FAS expression in SCC and EAC.**
Fatty acid synthase is expressed at high levels in human esophageal squamous cell carcinomas and adenocarcinomas. In addition, FAS is expressed at high levels in Barrett's esophagus with dysplasia.

In addition to being overexpressed in malignant tissues, increased FAS levels can also be detected in the circulation in cancer patients (30, 31), and our group has found that serum FAS levels could potentially be used as tumor marker. Figure2 shows the data of FAS serum in several cancers, where each cancer shows high levels of FAS compared with control. For esophageal cancer, we compared levels FAS in serum from 150 patients with invasive squamous cell carcinoma and 4 with invasive adenocarcinoma to those of 153 normal healthy individuals (Figure 3). The significantly higher levels in cancer patients than control patients suggest that measurements of FAS might be a useful tumor marker.

To explore anti-FAS therapy for esophageal cancer, we first confirmed that FAS expression is also high in xenografts of human esophageal squamous cell cancer cells, with levels that are similar to human tumors. A number of agents are available to inhibit FAS; previous laboratory studies have shown that cancer cell growth can be suppressed by inhibiting the activity of this enzyme FAS with cerulenin (a natural antibiotic), small interfering RNA specific for the FAS gene transcript [99], orlistat, a pancreatic lipase inhibitor developed for obesity treatment [100], or C75, a first-generation synthetic small-molecule developed specifically for inhibiting type 1 mammalian FAS, based on the known mechanism of action of cerulenin[101, 102].

However, efforts to treat xenograft cancers with C75 [103-105] have been hampered by transient, but severe, anorexia and weight loss caused by drug treatment, an effect that could also limit the use of this compound in the clinical setting [106]. C75 is a mimetic of malonyl-CoA, and in addition to inhibiting FAS, C75 stimulates fatty acid oxidation [most likely by activating carnitine Opalmitoyltransferase-1 (CPT1); ref.[107]]. This, in turn, seems to contribute to the reduction of neuropeptide Y expression in the hypothalamus [97, 106]. Based on these issues, we explored a second-generation drug, C93, which was designed to specifically inhibit FAS without affecting CPT1 activity [108]. Antineoplastic activity, without anorectic effects, can be achieved with this drug by selective pharmacologic inhibition of FAS without stimulation of CPT1, and we demonstrated effective treatment of mice bearing xenografts of the Colo680N squamous cell esophageal cancer cell line using this drug (figure4). Other animal experiments have also found C93 to work well for treatment of cancer xenografts in a variety of other tumor types [98, 109-112], and encouraging results have been seen in cancer chemoprevention experiments [113, 114].

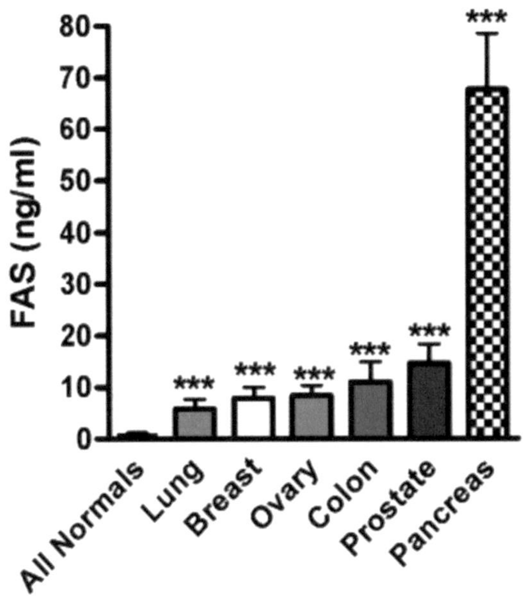

Normals & Cancer	*n*	Average FAS (ng/ml)	Standard Error	p Value (normals)
All Normals	119	0.97	0.18	n.a.
Lung	11	5.76	1.84	p<0.0001
Breast	12	7.85	2.21	p<0.0001
Ovary	13	8.39	1.93	p<0.0001
Colon	10	11.05	3.83	p<0.0001
Prostate	13	14.6	3.68	p<0.0001
Pancreas	20	67.7	10.82	p<0.0001

Fig. 2. **FAS-detect™ IHC serum levels in normal individuals and cancer patients.**

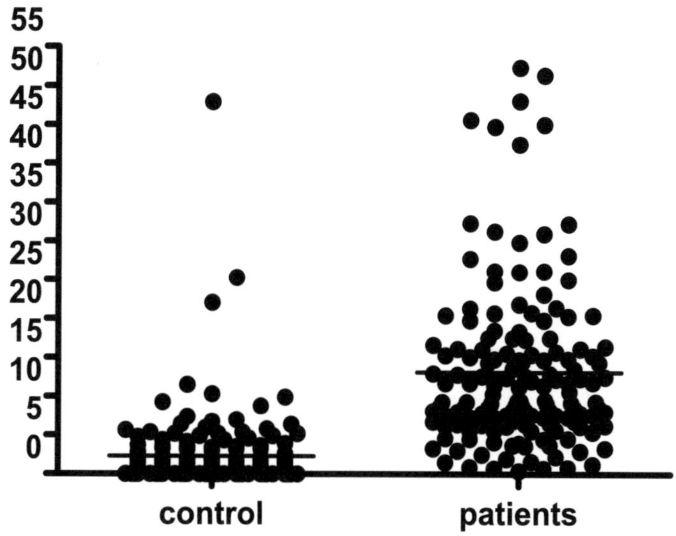

Fig. 3. **Serum FAS level in Esophageal cancer patients are significantly higher than control.**

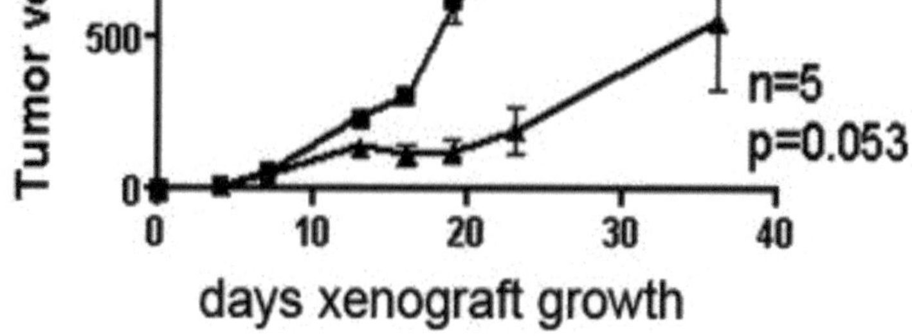

Fig. 4. **Treatment of esophageal cancer xenografts with C93.**

Growth facter
Epidermal growth factor receptor
Her-2/Neu
TKIs
Angiogenesis
Vascular endothelial growth factor
Metabolism target
Metformin
Fatty acid synthase

Table 1. Esophageal cancer: potential targets and markers.

6. Conclusions

In summary, it is well accepted that new targeted drug therapies need to be developed for advanced esophageal cancer due to the poor prognosis of this type of cancer. In this chapter, we have described the current clinical trial molecule targeted agents and metabolic pathways as targets for cancer therapy in esophageal cancer.

Most obviously, high expression levels of EGFR and VGFR in esophageal cancer make antibodies directed against these molecules logical choices for clinical testing. Several phase II studies are now assessing the efficacy of these agents in combination with standard therapy for treatment of esophageal cancer.

Already, the combination of bevacizumab and cetuximab/Panitumumab for patients with metastatic colorectal cancer has shown meaningful clinical benefit, and significant numbers of patients are experiencing prolonged survival with a reasonable quality of life due to these new agents. Within the coming years, several clinical trials will be completed to evaluate these agents for treatment of esophageal cancer. In Head and neck cancer, Cetuximab has also shown efficacy in the treatment. Because of many expressions, we expect this drug for improvement for the treatment of esophageal cancer.

Drugs targeting cellular metabolic pathways are also now attracting great attention for chemotherapy and chemoprevention. In this review, we have described the possibility of metformin for treatment of esophageal cancer based in part on evidence that diabetic patients have increased risks for developing many different types of cancers and clinical data indicating that diabetic patients taking metformin have improved responses to chemotherapy. Finally, fatty acid synthase (FAS) as a novel target for treatment of esophageal cancer was discussed. While clinical data is not yet available for anti-FAS therapy, promising preclinical data warrants attention to this area of investigation.

7. Acknowledgements

Declaration of personal and funding interests: None.

8. References

[1] Eslick, G.D., *Epidemiology of esophageal cancer.* Gastroenterology clinics of North America, 2009. 38(1): p. 17-25, vii.

[2] Herszenyi, L. and Z. Tulassay, *Epidemiology of gastrointestinal and liver tumors.* European review for medical and pharmacological sciences, 2010. 14(4): p. 249-58.

[3] Corley, D.A. and P.A. Buffler, *Oesophageal and gastric cardia adenocarcinomas: analysis of regional variation using the Cancer Incidence in Five Continents database.* International journal of epidemiology, 2001. 30(6): p. 1415-25.

[4] Shimada, H. and T. Ochiai, *Gene therapy for esophageal squamous cell carcinoma.* Frontiers in bioscience : a journal and virtual library, 2008. 13: p. 3364-72.

[5] Herbst, R.S., *Review of epidermal growth factor receptor biology.* International journal of radiation oncology, biology, physics, 2004. 59(2 Suppl): p. 21-6.

[6] Carpenter, G., et al., *Characterization of the binding of 125-I-labeled epidermal growth factor to human fibroblasts.* The Journal of biological chemistry, 1975. 250(11): p. 4297-304.

[7] Rothenberg, M.L., et al., *Randomized phase II trial of the clinical and biological effects of two dose levels of gefitinib in patients with recurrent colorectal adenocarcinoma.* Journal of clinical oncology : official journal of the American Society of Clinical Oncology, 2005. 23(36): p. 9265-74.

[8] Yu, W.W., et al., *Clinicopathological and prognostic significance of EGFR over-expression in esophageal squamous cell carcinoma: a meta-analysis.* Hepato-gastroenterology, 2011. 58(106): p. 426-31.

[9] Cronin, J., et al., *Epidermal growth factor receptor (EGFR) is overexpressed in high-grade dysplasia and adenocarcinoma of the esophagus and may represent a biomarker of histological progression in Barrett's esophagus (BE).* The American journal of gastroenterology, 2011. 106(1): p. 46-56.

[10] Friess, H., et al., *Concomitant analysis of the epidermal growth factor receptor family in esophageal cancer: overexpression of epidermal growth factor receptor mRNA but not of c-erbB-2 and c-erbB-3.* World journal of surgery, 1999. 23(10): p. 1010-8.

[11] Laskin, J.J. and A.B. Sandler, *Epidermal growth factor receptor: a promising target in solid tumours.* Cancer treatment reviews, 2004. 30(1): p. 1-17.

[12] Scagliotti, G.V., et al., *The biology of epidermal growth factor receptor in lung cancer.* Clinical cancer research : an official journal of the American Association for Cancer Research, 2004. 10(12 Pt 2): p. 4227s-4232s.

[13] Ang, K.K., et al., *Impact of epidermal growth factor receptor expression on survival and pattern of relapse in patients with advanced head and neck carcinoma.* Cancer research, 2002. 62(24): p. 7350-6.

[14] Gibault, L., et al., *Diffuse EGFR staining is associated with reduced overall survival in locally advanced oesophageal squamous cell cancer.* British journal of cancer, 2005. 93(1): p. 107-15.

[15] Hirsch, F.R., et al., *Epidermal growth factor receptor in non-small-cell lung carcinomas: correlation between gene copy number and protein expression and impact on prognosis.* Journal of clinical oncology : official journal of the American Society of Clinical Oncology, 2003. 21(20): p. 3798-807.

[16] Chung, C.H., et al., *Increased epidermal growth factor receptor gene copy number is associated with poor prognosis in head and neck squamous cell carcinomas.* Journal of clinical oncology : official journal of the American Society of Clinical Oncology, 2006. 24(25): p. 4170-6.
[17] Baselga, J., *Monoclonal antibodies directed at growth factor receptors.* Annals of oncology : official journal of the European Society for Medical Oncology / ESMO, 2000. 11 Suppl 3: p. 187-90.
[18] Cunningham, D., et al., *Cetuximab monotherapy and cetuximab plus irinotecan in irinotecan-refractory metastatic colorectal cancer.* The New England journal of medicine, 2004. 351(4): p. 337-45.
[19] Saltz, L.B., et al., *Phase II trial of cetuximab in patients with refractory colorectal cancer that expresses the epidermal growth factor receptor.* Journal of clinical oncology : official journal of the American Society of Clinical Oncology, 2004. 22(7): p. 1201-8.
[20] Cohen, R.B., *Epidermal growth factor receptor as a therapeutic target in colorectal cancer.* Clinical colorectal cancer, 2003. 2(4): p. 246-51.
[21] Joy, A.A. and C.A. Butts, *Extending outcomes: epidermal growth factor receptor-targeted monoclonal antibodies in non-small-cell lung cancer.* Clinical lung cancer, 2009. 10 Suppl 1: p. S24-9.
[22] Chung, C.H., et al., *Detection of tumor epidermal growth factor receptor pathway dependence by serum mass spectrometry in cancer patients.* Cancer epidemiology, biomarkers & prevention : a publication of the American Association for Cancer Research, cosponsored by the American Society of Preventive Oncology, 2010. 19(2): p. 358-65.
[23] Ibrahim, E.M., et al., *Cetuximab-based Therapy is Effective in Chemotherapy-naive Patients with Advanced and Metastatic Non-small-cell Lung Cancer: A Meta-analysis of Randomized Controlled Trials.* Lung, 2011. 189(3): p. 193-8.
[24] Stinchcombe, T.E. and M.A. Socinski, *Targeted therapies: Biomarkers in NSCLC for selecting cetuximab therapy.* Nature reviews. Clinical oncology, 2010. 7(8): p. 426-8.
[25] Ademuyiwa, F.O. and N. Hanna, *Cetuximab in non-small cell lung cancer.* Expert opinion on biological therapy, 2008. 8(1): p. 107-13.
[26] Bonner, J.A., et al., *Epidermal growth factor receptor as a therapeutic target in head and neck cancer.* Seminars in radiation oncology, 2002. 12(3 Suppl 2): p. 11-20.
[27] Licitra, L., et al., *Role of EGFR family receptors in proliferation of squamous carcinoma cells induced by wound healing fluids of head and neck cancer patients.* Annals of oncology : official journal of the European Society for Medical Oncology / ESMO, 2011.
[28] Smith, D., C. Bosacki, and Y. Merrouche, *[Use of anti-EGFR antibodies (cetuximab and panitumumab) in the treatment of metastatic colorectal cancer in KRAS wild type patients].* Bulletin du cancer, 2009. 96 Suppl: p. S31-40.
[29] Russo, A., et al., *The long and winding road to useful predictive factors for anti-EGFR therapy in metastatic colorectal carcinoma: the KRAS/BRAF pathway.* Oncology, 2009. 77 Suppl 1: p. 57-68.
[30] Lopez-Gomez, M., et al., *Different patterns of toxicity after sequential administration of two anti-EGFR monoclonal antibodies.* Clinical & translational oncology : official

publication of the Federation of Spanish Oncology Societies and of the National Cancer Institute of Mexico, 2010. 12(11): p. 775-7.

[31] Rother, M., *Impact of a pre-emptive skin treatment regimen on skin toxicities of anti-epidermal growth factor receptor monoclonal antibodies: more questions than answers.* Journal of clinical oncology : official journal of the American Society of Clinical Oncology, 2010. 28(27): p. e474; author reply e475-6.

[32] Zhang, W., M. Gordon, and H.J. Lenz, *Novel approaches to treatment of advanced colorectal cancer with anti-EGFR monoclonal antibodies.* Annals of medicine, 2006. 38(8): p. 545-51.

[33] Benvenuti, S., et al., *Oncogenic activation of the RAS/RAF signaling pathway impairs the response of metastatic colorectal cancers to anti-epidermal growth factor receptor antibody therapies.* Cancer research, 2007. 67(6): p. 2643-8.

[34] Karapetis, C.S., et al., *K-ras mutations and benefit from cetuximab in advanced colorectal cancer.* The New England journal of medicine, 2008. 359(17): p. 1757-65.

[35] Amado, R.G., et al., *Wild-type KRAS is required for panitumumab efficacy in patients with metastatic colorectal cancer.* Journal of clinical oncology : official journal of the American Society of Clinical Oncology, 2008. 26(10): p. 1626-34.

[36] Markman, B., et al., *EGFR and KRAS in colorectal cancer.* Advances in clinical chemistry, 2010. 51: p. 71-119.

[37] De Vita, F., et al., *A multicenter phase II study of induction chemotherapy with FOLFOX-4 and cetuximab followed by radiation and cetuximab in locally advanced oesophageal cancer.* British journal of cancer, 2011. 104(3): p. 427-32.

[38] Gold, P.J., et al., *Cetuximab as second-line therapy in patients with metastatic esophageal adenocarcinoma: a phase II Southwest Oncology Group Study (S0415).* Journal of thoracic oncology : official publication of the International Association for the Study of Lung Cancer, 2010. 5(9): p. 1472-6.

[39] Lorenzen, S., et al., *Cetuximab plus cisplatin-5-fluorouracil versus cisplatin-5-fluorouracil alone in first-line metastatic squamous cell carcinoma of the esophagus: a randomized phase II study of the Arbeitsgemeinschaft Internistische Onkologie.* Annals of oncology : official journal of the European Society for Medical Oncology / ESMO, 2009. 20(10): p. 1667-73.

[40] Janmaat, M.L., et al., *Predictive factors for outcome in a phase II study of gefitinib in second-line treatment of advanced esophageal cancer patients.* Journal of clinical oncology : official journal of the American Society of Clinical Oncology, 2006. 24(10): p. 1612-9.

[41] Zhao, Y., et al., *Preclinical evaluation of a potent novel DNA-dependent protein kinase inhibitor NU7441.* Cancer research, 2006. 66(10): p. 5354-62.

[42] Mok, T.S., et al., *Randomized, placebo-controlled, phase II study of sequential erlotinib and chemotherapy as first-line treatment for advanced non-small-cell lung cancer.* Journal of clinical oncology : official journal of the American Society of Clinical Oncology, 2009. 27(30): p. 5080-7.

[43] Rodriguez, C.P., et al., *A phase II study of perioperative concurrent chemotherapy, gefitinib, and hyperfractionated radiation followed by maintenance gefitinib in locoregionally advanced esophagus and gastroesophageal junction cancer.* Journal of thoracic oncology :

official publication of the International Association for the Study of Lung Cancer, 2010. 5(2): p. 229-35.
[44] Altiok, S., et al., *A novel pharmacodynamic approach to assess and predict tumor response to the epidermal growth factor receptor inhibitor gefitinib in patients with esophageal cancer.* International journal of oncology, 2010. 36(1): p. 19-27.
[45] Ilson, D.H., et al., *A phase 2 trial of erlotinib in patients with previously treated squamous cell and adenocarcinoma of the esophagus.* Cancer, 2011. 117(7): p. 1409-14.
[46] Burris, H.A., 3rd, *Dual kinase inhibition in the treatment of breast cancer: initial experience with the EGFR/ErbB-2 inhibitor lapatinib.* The oncologist, 2004. 9 Suppl 3: p. 10-5.
[47] Higa, G.M. and J. Abraham, *Lapatinib in the treatment of breast cancer.* Expert review of anticancer therapy, 2007. 7(9): p. 1183-92.
[48] Bouchalova, K., et al., *Triple negative breast cancer--current status and prospective targeted treatment based on HER1 (EGFR), TOP2A and C-MYC gene assessment.* Biomedical papers of the Medical Faculty of the University Palacky, Olomouc, Czechoslovakia, 2009. 153(1): p. 13-7.
[49] Hurvitz, S.A. and R.S. Finn, *What's positive about 'triple-negative' breast cancer?* Future oncology, 2009. 5(7): p. 1015-25.
[50] Hector, A., et al., *The Axl receptor tyrosine kinase is an adverse prognostic factor and a therapeutic target in esophageal adenocarcinoma.* Cancer biology & therapy, 2010. 10(10): p. 1009-18.
[51] Hung, M.C. and Y.K. Lau, *Basic science of HER-2/neu: a review.* Seminars in oncology, 1999. 26(4 Suppl 12): p. 51-9.
[52] Coussens, L., et al., *Tyrosine kinase receptor with extensive homology to EGF receptor shares chromosomal location with neu oncogene.* Science, 1985. 230(4730): p. 1132-9.
[53] Lee, K.F., et al., *Requirement for neuregulin receptor erbB2 in neural and cardiac development.* Nature, 1995. 378(6555): p. 394-8.
[54] Crone, S.A., et al., *ErbB2 is essential in the prevention of dilated cardiomyopathy.* Nature medicine, 2002. 8(5): p. 459-65.
[55] Olayioye, M.A., *Update on HER-2 as a target for cancer therapy: intracellular signaling pathways of ErbB2/HER-2 and family members.* Breast cancer research : BCR, 2001. 3(6): p. 385-9.
[56] Jung, S.Y., et al., *Worse prognosis of metaplastic breast cancer patients than other patients with triple-negative breast cancer.* Breast cancer research and treatment, 2010. 120(3): p. 627-37.
[57] Kim, K.C., et al., *Evaluation of HER2 Protein Expression in Gastric Carcinomas: Comparative Analysis of 1414 Cases of Whole-Tissue Sections and 595 Cases of Tissue Microarrays.* Annals of surgical oncology, 2011.
[58] Lin, C.K., et al., *Assessing the Impact of Polysomy-17 on HER2 Status and the Correlations of HER2 Status With Prognostic Variables (ER, PR, p53, Ki-67) in Epithelial Ovarian Cancer: A Tissue Microarray Study Using Immunohistochemistry and Fluorescent In Situ Hybridization.* International journal of gynecological pathology : official journal of the International Society of Gynecological Pathologists, 2011. 30(4): p. 372-379.

[59] Stoecklein, N.H., et al., *Copy number of chromosome 17 but not HER2 amplification predicts clinical outcome of patients with pancreatic ductal adenocarcinoma.* Journal of clinical oncology : official journal of the American Society of Clinical Oncology, 2004. 22(23): p. 4737-45.

[60] Yamanaka, Y., et al., *Overexpression of HER2/neu oncogene in human pancreatic carcinoma.* Human pathology, 1993. 24(10): p. 1127-34.

[61] Yentz, S. and T.D. Wang, *Molecular imaging for guiding oncologic prognosis and therapy in esophageal adenocarcinoma.* Hospital practice, 2011. 39(2): p. 97-106.

[62] Safran, H., et al., *Phase I/II study of trastuzumab, paclitaxel, cisplatin and radiation for locally advanced, HER2 overexpressing, esophageal adenocarcinoma.* International journal of radiation oncology, biology, physics, 2007. 67(2): p. 405-9.

[63] Szentirmay, Z., *[Effect of learning about the human genome on the development of pathology].* Orvosi hetilap, 2003. 144(51): p. 2499-508.

[64] Wei, Q., et al., *EGFR, HER2 and HER3 expression in esophageal primary tumours and corresponding metastases.* International journal of oncology, 2007. 31(3): p. 493-9.

[65] Zhan, N., et al., *Analysis of HER2 gene amplification and protein expression in esophageal squamous cell carcinoma.* Medical oncology, 2011.

[66] Baselga, J., et al., *Phase II study of weekly intravenous recombinant humanized anti-p185HER2 monoclonal antibody in patients with HER2/neu-overexpressing metastatic breast cancer.* Journal of clinical oncology : official journal of the American Society of Clinical Oncology, 1996. 14(3): p. 737-44.

[67] Slamon, D.J., et al., *Use of chemotherapy plus a monoclonal antibody against HER2 for metastatic breast cancer that overexpresses HER2.* The New England journal of medicine, 2001. 344(11): p. 783-92.

[68] Le, X.F., F. Pruefer, and R.C. Bast, Jr., *HER2-targeting antibodies modulate the cyclin-dependent kinase inhibitor p27Kip1 via multiple signaling pathways.* Cell cycle, 2005. 4(1): p. 87-95.

[69] Bang, Y.J., et al., *Trastuzumab in combination with chemotherapy versus chemotherapy alone for treatment of HER2-positive advanced gastric or gastro-oesophageal junction cancer (ToGA): a phase 3, open-label, randomised controlled trial.* Lancet, 2010. 376(9742): p. 687-97.

[70] Senger, D.R., et al., *Tumor cells secrete a vascular permeability factor that promotes accumulation of ascites fluid.* Science, 1983. 219(4587): p. 983-5.

[71] Kulke, M.H., et al., *Prognostic significance of vascular endothelial growth factor and cyclooxygenase 2 expression in patients receiving preoperative chemoradiation for esophageal cancer.* The Journal of thoracic and cardiovascular surgery, 2004. 127(6): p. 1579-86.

[72] Coughlin, S.S., et al., *Diabetes mellitus as a predictor of cancer mortality in a large cohort of US adults.* American journal of epidemiology, 2004. 159(12): p. 1160-7.

[73] Levine, W., et al., *Post-load plasma glucose and cancer mortality in middle-aged men and women. 12-year follow-up findings of the Chicago Heart Association Detection Project in Industry.* American journal of epidemiology, 1990. 131(2): p. 254-62.

[74] Saydah, S.H., et al., *Abnormal glucose tolerance and the risk of cancer death in the United States.* American journal of epidemiology, 2003. 157(12): p. 1092-100.

[75] Steevens, J., et al., *A prospective cohort study on overweight, smoking, alcohol consumption, and risk of Barrett's esophagus.* Cancer epidemiology, biomarkers & prevention : a publication of the American Association for Cancer Research, cosponsored by the American Society of Preventive Oncology, 2011. 20(2): p. 345-58.

[76] Bechade, D., et al., *[Review of the association between obesity and gastroesophageal reflux and its complications].* Gastroenterologie clinique et biologique, 2009. 33(3): p. 155-66.

[77] El-Serag, H., *The association between obesity and GERD: a review of the epidemiological evidence.* Digestive diseases and sciences, 2008. 53(9): p. 2307-12.

[78] Lee, M.S., et al., *Type 2 diabetes increases and metformin reduces total, colorectal, liver and pancreatic cancer incidences in Taiwanese: a representative population prospective cohort study of 800,000 individuals.* BMC cancer, 2011. 11: p. 20.

[79] Guh, D.P., et al., *The incidence of co-morbidities related to obesity and overweight: a systematic review and meta-analysis.* BMC public health, 2009. 9: p. 88.

[80] Cheng, K.K., et al., *A case-control study of oesophageal adenocarcinoma in women: a preventable disease.* British journal of cancer, 2000. 83(1): p. 127-32.

[81] Rubenstein, J.H., et al., *Relationship between diabetes mellitus and adenocarcinoma of the oesophagus and gastric cardia.* Alimentary pharmacology & therapeutics, 2005. 22(3): p. 267-71.

[82] Neale, R.E., et al., *Does type 2 diabetes influence the risk of oesophageal adenocarcinoma?* British journal of cancer, 2009. 100(5): p. 795-8.

[83] Yang, Y.X., *Do diabetes drugs modify the risk of pancreatic cancer?* Gastroenterology, 2009. 137(2): p. 412-5.

[84] Yang, Y.X., S. Hennessy, and J.D. Lewis, *Insulin therapy and colorectal cancer risk among type 2 diabetes mellitus patients.* Gastroenterology, 2004. 127(4): p. 1044-50.

[85] Chong, C.R. and B.A. Chabner, *Mysterious metformin.* The oncologist, 2009. 14(12): p. 1178-81.

[86] Nathan, D.M., et al., *Medical management of hyperglycemia in type 2 diabetes: a consensus algorithm for the initiation and adjustment of therapy: a consensus statement of the American Diabetes Association and the European Association for the Study of Diabetes.* Diabetes care, 2009. 32(1): p. 193-203.

[87] Evans, J.M., et al., *Metformin and reduced risk of cancer in diabetic patients.* BMJ, 2005. 330(7503): p. 1304-5.

[88] Bowker, S.L., et al., *Increased cancer-related mortality for patients with type 2 diabetes who use sulfonylureas or insulin.* Diabetes care, 2006. 29(2): p. 254-8.

[89] Zhou, K., et al., *Common variants near ATM are associated with glycemic response to metformin in type 2 diabetes.* Nature genetics, 2011. 43(2): p. 117-20.

[90] Lizcano, J.M., et al., *LKB1 is a master kinase that activates 13 kinases of the AMPK subfamily, including MARK/PAR-1.* The EMBO journal, 2004. 23(4): p. 833-43.

[91] Jiralerspong, S., et al., *Metformin and pathologic complete responses to neoadjuvant chemotherapy in diabetic patients with breast cancer.* Journal of clinical oncology : official journal of the American Society of Clinical Oncology, 2009. 27(20): p. 3297-302.

[92] Hirsch, H.A., et al., *Metformin selectively targets cancer stem cells, and acts together with chemotherapy to block tumor growth and prolong remission.* Cancer research, 2009. 69(19): p. 7507-11.

[93] 93. Kuhajda, F.P., *Fatty-acid synthase and human cancer: new perspectives on its role in tumor biology.* Nutrition, 2000. 16(3): p. 202-8.

[94] Nemoto, T., et al., *Overexpression of fatty acid synthase in oesophageal squamous cell dysplasia and carcinoma.* Pathobiology : journal of immunopathology, molecular and cellular biology, 2001. 69(6): p. 297-303.

[95] Weiss, L., et al., *Fatty-acid biosynthesis in man, a pathway of minor importance. Purification, optimal assay conditions, and organ distribution of fatty-acid synthase.* Biological chemistry Hoppe-Seyler, 1986. 367(9): p. 905-12.

[96] Ishimura, N., et al., *Fatty Acid Synthase Expression in Barrett's Esophagus: Implications for Carcinogenesis.* Journal of clinical gastroenterology, 2011.

[97] Crispino, P., et al., *Evaluation of fatty acid synthase expression in oesophageal mucosa of patients with oesophagitis, Barrett's oesophagus and adenocarcinoma.* Journal of cancer research and clinical oncology, 2009. 135(11): p. 1533-41.

[98] Orita, H., et al., *High levels of fatty acid synthase expression in esophageal cancers represent a potential target for therapy.* Cancer biology & therapy, 2010. 10(6): p. 549-54.

[99] De Schrijver, E., et al., *RNA interference-mediated silencing of the fatty acid synthase gene attenuates growth and induces morphological changes and apoptosis of LNCaP prostate cancer cells.* Cancer research, 2003. 63(13): p. 3799-804.

[100] Kridel, S.J., et al., *Orlistat is a novel inhibitor of fatty acid synthase with antitumor activity.* Cancer research, 2004. 64(6): p. 2070-5.

[101] Kuhajda, F.P., et al., *Fatty acid synthesis: a potential selective target for antineoplastic therapy.* Proceedings of the National Academy of Sciences of the United States of America, 1994. 91(14): p. 6379-83.

[102] Kuhajda, F.P., et al., *Synthesis and antitumor activity of an inhibitor of fatty acid synthase.* Proceedings of the National Academy of Sciences of the United States of America, 2000. 97(7): p. 3450-4.

[103] Gabrielson, E.W., et al., *Increased fatty acid synthase is a therapeutic target in mesothelioma.* Clinical cancer research : an official journal of the American Association for Cancer Research, 2001. 7(1): p. 153-7.

[104] Pizer, E.S., et al., *Increased fatty acid synthase as a therapeutic target in androgen-independent prostate cancer progression.* The Prostate, 2001. 47(2): p. 102-10.

[105] Wang, H.Q., et al., *Positive feedback regulation between AKT activation and fatty acid synthase expression in ovarian carcinoma cells.* Oncogene, 2005. 24(22): p. 3574-82.

[106] Loftus, T.M., et al., *Reduced food intake and body weight in mice treated with fatty acid synthase inhibitors.* Science, 2000. 288(5475): p. 2379-81.

[107] Thupari, J.N., et al., *C75 increases peripheral energy utilization and fatty acid oxidation in diet-induced obesity.* Proceedings of the National Academy of Sciences of the United States of America, 2002. 99(14): p. 9498-502.

[108] McFadden, J.M., et al., *Application of a flexible synthesis of (5R)-thiolactomycin to develop new inhibitors of type I fatty acid synthase.* Journal of medicinal chemistry, 2005. 48(4): p. 946-61.

[109] Orita, H., et al., *Selective inhibition of fatty acid synthase for lung cancer treatment.* Clinical cancer research : an official journal of the American Association for Cancer Research, 2007. 13(23): p. 7139-45.

[110] Ueda, S.M., et al., *Trophoblastic neoplasms express fatty acid synthase, which may be a therapeutic target via its inhibitor C93.* The American journal of pathology, 2009. 175(6): p. 2618-24.

[111] Ueda, S.M., et al., *Expression of Fatty Acid Synthase Depends on NAC1 and Is Associated with Recurrent Ovarian Serous Carcinomas.* Journal of oncology, 2010. 2010: p. 285191.

[112] Zhou, W., et al., *Fatty acid synthase inhibition activates AMP-activated protein kinase in SKOV3 human ovarian cancer cells.* Cancer research, 2007. 67(7): p. 2964-71.

[113] Orita, H., et al., *Inhibiting fatty acid synthase for chemoprevention of chemically induced lung tumors.* Clinical cancer research : an official journal of the American Association for Cancer Research, 2008. 14(8): p. 2458-64.

[114] Alli, P.M., et al., *Fatty acid synthase inhibitors are chemopreventive for mammary cancer in neu-N transgenic mice.* Oncogene, 2005. 24(1): p. 39-46.

10

Multiple Early-Stage Malignant Melanoma of the Esophagus with a Long Follow-Up Period After Endoscopic Treatment: Report of a Case and a Literature Review

Shin'ichi Miyamoto, Shuko Morita and Manabu Muto
Department of Gastroenterology and Hepatology, Graduate School of Medicine, Kyoto University, Sakyo, Kyoto, Japan

1. Introduction

Primary malignant melanoma of the esophagus (PMME) accounts for 0.1–0.2% of all malignant disease of the esophagus. Ninety-five percent of all melanomas are found in the derma, and only 0.5% are localized in the esophagus (Bisceglia et al. 2011). The prognosis of PMME is unfavorable because most patients are in the advanced stage at diagnosis and rapidly develop lymph node and distant metastases. Nine cases of early-stage PMME have been reported in eight papers (Minami et al. 2011; Miyatani et al. 2009; Morita et al. 2009; Suzuki et al. 2008; Kimura et al. 2005; Hara et al. 2003; Mikami et al. 2001; Kido et al. 2000). Only two of them were treated curatively by endoscopic mucosal resection (EMR) (Miyatani et al. 2009; Kimura et al. 2005). We now report on a rare case of multiple early-stage PMME, which could obtain prolonged survival for ten years by the combination of systemic chemotherapy, repeated endoscopic treatment, and transarterial chemoembolization.

2. Case report

A 75-year-old previously healthy man underwent an esophagogastroduodenoscopy (EGD) for screening. Three black-pigmented flat lesions were detected in the middle and lower thoracic esophagus (Fig. 1), and biopsy specimens revealed features of malignant melanoma. The patient refused esophagectomy, and endoscopic mucosal resection (EMR) was tried in August 2001. The resected specimen revealed that the tumor had invaded the lamina propria (Fig. 2) with no lymphatic or venous invasion and that the horizontal margin was positive. The patient again refused esophagectomy and was followed up closely in the outpatient clinic.

Five months after the first EMR, a recurrence was suspected near the EMR scar. The patient was referred to our hospital. As an alternative treatment to the esophagectomy, six courses of systemic chemotherapy comprising dacarbazine (100 mg/body on day 1, 200 mg/body on days 2–5), nimustine hydrochloride (100 mg/body on day 1), and vincristine (1 mg/body on day 1) were scheduled every four weeks. However, he was forced to discontinue the

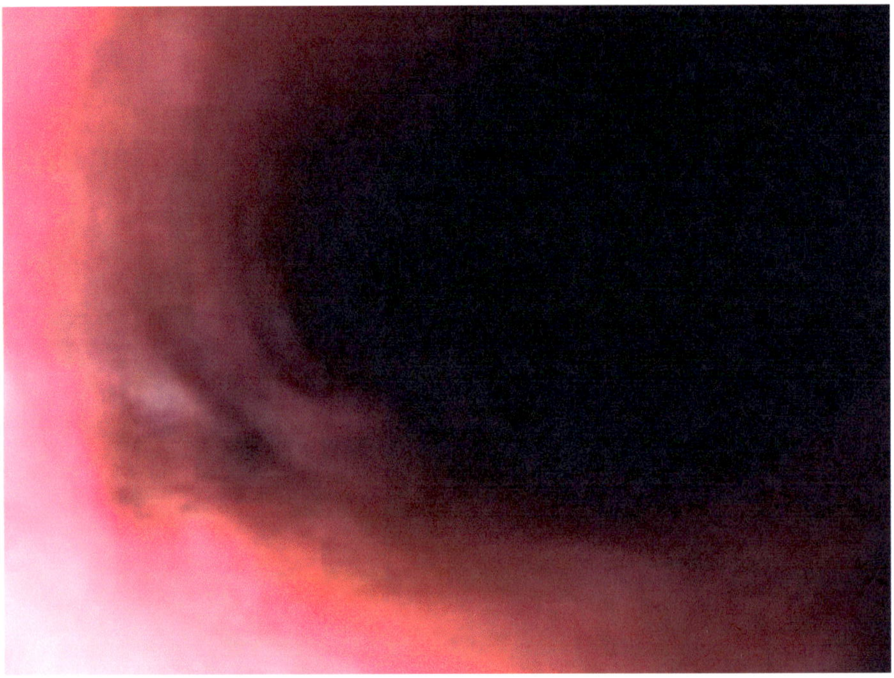

Fig. 1. Esophagogastroduodenoscopy showed a black-pigmented flat lesion in the lower esophagus.

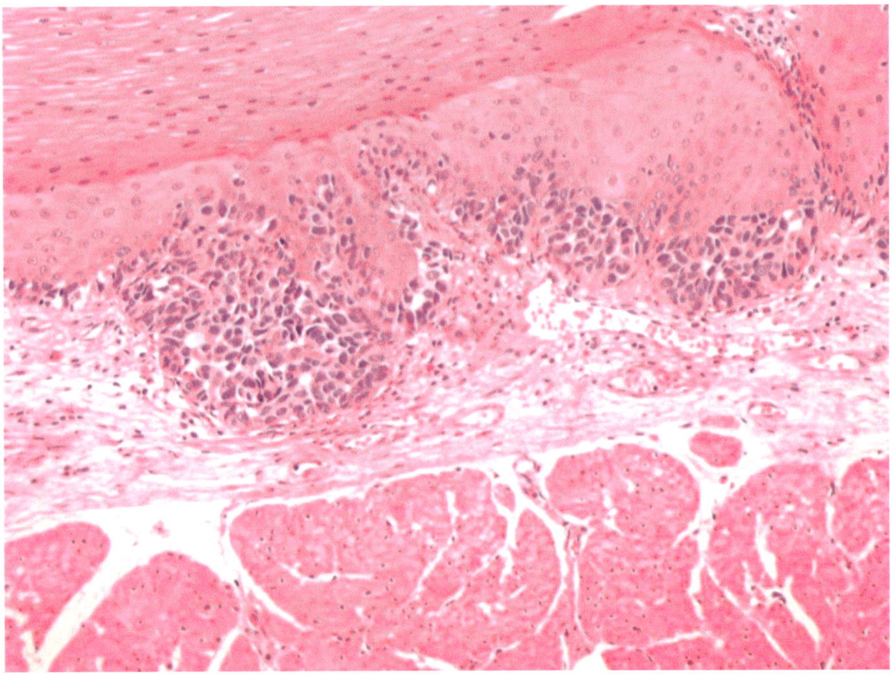

Fig. 2. A specimen from an endoscopic mucosal resection revealed that the melanoma cells had invaded the lamina propria.

treatment after four courses of chemotherapy because of severe thrombocytopenia. He then underwent an EGD every two or three months, and small black-pigmented spots resembling lentigo were detected frequently (Fig. 3). A biopsy specimen revealed the typical histological pattern of melanoma, suggesting metachronous multiple lesions. Because no lymph nodes were involved and no distant metastasis developed, endoscopic treatment including EMR (six times for nine lesions) and tumor ablation using argon plasma coagulation (four times for nine lesions) or bipolar coagulation probe (four times for six lesions) were performed until June 2009. The pathological diagnoses for all EMR specimens were in situ or microinvasive PMME with no lymphatic or venous invasion. Tumor cells were positive for melan A and HMB45 according to immunohistochemistry. A representative case of microinvasive PMME is shown in Fig. 4A and B. Three specimens of nine lesions resected by EMR showed clearly that the black-pigmented area was only part of the whole tumor, and the horizontal margin was positive. A representative horizontal-margin-positive case of PMME is shown in Fig. 5.

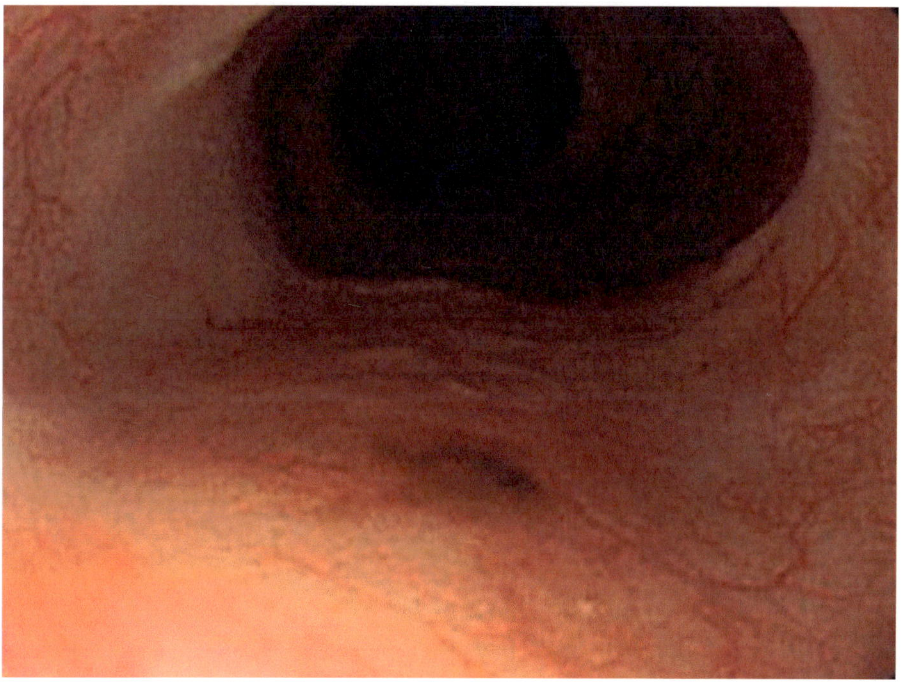

Fig. 3. Small black-pigmented spots resembling lentigo were detected frequently after the initial endoscopic treatment.

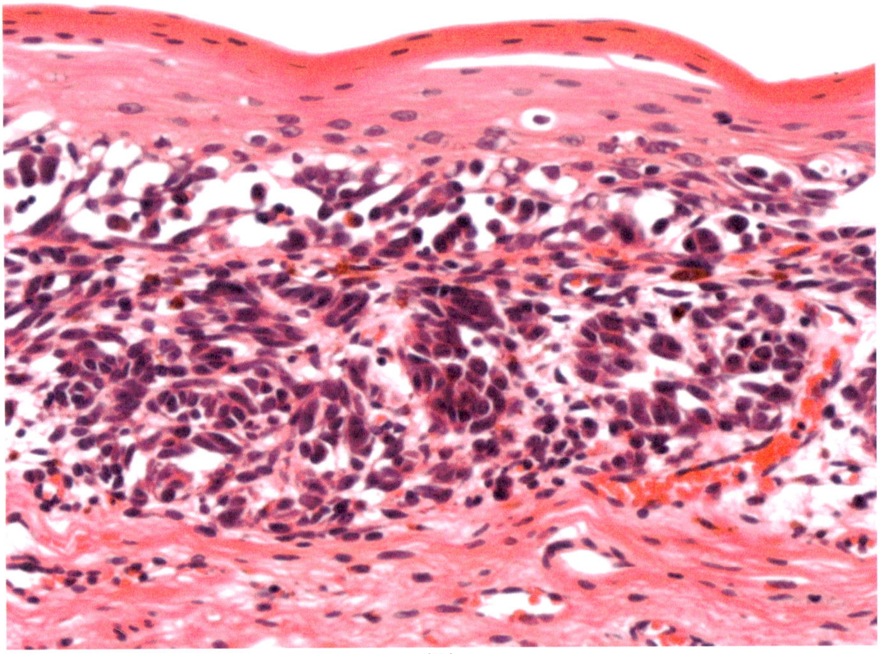

(A)

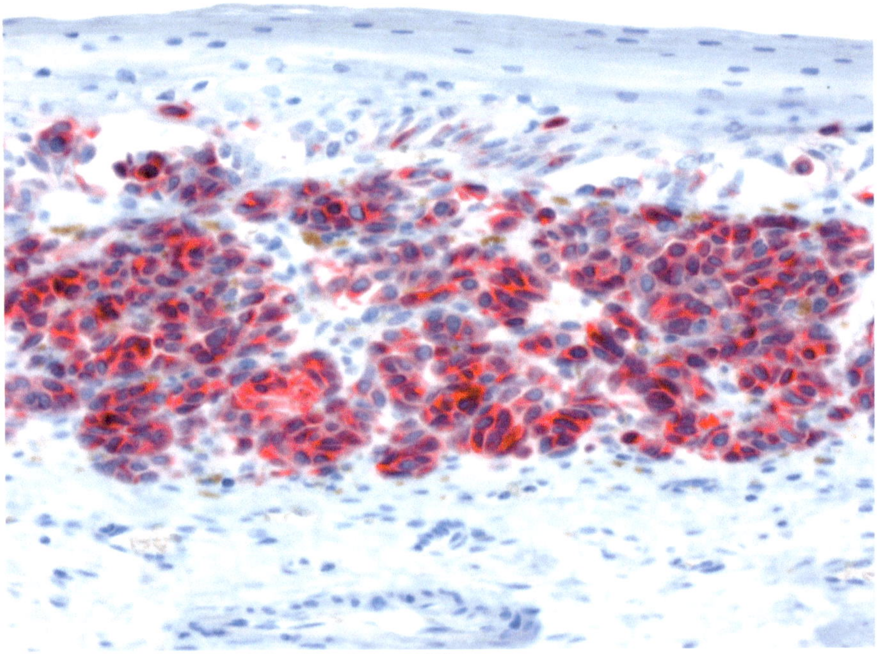

(B)

Fig. 4. A specimen from an endoscopic mucosal resection revealed a histological pattern typical of microinvasive PMME (A) and was immunohistochemically positive for melan A (B). A chromogenic reaction was developed using alkaline phosphatase.

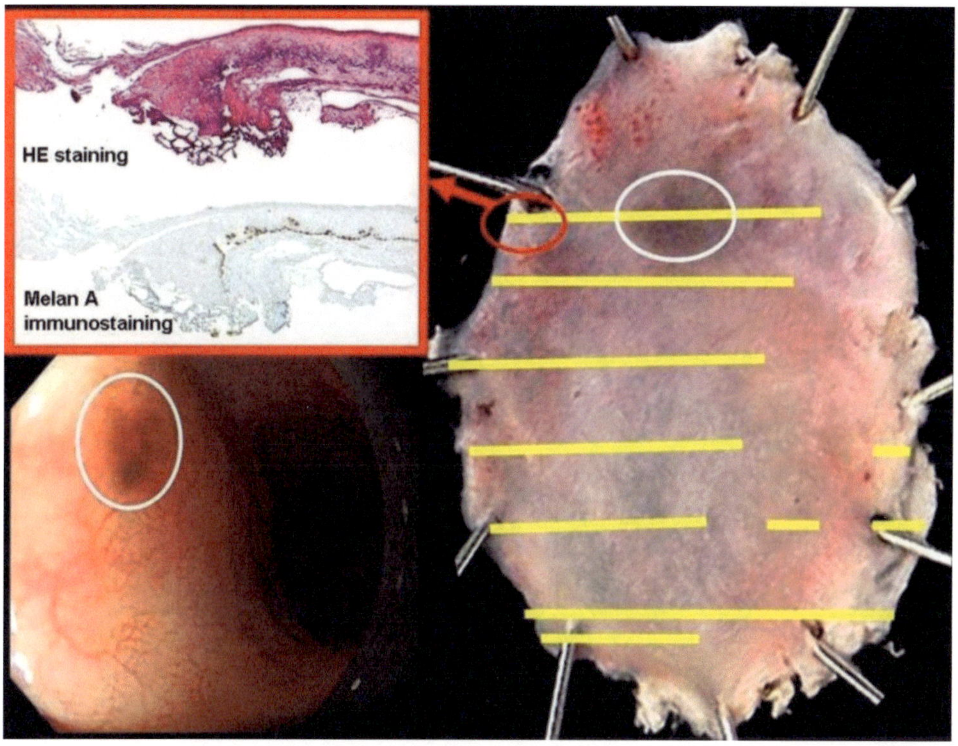

Fig. 5. A specimen from an endoscopic mucosal resection showed that the black-pigmented area was only part of the whole tumor, and the horizontal margin was positive.

Seven years after the first diagnosis of PMME, multiple hepatic tumors (in S4, S6, and S8) were detected by screening abdominal computed tomography (CT) in December 2007 (Fig. 6A). To make a definite diagnosis, a liver needle biopsy was performed in April 2008. The needle biopsy specimens revealed the same histological pattern of PMME (Fig. 6B) and were positive for melan A and HMB45. Then, hepatic metastasis was confirmed. The primary lesion was well controlled, and no other distant metastasis was observed. Because the patient was too old to reintroduce systemic chemotherapy and the dynamic CT image suggested a hypervascular liver tumor, transarterial chemoembolization (TACE) was selected. The hepatic metastases gradually progressed even though he received TACE in June 2008 and April 2010. He died in August 2011 of hepatic failure because of progression of hepatic metastases. The clinical course of this case is summarized in Fig. 7.

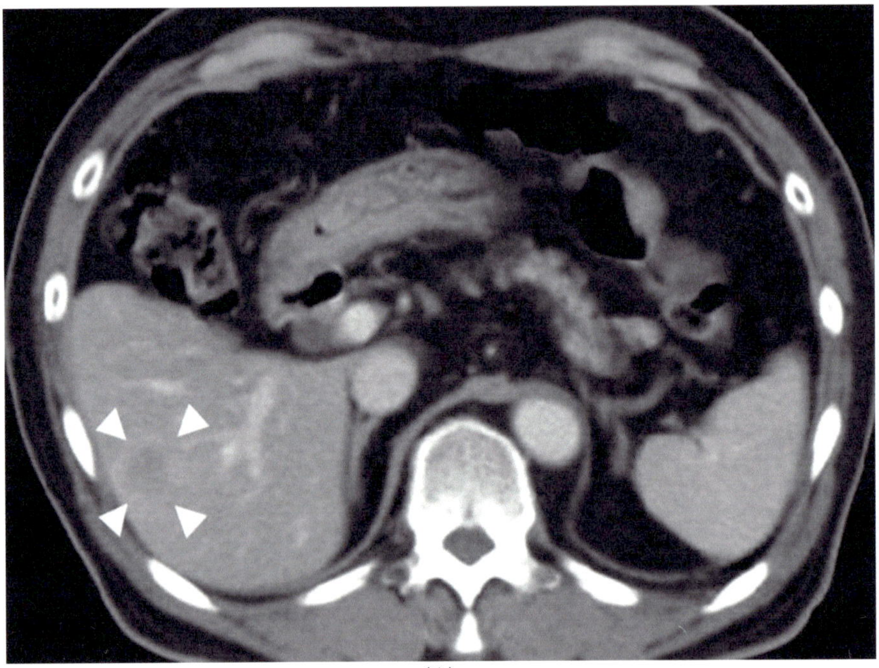

(A)

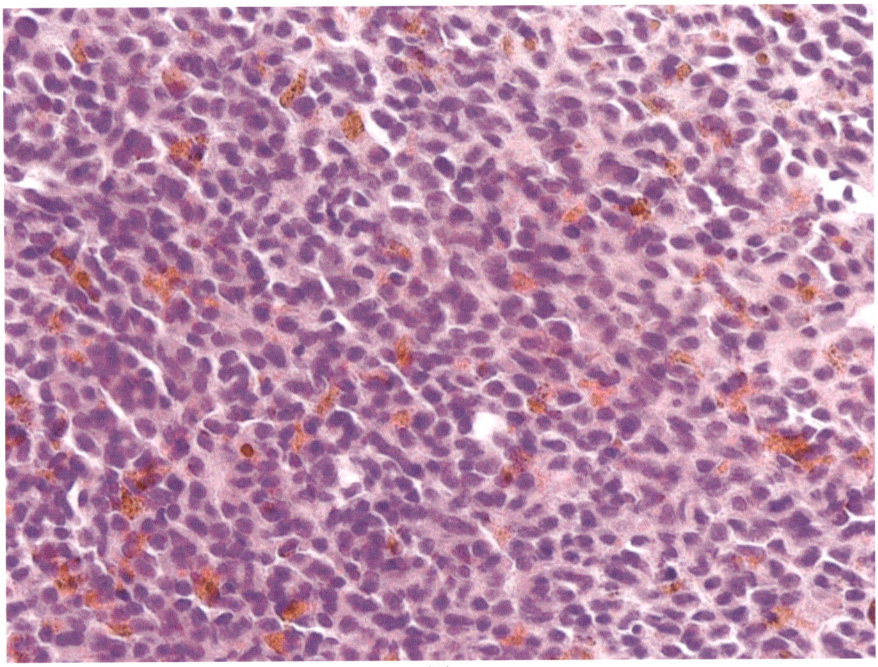

(B)

Fig. 6. (A) Seven years after the first diagnosis, multiple liver tumors were detected by screening abdominal computed tomography (*arrow in S6*). (B) A needle biopsy specimen from the liver tumor revealed a histological pattern typical of malignant melanoma.

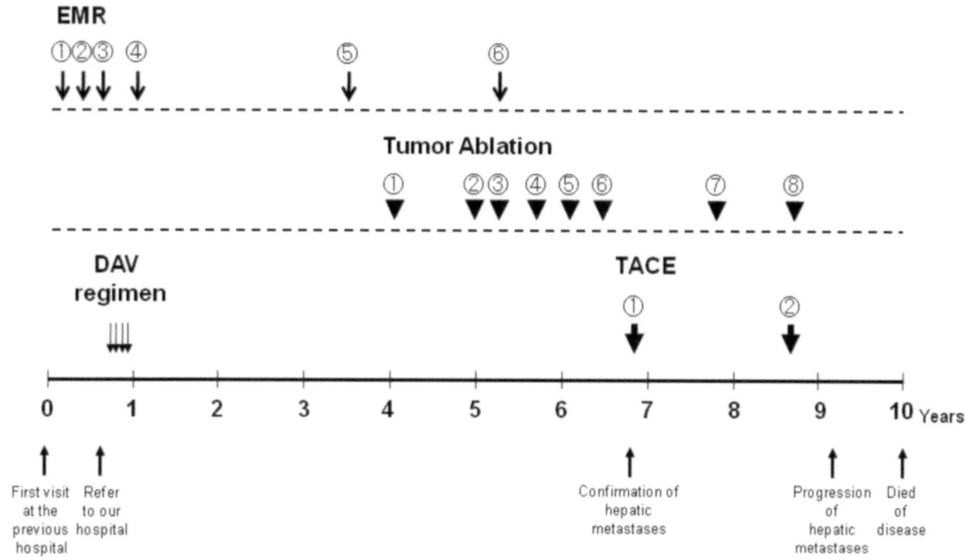

TACE; transarterial chemoembolization
DAV; dacarbazine, nimustine hydrochloride, and vincristine

Fig. 7. Clinical course of this case. Local control of multiple early-stage PMME was achieved mainly by endoscopic treatment (six endoscopic mucosal resections (EMRs) for nine lesions and eight instances of tumor ablation therapy with argon plasma coagulation or a bipolar coagulation probe for 15 lesions).

3. Discussion

The following diagnostic histological criteria for PMME have been suggested by Allen and Spitz (Allen & Spitz. 1953): (1) a typical histological pattern of melanoma and the presence of melanin granules within the tumor cells, (2) origin in an area of junctional change within the squamous epithelium, and (3) junctional activity with melanotic cells in the adjacent epithelium. The melanoma cells were immunohistochemically positive for melan A, HMB45, and S-100 protein. These stains are useful for diagnosing amelanotic melanomas in which the tumor cells show no evident melanin granules (Fenoglio-Preiser et al. 2008).

The prognosis of PMME is extremely poor because of its rapid metastatic spread via the lymphatic and blood vessels. Early death from widespread metastases is the usual clinical course. The average overall survival is only 10–13 months, and only one-third of all patients survive for longer than one year after diagnosis (Bisceglia et al. 2011). Surgical resection is considered the best method for treating PMME (Adili & Moning 1997; Kato et al. 1991; Chalkiadakis et al. 1985; Ludwig et al. 1981). Smaller satellite nodules may present around the main tumor, and wider margins of resection are required for treating PMME than with other esophageal tumors. However, even if only the patients whom undergone radical esophageal resection are analyzed, the five-year survival rate is less than 5% (Simpson et al. 1990; Sabanathan et al. 1989). Therapeutic options such as radiotherapy, chemotherapy, and immunotherapy provide limited benefits, even when used in conjunction with surgery.

Table 1 summarizes nine cases of early-stage PMME previously published in the English literature. This table demonstrates that PMME has a relatively good prognosis as long as it is detected early. However, it remains to be fully elucidated whether these minute lesions are true premalignant lesions of advanced PMME.

Case	Reference	Age/ Gender	Location	Macroscopic type	Number of lesions	Depth of invasion	Treatment	Survival/ Outcome
1	Kido, et al. 2000	60/male	lower	flat	solitary	LPM[a]	surgery	unknown
2	Mikami, et al. 2001	42/female	middle	polypoid	solitary	LPM	surgery+chemotherapy	2y7m[e]/alive
3	Hara, et al. 2003	52/male	middle	flat	solitary	EP[b]	surgery+chemotherapy	1 y3m/alive
4	Kimura, et al. 2005	73/male	lower	flat	solitary	EP	EMR[c]	1y3m/alive
5	Suzuki, et al. 2008	62/male	upper to middle	flat	solitary	EP	surgery	2y9m/alive
6		67/male	lower	flat	solitary	LPM	surgery	4y5m/alive
7*	Morita, et al. 2009	75/male	lower	flat	multiple	LPM	EMR+chemotherapy → TACE[d]	10y/dead
8	Miyatani, et al. 2009	64/female	lower	flat	solitary	LPM	EMR	2y6m/alive
9	Minami, et al. 2011	72/male	lower	flat	solitary	EP	surgery	2y1m/alive

*The same case of this chapter.
[a]LPM, Tumor invades lamina propria muscle; [b]EP, carcinoma in situ; [c]EMR, endoscopic mucosal resection; [d]TACE, transarterial chemoembolization for hepatic metastases
[e]y; year, m; month

Table 1. Features and outcome of early-stage (intramucosal) malignant melanoma of the esophagus published in the literaure.

Endoscopically, PMME lesions appear as intraluminal, polypoid, and (usually, but not necessarily) pigmented, irregular masses, which might also be ulcerated. However, only one of nine reported cases of early-stage PMME was the polypoid type (Mikami et al. 2001), and the other eight cases were all the flat type (Minami et al. 2011; Miyatani et al. 2009; Morita et al. 2009; Suzuki et al. 2008; Kimura et al. 2005; Hara et al. 2003; Kido et al. 2000) (Table 1). In contrast, no report is available about the flat-type submucosal invasive PMME. In the present case, many satellite lesions occurred in separate areas, and all lesions were the flat type. In almost 90% of patients, the lesions occur in the middle or distal one-third of the esophagus, usually as a solitary tumor, but multiple lesions have been reported in 12% of patients (Sabanathan et al. 1989; Joob et al. 1995). To our knowledge, present case is the first report of multiple early-stage PMME.

Especially in cases of the flat-type PMME, it is difficult to accurately define the tumor area macroscopically. Because the melanoma cells originated from the basal/deeper layers of the epithelium, it is likely that the size of the black-pigmented area depends on the number and density of the melanoma cells and does not reflect the true size of the tumor. Narrow-band imaging and/or magnifying endoscopy (Cohen, 2007) were not useful for accurately determining the tumor area in the present case (Fig. 8A–C).

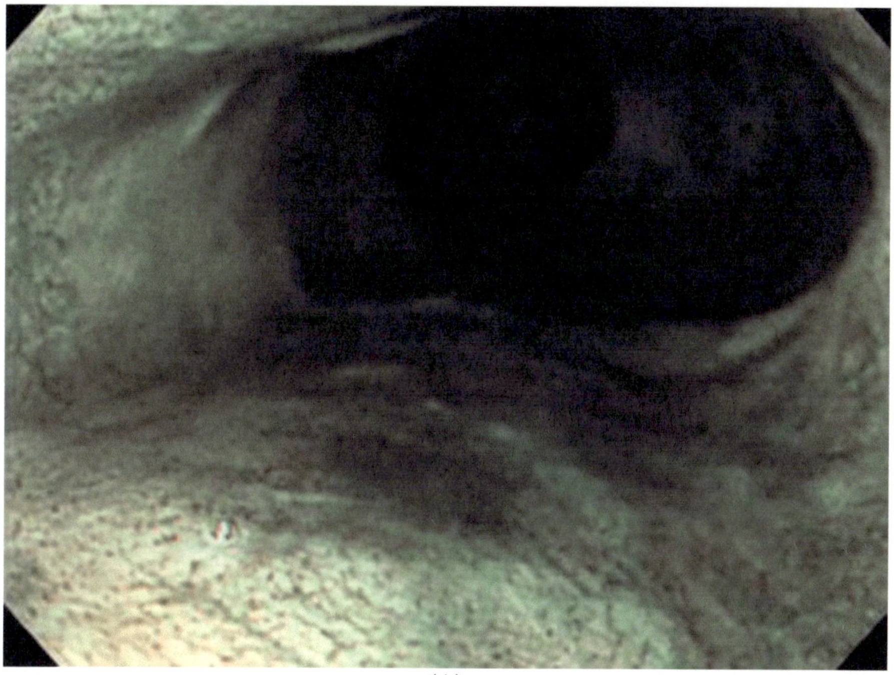

(A)

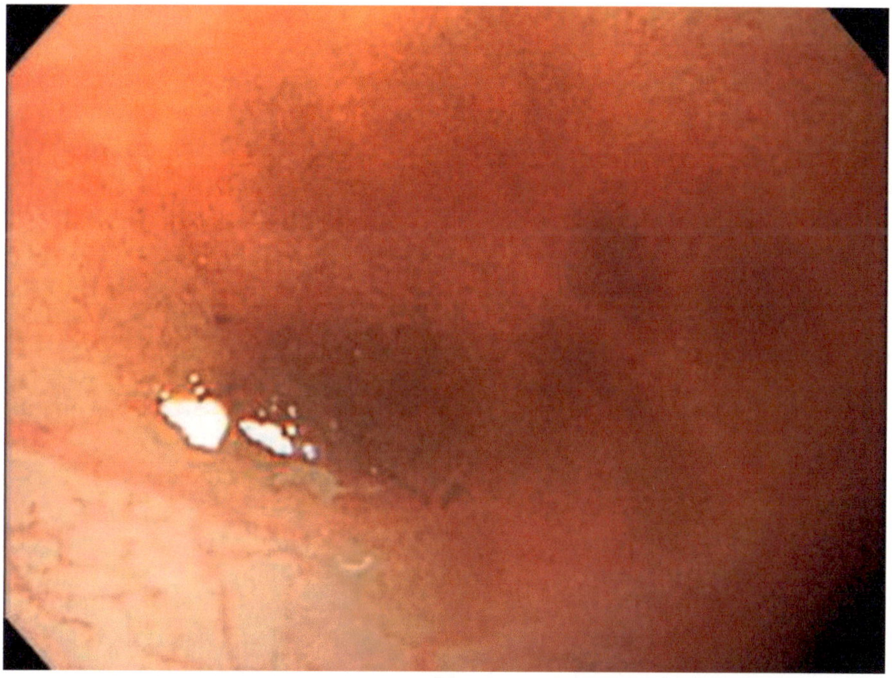

(B)

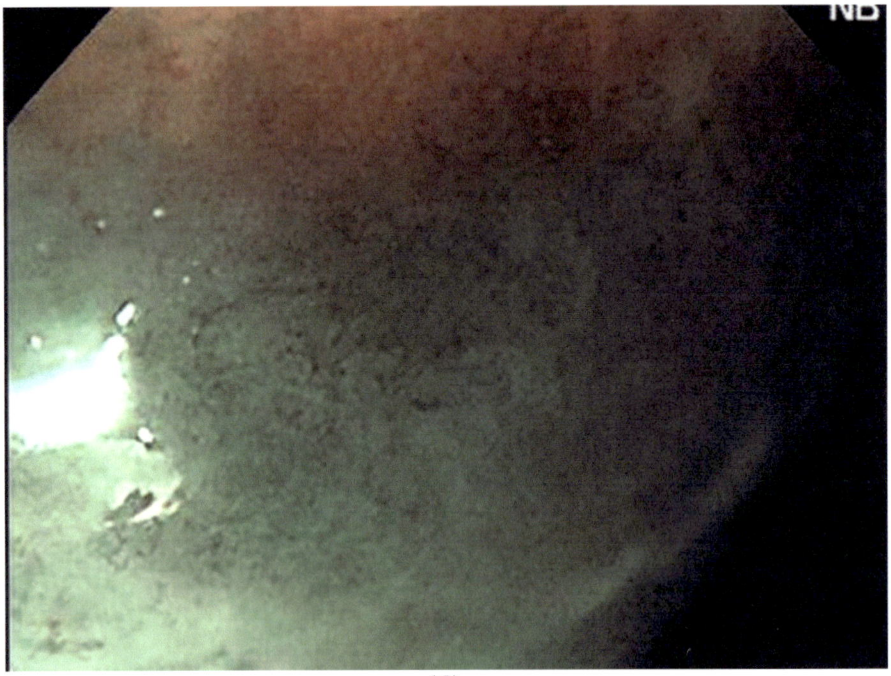

(C)

Fig. 8. Narrow-band imaging (A), magnifying endoscopy (B), and magnifying endoscopy with narrow-band imaging (C) were not useful for accurately determining the tumor area.

Endoscopic treatment for PMME should be considered for diagnostic purposes (Hirose et al. 2002) and for treatment purposes in limited cases (Miyatani et al. 2009; Morita et al. 2009; Kimura et al. 2005). PMME, especially the polypoid type, can be removed technically by endoscopic treatment (Ho et al. 2007; Herman et al. 2001; Xinopoulos et al. 2001; the depth of the tumor invasion was not mentioned in these three papers); however, indications for local therapy for this disease are still controversial because of the inaccurate diagnosis of the tumor area and the possibility of synchronous multiple lesions (Morita et al. 2009; Ho et al. 2007; Xinopoulos et al. 2001). Further accumulation of early-stage PMME data is required to clarify the tumor behavior of this rare disease.

4. References

Adili F., and Moning S.P. (1997) Surgical therapy of primary malignant melanoma of the esophagus. *Ann Thorac Surg.* 63(5):1461–1463.

Allen A.C., and Spitz S. (1953) Malignant melanoma: a clinic-pathological analysis of the criteria for diagnosis and prognosis. *Cancer.* 6(1):1–45.

Bisceglia M., Perri F., Tucci A., Tardio M., Panniello G., Vita G., and Pasquinelli G. (2011) Primary malignant melanoma of the esophagus: a clinicopathologic study of a case with comprehensive literature review. *Adv Anat Pathol.* 18(3):235–252.

Chalkiadakis G., Wihlm J.M., Morand G., Weill-Bousson M., and Witz J.P. (1985) Primary malignant melanoma of the esophagus. *Ann Thorac Surg.* 39(5):472–475.

Cohen J., editor. (2007) *Advanced digestive endoscopy: comprehensive atlas of high resolution endoscopy and narrow band imaging.* 1st ed. Massachusetts: Blackwell Publishing: pp. 49–66.

Fenoglio-Preiser C.M., Noffsinger A.E., Stemmermann G.N., Lantz P.E., and Isaacson P.G. (2008) *Gastrointestinal pathology. An atlas and text.* 3rd ed. Philadelphia: Lippincott Williams & Wilkins: pp. 125–126.

Hara S., Noguchi M., Sugiyama K., Yamaguchi M., Unakami M., Imatani A., Ohara S., and Shimosegawa T. (2003) A case of primary malignant melanoma of the esophagus in situ (in Japanese with English abstract). *Gastroenterol Endosc.* 45(5):935–939.

Herman J., Duda M., Lovecek M., and Svach I. (2001) Primary malignant melanoma of the esophagus treated by endoscopic ablation and interferon therapy. *Dis Esophagus.* 14:239–240.

Hirose T., Izue Y., Hanashi T., Yoshida M., Katoh H., Momma K., Funada N., and Koike M. (2002) Malignant melanoma of the esophagus, report of a case (in Japanese with English abstract). *Stomach and Intestine (Tokyo)* 37(10):1361–1365.

Ho K.Y., Cheng J., Wee A., and Soo K.C. (2007) Primary malignant melanoma of the esophagus with multiple esophageal lesions. *Nat Clin Pract Gastroenterol Hepatol.* 4(3):171–174.

Joob A.W., Haines G.K. 3rd, Kies M.S., and Shields T.W. (1995) Primary malignant melanoma of the esophagus. *Ann Thorac Surg.* 60(1):217–222.

Kato H., Watanabe H., Tachimori Y., Watanabe H., Iizuka T., Yamaguchi H., Ishikawa T., and Itabashi M. (1991) Primary malignant melanoma of the esophagus: report of four cases. *Jpn J Clin Oncol.* 21(4):306–313.

Kido T., Morishima H, Nakahara M., Nakao K., Tanimura H., Nishimura R., and Tsujimoto M. (2000) Early stage primary malignant melanoma of the esophagus. *Gastrointest Endosc.* 51(1):90–91.

Kimura H., Kato H., Sohda M., Nakajima M., Fukai Y., Miyazaki T., Masuda N., Manda R., Fukuchi M., Ojima H., Tsukada K., and Kuwano H. (2005) Flat-type primary malignant melanoma of the esophagus treated by EMR: case report. *Gastrointest Endosc.* 61(6):787–789.

Ludwig M.E., Shaw R., and de Suto-Nagy G. (1981) Primary malignant melanoma of the esophagus. *Cancer.* 48(11):2528–2534.

Mikami T., Fukuda S., Shimoyama T., Yamagata R., Nishiya D., Sasaki Y., Uno Y., Saito H., Takaya S., Kamata Y., and Munakata A. (2001) A case of early-stage primary malignant melanoma of the esophagus. *Gastrointest Endosc.* 53(3):365–367.

Minami H., Inoue H., Satodate H., Hamatani S., and Shin-Ei K. (2011) A case of primary malignant melanoma in situ in the esophagus. *Gastrointest Endosc.* 73(4):814–815.

Miyatani H., Yoshida Y., Ushimaru S., Sagihara N., and Yamada S. (2009) Slow growing flat-type primary malignant melanoma of the esophagus treated with cap-assisted EMR. *Dig Endosc.* 21:255–257.

Morita S., Miyamoto S., Matsumoto S., Manabu M., and Chiba T. (2009) Multiple early-stage malignant melanoma of the esophagus with long follow-up period after endoscopic treatment: report of a case. *Esophagus.* 6:249–252.

Sabanathan S., Eng J., and Pradhan G.N. (1989) Primary malignant melanoma of the esophagus. *Am J Gastroenterol.* 84(12):1475–1481.

Simpson N.S., Spence R.A., Biggart J.D., and Cameron C.H. (1990) Primary malignant melanoma of the oesophagus. *J Clin Pathol.* 43(1):82–83.

Suzuki H., Nakanishi Y., Taniguchi H., Shimoda T., Yamaguchi H., Igaki H., Tachimori Y. and Kato H. (2008) Two cases of early-stage esophageal malignant melanoma with long-term survival. *Pathol Int.* 58:432–435.

Xinopoulos D., Archavlis E.M., Kontou M., Tsamakidis K., Dimitroulopoulos D., Soutos D, and Paraskevas E.M. (2001) Primary melanoma of the oesophagus treated endoscopically. A case report. *Dig Liver Dis.* 33:254–257.

11

Pulmonary Edema Induced by Esophagectomy

Yusuke Sato, Satoru Motoyama and Junichi Ogawa
Department of Surgery, Akita University School of Medicine, Japan

1. Introduction

Esophageal cancer is the seventh leading cause of cancer deaths worldwide (410,000 new cases annually)(1). Asian, Middle Eastern, and East African countries have a markedly higher incidence of esophageal cancer than other areas. In the United States, the incidence of adenocarcinoma of the distal esophagus and gastroesophageal junction has progressively increased to approximately 70% of all esophageal cancers over the last two decades. It affects mostly Caucasian men, and its pathogenesis is linked to gastroesophageal reflux disease (GERD) and the development of Barrett's esophagus. On the other hand, squamous cell carcinoma is responsible for 95% of all esophageal cancers worldwide. It arises from whole esophagus, from the cervical esophagus to the gastroesophageal junction, and spreads to the cervical, thoracic, and abdominal lymph nodes with relative ease because of the abundant and complex lymphatic network (2). Therefore, esophagectomy with extensive neck, thoracic, and abdominal lymph node dissection, the so-called "3-field lymph node dissection," is needed for curative surgery for esophageal squamous cell carcinoma (3). Though chemotherapy, radiotherapy, and combination therapy of both have been substantially developed as treatments for esophageal squamous cell carcinoma in recent years, these treatments are still inferior in survival rate and late toxicity compared to surgery (4).

Esophagectomy with 3-field lymph node dissection is one of the most invasive surgical procedures. This highly invasive surgery is currently still associated with high morbidity, despite improvements in surgical techniques and perioperative managements. A "cytokine storm" during and after esophagectomy induces severe hemodynamic changes involving loss of circulating blood volume and filling of the third space. Furthermore, extensive lymph node dissection and ligation or excision of the thoracic duct have a causal influence on mediastinal lymphostasis, which disturbs drainage of extravascular lung water (EVLW) from the lungs and causes pulmonary edema. Pulmonary edema may form the base of pulmonary complications such as atelectasis and pneumonia, the most common complications after esophagectomy.

Monitoring of EVLW in cases of critically ill patients with acute lung injury (ALI) or acute respiratory distress syndrome (ARDS) has proved to be very informative and useful for predicting outcome (5.6).

Based on these findings, we monitored perioperative changes in EVLW using the recently developed single transpulmonary thermodilution technique to determine whether EVLW correlates with respiratory function and predicts pulmonary complications. In this chapter, we expound on the importance of recognizing and monitoring EVLW during perioperative managements of esophagectomy for thoracic esophageal squamous cell carcinoma.

2. Extravascular Lung Water (EVLW)

EVLW is the amount of water that is present in the lungs outside of the pulmonary vasculature, put simply, the alveoli and interstitium of the lungs. Thus, EVLW is a quantitative term describing pulmonary edema. EVLW is expressed using the formulas described in **Fig.1**. Intrathoracic thermal volume (ITTV) is computed by multiplying cardiac output (CO) by mean transit time (MTt), which is the time when half of the indicator has passed the point of detection of the artery. Pulmonary thermal volume (PTV) is computed by multiplying CO by downslope time (DSt), which is the exponential downslope time of the thermodilution curve. Global end diastolic volume (GEDV) is calculated by subtracting PTV from ITTV. Intrathoracic blood volume (ITBV) is expressed as GEDV x 1.25. Finally, EVLW is calculated by subtracting ITBV from ITTV. Extravascular lung water index (EVLWI, EVLW/body surface area, ml/m^2) is a more precise parameter than EVLW and provides more accurate results, particularly in overweight patients.

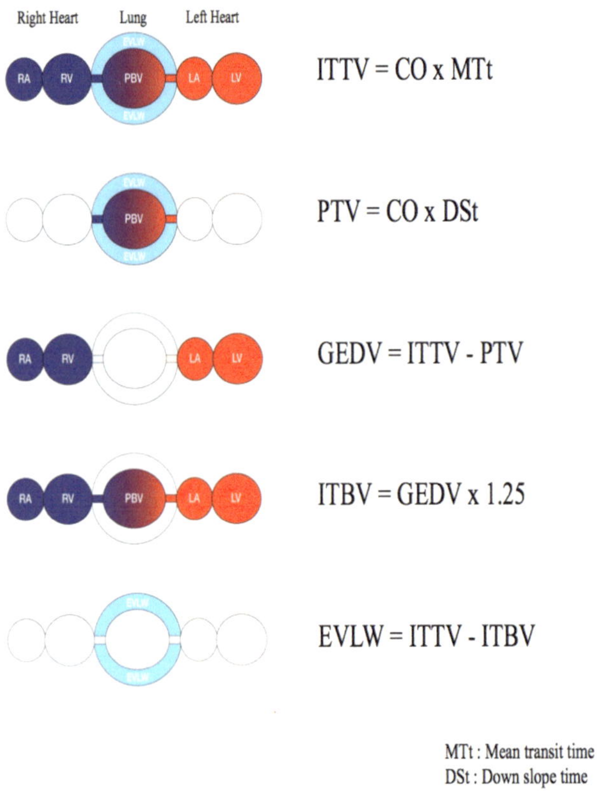

Fig. 1. EVLW and other parameters such as intrathoracic thermal volume (ITTV), pulmonary thermal volume (PTV), global end diastolic volume (GEDV), and intrathoracic blood volume (ITBV) are described with these formulas.

3. PiCCO

PiCCO (Pulsion Medical Systems, Munich, Germany, http://www.pulsion.com) is a less invasive advanced hemodynamic monitoring system employing the single transpulmonary thermodilution technique **(Fig.2)**. It requires only a standard central venous catheter and a femoral, axillary, brachial, or radial artery catheter (but not a pulmonary artery catheter). This system enables monitoring of cardiac function, vascular tone, and fluid distribution, including EVLW. EVLW and EVLWI are automatically calculated after a bolus infusion of cold saline via the central venous catheter. As mentioned above, monitoring EVLW using this system in critically ill patients with ALI/ARDS has proved to be very informative and useful for predicting outcome. The current PiCCO2 system is employed for management of patients not only with ALI / ARDS but also septic shock, burns, major surgery, and cardiac surgery, among others.

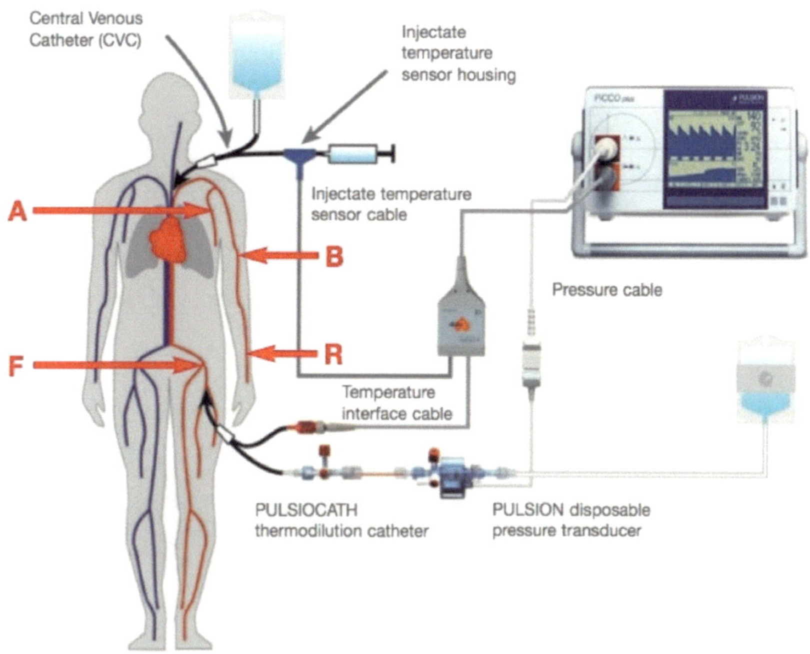

Fig. 2. General outline of the PiCCO system, which requires only a standard central venous catheter and a femoral, axillary, brachial, or radial artery catheter, but not a pulmonary artery catheter.

4. EVLW monitoring predicts pulmonary complications after esophagectomy

To determine whether EVLW correlates with respiratory function and predicts pulmonary complications after esophagectomy, we enrolled 23 patients with thoracic esophageal cancer in a prospective observational clinical trial (8). Informed consent was obtained from all patients.

All of these patients underwent esophagectomy with extensive lymph node dissection and reconstruction involving insertion of a gastric tube via the posterior mediastinal route. They were also monitored perioperatively using PiCCO from the day prior to surgery through postoperative day (POD) two. Our standard operative procedure is right transthoracic esophagectomy and resection of the lesser curvature with dissection of the mediastinal (involving the periesophageal region and areas around trachea and bilateral main bronchus), the abdominal (involving the perigastric region and areas around the celiac axis), and the bilateral neck lymph nodes (areas around common carotid artery, internal jugular vein and transverse cervical artery), the so-called "three-field lymph node dissection". Following surgery, the extubation criteria for the intratracheal tube were PaO_2 >100 Torr with a <40% inspired fraction of oxygen (FiO_2), forced vital capacity >800 ml, and no pulmonary complications. Based on these extubation criteria, the tracheal tubes were removed from 11 patients on the morning of POD one (extubation group); the remaining 12 patients remained intubated (intubation group). The respiratory Index was calculated using the following equation: respiratory index = $(PAO_2 - PaO_2)/PaO_2$, where $PAO_2 = [(760 - 47 \text{ (atmospheric pressure)}) \times FiO_2 - PaCO_2/0.8]$. The respiratory index essentially reflects the ability to oxygenate the lung.

In all patients, EVLW correlated significantly with the respiratory index ($r = 0.638$, $p < 0.0001$) at all measurement points after surgery (**Fig. 3**). The changes in EVLW and respiratory index during the perioperative period in the extubation and intubation groups are shown separately in **Fig.4**. In the extubation group, EVLW was clearly reduced immediately after surgery ($p = 0.0068$), but it recovered to preoperative levels within 12 h after surgery and remained at that

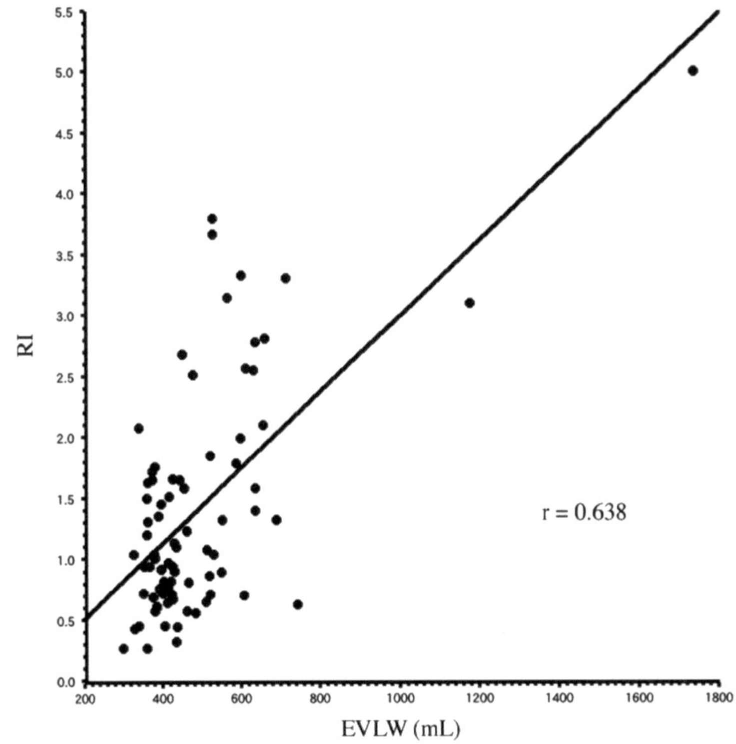

Fig. 3. EVLW correlated significantly with the respiratory index (RI) (r = 0.638, p <0.0001) at all measurement points after esophagectomy.

level through POD two. By contrast, in the intubation group, both EVLW and respiratory index were elevated 12 h after surgery and were even higher 24 h after surgery. All of the patients in the extubation group recovered with no pulmonary complications, whereas four patients (33%) in the intubation group developed pneumonia or atelectasis that required artificial respiration managements. In all four patients that developed pulmonary complications, an increase in EVLW preceded their onset.

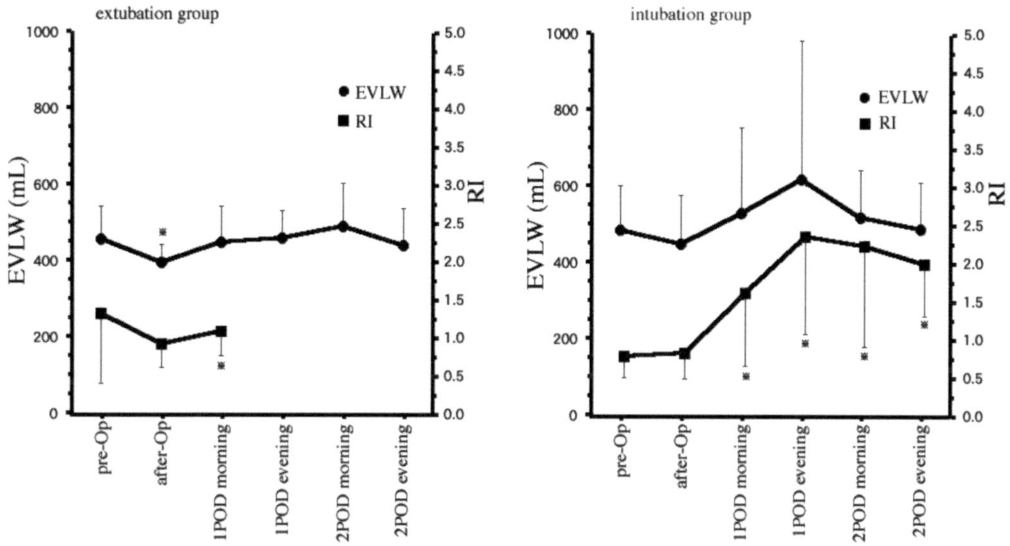

Fig. 4. The changes in EVLW and the respiratory index (RI) during the perioperative period in the extubation and intubation groups. In the intubation group, both EVLW and respiratory index were elevated 12 h after surgery and were even higher 24 h after surgery.

5. Conclusion

We have shown that EVLW measured using the PiCCO system reflects the level of postoperative pulmonary edema induced by esophagectomy with extended lymph node dissection. Patients who showed no significant postoperative changes in EVLW or respiratory index recovered without pulmonary complications. By contrast, those patients who showed an increase in EVLW on POD one showed a substantial increase in their respiratory index, and some developed pulmonary complications. Measurement of the EVLW using the PiCCO system thus proved to be a useful method for monitoring the pulmonary edema and was predictive of the pulmonary complications that subsequently occurred. This PiCCO system enables us to begin early managements of patients who develop pulmonary edema following esophagectomy with extensive lymph node dissection.

6. References

[1] "WHO Disease and injury country estimates". World Health Organization. 2009. Retrieved Nov. 11, 2009.

[2] Motoyama S, Maruyama K, Sato Y et al. Status of involved lymph nodes and direction of metastatic lymphatic flow between submucosal and t2-4 thoracic squamous cell esophageal cancers. World J Surg. 2009 Mar;33(3):512-7.

[3] Akiyama H, Tsurumaru M, Udagawa H et al. Radical lymph node dissection for cancer of the thoracic esophagus. Ann Surg. 1994 September; 220(3): 364–373.

[4] Kato K, Muro K, Minashi K et al. Phase II Study of Chemoradiotherapy with 5-Fluorouracil and Cisplatin for Stage II-III Esophageal Squamous Cell Carcinoma: JCOG Trial (JCOG 9906). Int J Radiat Oncol Biol Phys. 2010 Oct 5.

[5] Martin GS, Eaton S, Mealer M et al. Extravascular lung water in patients with severe sepsis: a prospective cohort study. Crit Care 2005;9:R74–R82.

[6] Michard F, Schachtrupp A, Toens C. Factors influencing the estimation of extravascular lung water by transpulmonary thermodilution in critically ill patients. Crit Care Med 2005;33:1243–1247.

[7] Abo S, Kitamura M, Hashimoto M et al. Analysis of results of surgery performed over a 20-year period on 500 patients with cancer of the thoracic esophagus. Surg Today 1996;26:77–82.

[8] Sato Y, Motoyama S, Maruyama K et al. Extravascular Lung Water Measured Using Single Transpulmonary Thermodilution Reflects Perioperative Pulmonary Edema Induced by Esophagectomy. Eur Surg Res 2007;39:7-13.